Every Heart Attack Is Preventable

*How to Take Control of
the 20 Risk Factors
and Save Your Life*

Michael Mogadam, M.D.

LifeLine
Press

A REGNERY COMPANY • WASHINGTON, DC

Library of Congress Cataloging-in-Publication Data

Mogadam, Michael.
   Every heart attack is preventable : how to take control of the 20 risk factors and save your life / by Michael Mogadam.
      p. cm.
   Includes index.
   ISBN 0-89526-207-X
   1. Myocardial infarction—Risk factors. 2. Coronary heart disease—Risk factors.
3. Myocardial infarction—Prevention. I. Title

RC685.I6 M576 2001
616.1'2305—dc21   2001029323

Published in the United States by
Lifeline Press
A Regnery Publishing Company
One Massachusetts Avenue, NW
Washington, DC 20001

Visit us at www.regnery.com

Distributed to the trade by
National Book Network
4720-A Boston Way
Lanham, MD 20706

Printed on acid-free paper
Manufactured in the United States of America

10 9 8 7 6 5 4 3 2 1

BOOK DESIGN BY AMY CADE
SET IN JANSON

Books are available in quantity for promotional or premium use. Write to Director of Special Sales, Regnery Publishing, Inc., One Massachusetts Avenue, NW, Washington, DC 20001, for information on discounts and terms or call (202) 216-0600.

To Eve, Roya, and Ryan, for being so patient
while I completed this book.

Contents

Introduction
Why This Book?

I began this project five years ago out of a deep concern that the prevailing wisdom concerning the prevention of heart disease was woefully inadequate. It remains so today.

We have a disease-oriented society. We wait until people have heart attacks, then aggressively treat them with every advanced technology available to "save" them; but we do very little to prevent these almost always preventable tragedies. Each year, more than one-and-a-half million Americans suffer heart attacks, many in their thirties, forties, and fifties. Of the 500,000 who die from heart attacks each year, more than a third won't even make it to a hospital; for them, all the sophisticated, hospital-based technology is worthless.

For more than three decades the medical community has promoted a flawed and outdated notion that elevated blood cholesterol is the principal cause of coronary artery disease, and that low-fat, low-cholesterol diets significantly lower blood cholesterol and therefore reduce the risk of heart attacks and strokes. Although an elevated blood cholesterol level is a major risk factor for coronary artery disease, so are nineteen other major (and twenty minor) risk factors, most of which are not affected by low-fat, low-cholesterol diets.

A recent episode illustrated the sad state of misinformation that prevails in the media concerning the causes of heart disease. During the post-presidential election media frenzy of 2000, it was reported that Richard Cheney, the fifty-four-year-old Republican vice presidential candidate, had suffered a heart attack, his fourth. As part of their coverage, newspapers across the country ran feature stories on the factors that contribute to coronary artery disease, and the "medical experts" on the television networks talked about the "major risk factors for heart attacks." Without exception, all of these reports parroted the conventional wisdom about coronary artery disease, citing only high cholesterol, high blood pressure, smoking, and sedentary lifestyle as risk factors for heart attacks, with a few mentioning diabetes as an added risk. None even hinted at the other fifteen major coronary risk factors, some of which were, evidently, relevant to Mr. Cheney's case.

Regrettably, this comes as no surprise. Despite the fact that the science of coronary care has advanced by leaps and bounds in the past decade, most of the general public (and much of the medical community) is operating on the basis of information and recommendations that are dated, ineffective, and even harmful. There are hopeful signs that this situation may be changing, particularly in the area of dietary recommendations. After more than three decades of promoting a low-fat, low-cholesterol diet to combat coronary artery disease, the American Heart Association published a science advisory on April 3, 2001, acknowledging that its previous recommendations have not been very successful. Based on a large number of studies published over the past decade, the AHA now supports a Mediterranean-style diet as an antidote to the epidemic of coronary artery disease. The Twenty Risk Factor Diet, introduced in Chapter 3 of this book, is a refined and contemporary version of the Mediterranean diet, which now has the belated blessings of the AHA.

Because of the prevailing misinformation about the factors that contribute to coronary artery disease, I felt it was necessary to write a book that educates people about *all* the risk factors and tells them exactly what they can do to prevent those risk factors from developing (or to treat them after they have already developed). As they say, a little knowledge is a dangerous thing, and when it comes to the prevention of heart disease, it is vital to be fully informed.

Almost every day I see men and women in my practice, many in the prime of life, who have one or more undiagnosed or inadequately treated major coronary risk factors. According to the U.S. Census Bureau, more than 93 million Americans are forty-five years of age or older. At least one half of this population has coronary artery disease in various stages of development; almost everyone in this group has multiple identifiable coronary risk factors. If their risk factors were diagnosed early and treated appropriately, countless cardiac disabilities and deaths might be prevented.

In the United States, the annual death toll from heart attacks, strokes, and hardening of the arteries is over 920,000. This is equal to the next seven leading causes of death combined, including cancers, chronic lung diseases, AIDS and other infections, accidents, diabetes, suicides, and homicides. Yet most of the cardiovascular diseases are preventable (and it is quite possible to predict with a reasonable degree of accuracy who is at high risk). As seen in Table 1, coronary artery disease does not occur in older persons only; it begins at a very young age and progresses slowly over the years before causing a fatal or nonfatal heart attack.

Table 1
Percent of Young Americans Who
Have Early Coronary Artery Disease*

	WHITE		AFRICAN AMERICAN	
AGE	MALES	FEMALES	MALES	FEMALES
15-19	24	7	24	18
20-24	28	15	32	12
25-29	39	21	42	25
30-34	51	32	49	38

* Based on autopsy data of 2,876 subjects who had died of external causes.
(Adapted from Strong, J.P., et al. Jama 1999; 281: 727-735)

Although during the 1980s and early 1990s death rates from heart attack and other cardiovascular events declined in the United States (and western Europe), in the past several years the trend has reversed. Today a global epidemic of cardiovascular diseases is underway; cardiovascular diseases, especially heart attacks, are now the leading cause of death worldwide. In the 1960s, heart attacks were primarily a disease of the affluent; today they are also rampant among the less affluent, both here and abroad.

This is an epidemic that demands action, and this book provides you with a personal battle plan. *Every Heart Attack Is Preventable* means what it says—and shows you how to protect yourself, practically, from the most important coronary risk factors.

Every Heart Attack Is Preventable is a compelling all-in-one book that gives you the latest science—science your doctor might not even know. It will show you how to save your heart—and perhaps your life.

How to Read This Book

For convenience, I have included numerous easy-to-read tables and figures that illustrate what is being discussed in the text. You will find cross-references throughout the text to other sections of the book where more information can be found about the subject under discussion. References to material in Part I are made by chapter—e.g., (Chapter 2, "Fruits, Vegetables, Herbs, and Nuts"); material in Part II is referenced according to the section on the risk factor being discussed—e.g., (Part II, (10)).

So as not to overwhelm readers with information—however useful—I have put some of the more detailed discussion of issues raised in the course of the book in a "notes" section at the back; it can be easily referenced by anyone interested in going a bit deeper into those subjects. Also in the back is a useful glossary of scientific and medical terms.

—Michael Mogadam, M.D.

Part I:
Nutrition and Heart Disease

Chapter 1
The ABCs of
Coronary Artery Disease

Blood Cholesterol

Right or wrong, the first item on the mind of everyone concerned about a heart attack or stroke is their blood cholesterol level. Although it is true that cholesterol particles circulating in the bloodstream have an essential role in the development of coronary artery disease, all cholesterol particles are not alike. Some are harmful and others carry significant benefits for the heart. So before we proceed with other issues, let's demystify and understand what it is we are talking about.

Cholesterol is a type of fat which is present only in animals. No plant or plant product contains cholesterol. Cholesterol is not a useless or harmful substance without any redeeming features. Nearly all animal and human cells have some cholesterol as a component of their cell wall or internal machinery. Without sufficient cholesterol, animal life could not exist. But as with blood sugar, calcium, and sodium, it is the excessive levels of blood cholesterol that are harmful.

Cholesterol cannot dissolve in the bloodstream. To move from the intestine and liver into other tissues, cholesterol needs a vehicle. These vehicles are called "lipoproteins" (*lipo*, from the word lipid, means fat, + proteins). The more protein and the less fat lipoproteins have, the heavier or "denser" they are. This is analogous to a lean steak being denser than a piece of steak with fatty streaks. On the basis of their protein content or density, lipoproteins fall into five major classes (Figure 1):

(1) Very low-density lipoproteins (VLDL)

(2) Intermediate-density lipoproteins (IDL)

(3) Low-density lipoproteins (LDL)

(4) High-density lipoproteins (HDL)

(5) Humans, primates, and a few other animals have another lipoprotein

Figure 1
Lipoprotein Cholesterol Particles

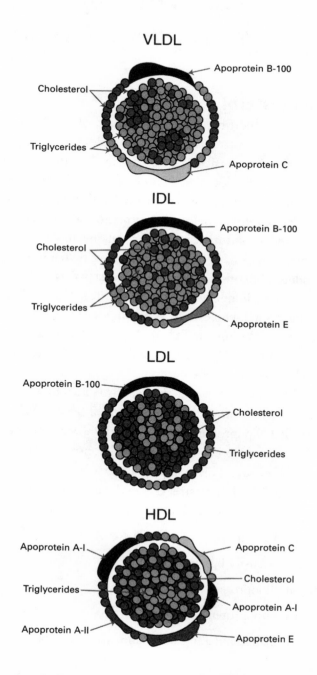

called "lipoprotein(a)." But lipoprotein(a) is not measured in a routine cholesterol panel.

Triglycerides (tri = three, glyceride = fatty acid) are the predominant form of fat in the bloodstream, especially soon after eating fatty meals. Triglycerides do not contain any cholesterol or protein; hence they are not lipoproteins. However, all lipoproteins, especially VLDL particles, carry some triglycerides in their core. With the exception of HDL (the "good" cholesterol), all other lipoproteins are coronary-unfriendly (the "bad" cholesterol).

The protein part of lipoproteins is called "apoprotein." Apoproteins are essentially the "brain" or conductor of lipoproteins, and are responsible for the good or the bad deeds of these little fat globules. The three important apoproteins are A-1, which makes HDL cardio-protective, B-100, which is responsible for the misdeeds of LDL, and apoprotein E, which determines whether people's blood cholesterol goes up in response to fatty foods (Part II, (18)).

At present, the National Cholesterol Education Program, which is composed of over twenty organizations including the American Heart Association, has set the following guidelines for blood levels of various lipoproteins and triglycerides (Table 2).

Table 2
Current Lipoprotein Categories
(mg/dl)

	TC	TG	LDL	VLDL*	HDL	TC/HDL
NORMAL	<200	<200	<130	<40	>35	<5
BORDERLINE HIGH	200-240	200-400	130-160	40-80	N/A	N/A
HIGH	>240	>400	>160	>80	N/A	N/A

TC = Total Cholesterol   TG = Triglycerides
LDL = LDL Cholesterol   VLDL = VLDL Cholesterol
HDL = HDL Cholesterol   TC/HDL = Total Cholesterol to HDL Ratio
* IDL is measured along with VLDL

The National Cholesterol Education Program guidelines were proposed over a decade ago, and were based on data available at that time. There is no doubt that these arbitrary levels are now outdated and must be revised. In fact, all "borderline" values are abnormal, and recent studies have shown that the majority of people who suffer heart attacks or strokes have cholesterol levels that actually fall in this so-called "borderline" range, as shown in Figure 2. In Table 3, I have introduced the desirable cholesterol levels, which are based on voluminous recent data and are applicable to all age groups, including children and the elderly, with or without coronary artery disease.

As seen in Figure 2, a large majority of people who suffer heart attacks or strokes have a total cholesterol that falls in the range of 180 to 240 mg/dl, values that the National Cholesterol Education Program and the American Heart Association consider "borderline." Obviously, these values are abnormal and you should not accept them because "my doctor said my cholesterol levels are fine." They are not. In fact, the closer your total cholesterol is to 150 (and the farther your LDL is below 100), the lower your risk of a future heart attack. Similarly, you should not settle for an HDL cholesterol level of less than 45 if you are a man, or less than 55 if you are a woman.

Table 3
Desirable Blood Levels of Cholesterol
(mg/dl)

TOTAL CHOLESTEROL	<180
"BAD" LDL CHOLESTEROL	<100
"BAD" VLDL CHOLESTEROL	<30
"GOOD" HDL CHOLESTEROL	
IN MEN	>45
IN WOMEN	>55
TOTAL CHOLESTEROL/HDL RATIO	<4
TRIGLYCERIDES	<150

Total Cholesterol measures both good and bad cholesterol particles. Thus, when the level of good HDL is high, i.e., 70-80 mg/dl, it will raise the Total Cholesterol but lower the ratio of Total Cholesterol/HDL Cholesterol.

> = GREATER THAN
< = LESS THAN

Figure 2
The Relation of Total Blood Cholesterol (mg/dl) to Risk of Heart Attack

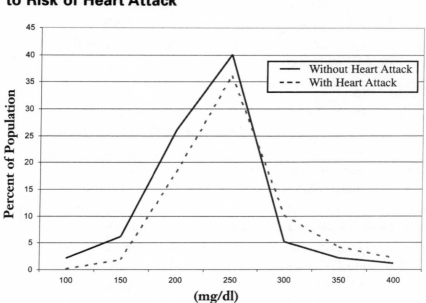

Anatomy of a Heart Attack:
The "Coronary Quartet"

Heart attacks do not suddenly strike people when they reach their forties or fifties. In most cases the process begins in childhood and adolescence (Table 1; Figure 3). Heart attacks are the end point or the last stage of this smoldering process which I have called the "Coronary Quartet."

Stage One

The arteries have a unique ability to constrict or relax like elastic tubes. They can do this indefinitely without experiencing any fatigue because of specialized smooth muscles in their walls (skeletal muscles, in contrast, are made of a different kind of muscle cells, and can experience fatigue with repetitive contractions). The inner lining of arteries (the endothelium) is made up of a single layer of cells (the endothelial cells) which protect the arterial wall like the durable interior layer of pipes and hoses. When these cells are damaged, they become leaky and allow white blood cells, platelets, and LDL cholesterol particles to pass into the artery's wall. The smooth muscle cells also become dysfunctional and cannot relax the arteries. The role of endothelial cells in protecting against coronary artery disease and heart attacks is so important that Dr. Robert Furchgott of the State University of New York in Brooklyn was awarded the 1998 Nobel Prize in Physiology and Medicine for his pioneering research in this area.

Stage Two

When we take a bite out of an apple and allow the apple to sit on the counter, it begins to turn brown within a short time. This is oxidization. A rusty nail is also the product of oxidization. In general, LDL cholesterol particles are not harmful unless they are oxidized, either in the bloodstream or inside the wall of coronary or other arteries. Once LDL particles trespass through a leaky arterial wall, they can become oxidized especially if there are very few or no antioxidants present to defend these particles (Figure 4). Oxidized LDL is the arsonist that sets the artery wall on fire, and then keeps fueling the flames.

Stage Three

Oxidized LDL is toxic to the arterial wall and causes a biochemical turmoil within it. Slowly, smooth muscle cells and collagen fibers begin to move into the area of turmoil and entrap a number of substances from the circulating blood, including calcium, iron, copper, magnesium, and fibrin. All of this "junk pile" thickens the arterial wall, and makes it bulge into the lumen of the artery. At this point, the junk pile is called a "plaque," or a "coronary lesion." When numerous coronary lesions are scattered throughout the arterial tree, the condition is called "atherosclerosis," or "hardening of the arteries."

The first three stages of a coronary quartet can be seen as early as childhood and adolescence. In fact, some autopsy data from infants who had died of noncardiac causes have shown early changes in the first few weeks of life, suggesting that the process of heart disease can begin at any time. But it usually takes many years for the progression of the first three stages of the coronary quartet, and the process sometimes spans thirty to fifty years. It is this slow progression that lulls people into inaction until the catastrophic fourth stage.

Tragically, for one-third of the people who reach it (or 500,000 Americans each year) the fourth stage is a fatal event. The goal is to prevent the progression of this deterioration long before its final stage.

Figure 3
Estimated Prevalence of Cardiovascular Disease
(By Age and Sex)

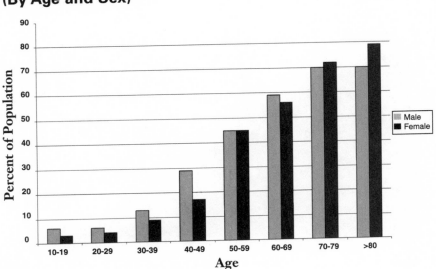

Stage Four

Fatty plaques are very fragile, unstable, and can crack or rupture easily. These "unstable plaques," or "vulnerable lesions," can rupture, and account for more than 80 percent of heart attacks (the other 20 percent are due to progressive clogging of the artery).

When a vulnerable plaque bursts, blood platelets quickly move in and clump together and form the core of a blood clot that gets larger and larger (within a few minutes to a few hours). This newly formed clot (or "thrombus") chokes off blood flow to the heart muscle (Figure 4). This is a heart attack or a "myocardial infarction." Depending on the size and the speed at which a coronary thrombosis expands, the individual may suffer a minor heart attack, or a massive and fatal one.

To prevent coronary artery disease and a subsequent heart attack, we must prevent the coronary quartet at the starting gate, or interrupt it as early as possible. Even among people with advanced coronary artery disease who have already suffered heart attacks, a future coronary event can be prevented by stopping the progression of the coronary quartet. Subsequent chapters will provide effective recommendations to achieve this goal by reducing major coronary risk factors and stabilizing existing coronary plaques.

Figure 4
Coronary Artery Disease Quartet

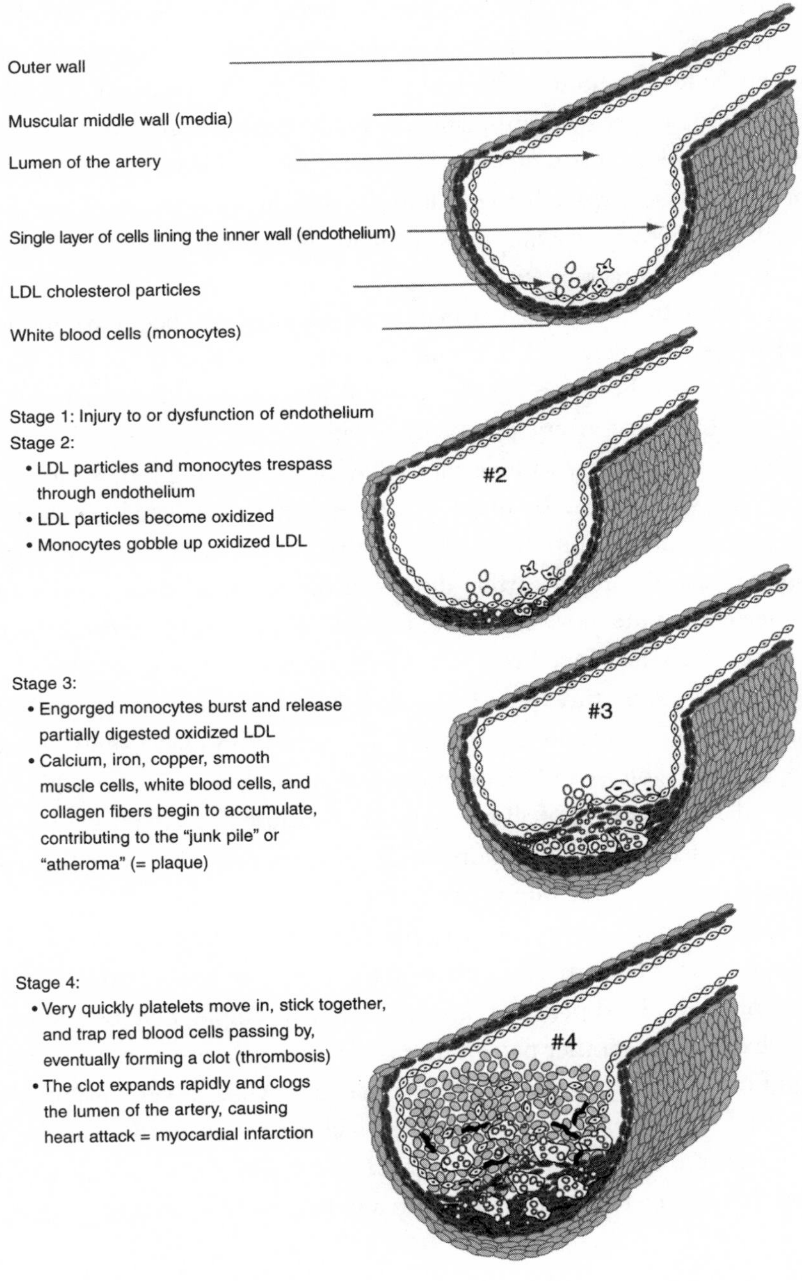

Outer wall

Muscular middle wall (media)

Lumen of the artery

Single layer of cells lining the inner wall (endothelium)

LDL cholesterol particles

White blood cells (monocytes)

Stage 1: Injury to or dysfunction of endothelium
Stage 2:
• LDL particles and monocytes trespass
  through endothelium
• LDL particles become oxidized
• Monocytes gobble up oxidized LDL

Stage 3:
• Engorged monocytes burst and release
  partially digested oxidized LDL
• Calcium, iron, copper, smooth
  muscle cells, white blood cells, and
  collagen fibers begin to accumulate,
  contributing to the "junk pile" or
  "atheroma" (= plaque)

Stage 4:
• Very quickly platelets move in, stick together,
  and trap red blood cells passing by,
  eventually forming a clot (thrombosis)
• The clot expands rapidly and clogs
  the lumen of the artery, causing
  heart attack = myocardial infarction

The Twenty Major Risk Factors

Heart attacks and strokes—unlike a strep throat or a broken wrist—do not have a single identifiable cause. A variety of risk factors are almost always involved. Driving down a tortuous mountain road on a rainy night at sixty miles per hour—with bad brakes, worn tire treads, and streaking windshield wipers—while dozing off behind the wheel, clearly involves numerous risk factors that lead to a catastrophic accident. A single risk factor is, of course, less likely to result in an accident. Similarly, multiple interacting risk factors over the course of many years dramatically increase the risk of a heart attack or stroke.

As noted, the process of coronary artery disease may begin in childhood and progress slowly and unevenly over the next twenty to forty years. Along the way, however, we can stop this process. In a few situations, the pace of coronary artery disease is greatly accelerated—especially after coronary angioplasty, with certain infections, including AIDS, or after a heart transplantation. In these situations, what usually takes twenty to forty years can be compressed into months. In each instance—whether the usual variety of coronary artery disease or the accelerated form—the more numerous and the more aggressive the risk factors are, the shorter the lagtime to a fully developed coronary artery disease and heart attack.

There are over three hundred risk factors for coronary artery disease. Among these, twenty are considered "major," and another twenty "minor" risk factors (Tables 4 and 5); the remainder are only trivial co-conspirators. More than 98 percent of all heart attacks are caused by the interaction and harmful effects of two or more major risk factors, with or without the added burden of some minor risk factors.

The impact of a given coronary risk factor is not the same for everyone. The response of a particular person to high levels of homocysteine or cholesterol, high blood pressure or smoking, for example, may be greater or less than that of another person. But the coexistence of several risk factors significantly increases the risk of coronary artery disease and eventually a heart attack. In subsequent chapters, I will demystify all the major coronary risk factors, in addition to providing you with a state-of-the-art road map that will enable you to deal with any risk factors you may have.

Table 4
The Twenty Major Coronary Risk Factors

RISK FACTOR	RELATIVE RISK*
LOW BIRTH WEIGHT	2
HIGH BLOOD PRESSURE	2
ABDOMINAL OBESITY	2
CHRONIC INFECTIONS (C. PNEUMONIA, HERPES, ETC.)	2
ELEVATED BLOOD FIBRINOGEN LEVEL	2
ABNORMAL BLOOD PLATELETS	2
TOO MANY RED BLOOD CELLS (HEMATOCRIT >48)	3
ELEVATED BLOOD HOMOCYSTEINE LEVEL	3
NEGATIVE AFFECT (DEPRESSION, ANGER, HOSTILITY)	3
SMOKING	3
SEDENTARY LIFESTYLE	3
ELEVATED BLOOD TRIGLYCERIDES 3	3
ELEVATED LDL CHOLESTEROL	3
ELEVATED LIPOPROTEIN(A)	3
LOW HDL CHOLESTEROL	3
AN ATHEROGENIC DIET (A TYPICAL WESTERN DIET)	3
DIABETES	3
AGE: >45 FOR MEN AND >55 FOR WOMEN**	3
PREMATURE CAD IN CLOSE FAMILY MEMBER < 55 YEARS OF AGE	10
PERSONAL (PREVIOUS) HISTORY OF A CORONARY EVENT	20

* For comparison, the Relative Risk of lung cancer in a long-term heavy smoker is 10 times higher than in a nonsmoker.
** Relative Risk for age >65 is 8 times higher, and for age >79 is 34 times higher than for age <35.

Table 5
The Twenty Minor Coronary Risk Factors*

1.	LONG-TERM ESTROGEN DEFICIENCY IN WOMEN
2.	CHRONIC KIDNEY DISEASES
3.	CHRONIC BRONCHITIS OR EMPHYSEMA
4.	AN UNDERACTIVE THYROID
5.	SYSTEMIC LUPUS, ESPECIALLY AMONG YOUNG WOMEN
6.	INFECTION WITH AIDS VIRUS
7.	CHRONIC ALCOHOL ABUSE (ALCOHOLISM)
8.	RAPID HEART RATE (>80 PER MINUTE) OR HIGH WHITE BLOOD CELLS (>9000/ML)
9.	SOFT WATER (CONTAINING LOW MAGNESIUM AND CALCIUM LEVELS)
10.	CERTAIN OCCUPATIONS SUCH AS BEING AN AIR TRAFFIC CONTROLLER, FIREMAN, POLICE OFFICER, MINISTER/RABBI
11.	OVERWORKING (OVER 60 HOURS PER WEEK), ALL WORK AND NO FUN
12.	DISSATISFACTION WITH WORK OR PERSONAL LIFE (INADEQUATE WORK RESPON-SIBILITY, NON-SUPPORTIVE SPOUSE OR BOSS, UNPLEASANT OR HOSTILE WORK ENVIRONMENT, ISOLATION, ETC.)
13.	POVERTY, MALNUTRITION, POOR ACCESS TO HEALTH CARE, CROWDING, AIR POLLUTION
14.	WIDOWS/WIDOWERS/DIVORCED PERSONS/LOVELESS LIFE
15.	BEING AFRICAN AMERICAN, NORTHERN EUROPEAN, SCOTTISH, OR WELSH
16.	SHORT STATURE, BALDNESS, OR EARLY GRAYING
17.	CERTAIN DRUGS OVER A LONG PERIOD SUCH AS CORTISONE AND OTHER IMMUNE SUPPRESSANTS, ANDROGENIC STEROIDS, BIRTH CONTROL PILLS AMONG SMOKERS, EXCESSIVE INTAKE OF VITAMIN A OR D (> TWICE RDA/DAY)
18.	BLOOD TYPE A OR AB, AND BLOOD LEWIS TYPE A - B -
19.	ABNORMAL BLOOD CLOTTING
20.	THERE ARE A LARGE NUMBER OF OTHER MINOR RISK FACTORS, INCLUDING SOME GENETIC DISORDERS WHOSE IMPACT IS NOT FULLY UNDERSTOOD OR VALIDATED

* Generally speaking, #19 and #20 are rarely tested for and collectively may account for <1% of all cases of CAD. Such tests are very expensive and should not be used for screening.

The Twenty Minor Risk Factors

As seen in Table 5, a large number of the minor risk factors are chronic diseases or socioeconomic factors. In most of these cases, their negative impact on coronary arteries is attributable to their association with, and contribution to, a variety of major risk factors. For example, chronic kidney diseases are associated with hypertension, elevated LDL cholesterol, and triglycerides, as well as a sedentary lifestyle. Chronic lung diseases are often due to long-term, heavy smoking or intercurrent infections, particularly chlamydia pneumoniae; they also contribute to sedentary lifestyle, poor oxygenation of blood, and lower blood antioxidant levels. An underactive thyroid gland can not only raise the LDL cholesterol by 30 to 50 percent, it can also cause hypertension and heighten the risk of coronary artery disease.

Socioeconomic factors contribute to poor access to, or lack of, medical care, and to undertreatment of major risk factors such as hypertension, abnormal blood cholesterol levels, diabetes, and stress or negative affect. Excessive drinking, smoking, lack of exercise, poor nutrition, and low intake of antioxidants may also be contributing factors. It is highly unlikely that poverty, overcrowding, or a given occupation—by themselves and independent of the twenty major risk factors—have a definite, as yet unknown, impact on coronary arteries.

Estrogen deficiency in women is a relatively easy risk factor to remedy for those who are motivated (Appendix B). Balding, early graying, and short stature are markers for a genetic predisposition to low HDL cholesterol, abdominal obesity, elevated blood cholesterol, and triglycerides. They are not associated with a stand-alone, genetic abnormality which can independently harm coronary arteries.

Certain blood types (such as Lewis a-negative or b-negative) can increase the risk of coronary artery disease, but the underlying mechanisms are not well defined. Presumably in these blood types, the risk of clot formation inside the coronary artery is somewhat increased. A combination of low-dose aspirin (81 milligrams per day) and vitamin E (400 IU per day) is often sufficient to counteract the negative impact of these blood types, provided there are no other associated major risk factors.

Systemic lupus and AIDS can cause an accelerated form of coronary artery disease, sometimes within a few short years (as opposed to twenty to thirty years). These diseases represent different impairments of the immune system which negatively impact the vascular system, but they are also associated with a wide range of complications and major coronary risk factors. The concern over the fast-track development of coronary artery disease in patients with systemic lupus or AIDS makes a more aggressive approach to treatment of major coronary risk factors even more compelling.

What You Should Do

Even though the contribution of minor risk factors to coronary artery disease may be relatively small, their presence should heighten your awareness and your doctor's effort to look for and correct any coexisting major risk factors. Although you should try to correct as many of these minor risk factors as you can, your main focus should still be on major risk factors.

Chapter 2
Debunking Dietary Myths

Should We Fear Dietary Cholesterol?

Cholesterol is a pearly fat that is present in animal flesh and animal products such as dairy products and eggs. Contrary to a common misconception, dietary cholesterol accounts for only 10 to 30 percent of blood cholesterol; the other 70 to 90 percent is made from the breakdown by-products of carbohydrates and proteins, mostly in the liver. Cattle, too, eat no cholesterol, get very little saturated fat from hay or feed, and have a diet that is rich in complex carbohydrates. Yet, cattle grow to huge sizes with plenty of saturated fat and cholesterol in their fat, meat, and milk. Chickens also have a rigid vegetarian diet, but do not lay fat-free or cholesterol-free eggs. Thus animals and humans are efficient factories that take in various nutrients, including carbohydrates and proteins, and convert them into other products such as fat, cholesterol, hormones, or other biological compounds.

Although practically every cell in the body needs cholesterol for its survival, dietary cholesterol is not essential. This explains why strict vegetarians can have perfectly normal functioning bodies, and normal or even high blood cholesterol levels, without receiving any cholesterol from outside sources. From the nutritional standpoint, dietary cholesterol is an unnecessary nutrient. It entered our diet about two-and-a-half-million years ago when Homo erectus, our distant ancestor, began eating meat. But dietary cholesterol is not necessarily harmful or evil. For the past thirty years many nutrition gurus and zealots have targeted dietary cholesterol for extinction, but always more out of emotion than scientific merit. Cutting back dietary cholesterol to less than 200 mg per day is neither practical nor relevant to cardiovascular diseases. Although a hundred million Americans have elevated blood cholesterol levels, in the majority, dietary cholesterol is not the main culprit. Surely, the other 180 million Americans who have "desirable" cholesterol levels are not all strict vegetarians.

Many studies over the past two decades have shown that long-term, low-cholesterol diets are unlikely to have a significant impact on lowering blood cholesterol levels or the risk of heart disease. Indeed, for every 100 mg reduction in dietary cholesterol intake, there is an average decrease of only 2 to 4 mg in blood cholesterol. So for most people, lowering their dietary cholesterol from 400 mg per day to 200 mg only lowers their blood cholesterol by 4 to 8 mg. This is simply too trivial and unimpressive to justify all the fuss surrounding dietary cholesterol.

The human body is not a passive dump-yard where dietary cholesterol piles up with every bite. Our bodies have two ways to control such a buildup:

First, the intestine absorbs only 30 to 50 percent of dietary cholesterol. But a large dietary load of cholesterol can overwhelm the absorptive capacity of the intestine, lowering the absorption of dietary cholesterol much further. This explains, in part, why the blood cholesterol level of one eighty-eight-year-old man was perfectly normal, even though for nearly twenty years he had the unusual dietary habit of eating about twenty-five eggs per day, amounting to approximately 6000 mg of dietary cholesterol daily.

Second, every liver cell has special gates or receptors on its surface that facilitate the entry of LDL cholesterol so that it can be converted to other needed compounds. A high number of LDL-receptors (six to eight receptor sites per cell, instead of two or three) will trap and remove more LDL particles from the blood circulation, thereby lowering blood cholesterol levels. Conversely, when the liver cells do not or cannot produce LDL-receptors, the "homeless" LDL particles stay in the blood circulation and keep the blood cholesterol level high.

In many people dietary cholesterol does not raise blood cholesterol levels. These individuals are referred to as "cholesterol nonresponders." In these individuals, their defensive systems—the liver and the intestines—work effectively to cope with dietary cholesterol load. For example, the man who ate twenty-five eggs every day for nearly twenty years was not only able to reduce his cholesterol absorption to less than 10 percent, but also trapped and disposed of more LDL particles by doubling or tripling the number of LDL-receptors in his liver cells (Part II, (18)).[1]

In some people one or both defense systems may be impaired, resulting in an elevated blood cholesterol level. Often the problem is not the number of LDL-receptors, but the inability of these receptors to function properly. Since LDL-receptors are primarily made up of proteins, even a minor genetic alteration can render them quite useless, or far less effective. So far, over 350 different defects in LDL-receptors have been identified, each affecting the ability of these receptors to various degrees. Individuals with these mutations of their LDL-receptors are almost always cholesterol-responders (their blood cholesterol goes up with dietary cholesterol and saturated fat intake).

It is estimated that nearly 70 percent of the population of the United States are cholesterol nonresponders, whereas 30 percent are cholesterol responders. Even in cholesterol responders the blood cholesterol level is not so fragile as to rise significantly after eating two eggs or a shrimp dinner. The kind of fat accompanying dietary cholesterol will have a significant impact on how the body responds to a given cholesterol load. Moreover, the absorption of cholesterol may be hindered by a number of dietary components, including fruits, vegetables, and legumes containing plant sterols (cholesterol look-alikes). Certain shellfish also contain cholesterol look-alikes which, very much like their plant counterparts, decrease the absorption of shellfish's cholesterol from the intestine (Chapter 2, "Omega-3 Polyunsaturated Fat").

A recent study examining the risk of coronary artery disease in middle-aged men of Japanese ancestry living in Japan, Honolulu, and San Francisco, showed that their dietary cholesterol was essentially similar. For example, dietary cholesterol intake of the Japanese was 464 mg per day, compared to 545 mg per day for Japanese Hawaiians, and 533 mg per day for men of Japanese ancestry living in San Francisco. Yet, death from coronary artery disease was twice higher among Japanese living in Hawaii and nearly three times higher among those living in San Francisco than among those residing in Japan. Dietary saturated fat intake of these three groups, on the other hand, was significantly different at 7 percent, 13 percent, and 16 percent of total fat intake for the Japan, Honolulu, and San Francisco groups, respectively.

Excessive intake of any nutrient is unhealthful and may even be harmful. No sensible nutritionist recommends excessive intake of vitamin A, vitamin C, cholesterol, proteins, or any other nutrient. On the other hand, the unrelenting criticism of dietary cholesterol also serves no purpose, and has created a considerable amount of dietary confusion. The failure to distinguish the impact of dietary cholesterol from saturated fat has contributed to identifying one with the other, and made dietary cholesterol guilty by association. People fear eating eggs when in fact eggs are nearly the perfect food, especially for children and older persons. Often people avoid eating shellfish, when in fact any shellfish (except squid) is preferable to chicken, turkey, or any other meat. The edible oil industry has further added to the anti-cholesterol campaign by perpetuating the myth that margarines and shortenings are healthy alternatives to butter—which they most certainly are not (Chapter 2, "Trans Fatty Acids")!

There is no scientifically valid evidence to suggest that moderate dietary cholesterol intake of about 300 to 400 mg per day—particularly when prepared with olive oil, hazelnut oil, canola oil, or other non-hydrogenated vegetable oils—contributes to cardiovascular diseases. In fact, if you have a low level of HDL cholesterol, severe dietary cholesterol restrictions may contribute to further lowering of HDL levels, making a bad situation even worse. Moreover, a single meal, or a day, or a week of dietary "indiscretion" in which cholesterol exceeds a certain arbitrary limit, would not cause irreparable harm to anyone's coronary arteries or provoke a heart attack. So, instead of focusing on drastically cutting back dietary cholesterol, the way to go is to reduce saturated fats and trans fatty acids (Chapter 2, "Saturated Fat" and "Trans Fatty Acids"). More importantly, the Twenty Risk Factor (TRF) scores of foods introduced in Chapter 3 obviate the need for any concern over cholesterol or fat content of foods, because these variables have already been calculated into the TRF scores.

Saturated Fat: Not Always Evil

Many people today recoil as soon as they see saturated fat on a food label and cringe at the thought of eating greasy food loaded with saturated fat (for a description of why a fat is called saturated or polyunsaturated, see Chapter 2, "Omega-6 Polyunsaturated Fat"). But in truth, saturated fat is not always an evil to be avoided at all costs. To be sure, saturated fat has the nasty habit of raising blood cholesterol level in some people, but in nearly 70 percent of the population, saturated fat does not have an appreciable cholesterol-raising effect.[2]

Because saturated fats are present in many foods, in the real world it is extremely difficult to avoid them altogether. It is quite frustrating, and even counterproductive, to embark on a search-and-avoid mission to locate every gram of saturated fat in one's diet. It is likely to make eating an unpleasant chore rather than a pleasant experience.

Rates of long-term adherence to rigid diets are, moreover, very poor and, in most studies, have ranged from zero to 4 percent. So it is counterproductive to be fanatical about avoiding any food containing saturated fat, just as it is with cholesterol. Your goal should be to reduce, not completely avoid, saturated fat. The Twenty Risk Factor scoring system (Chapter 3) has computed the saturated fat content of thousands of foods and snacks, taking away the worry and uncertainty about choosing healthful foods. Instead of focusing on the saturated fat or cholesterol, you can simply use the TRF scoring system for all your foods.

Monounsaturated Fat: The Heart Protector

A vast body of scientific evidence has consistently confirmed the long-term safety and health benefits of monounsaturated fats.[3] For instance, a recent study of 5,632 Italians, ages sixty-five to eighty-four, showed that among this population with a typical Mediterranean diet, higher intake of monounsaturated fat was associated with a significant protection against age-related cognitive decline. In sharp contrast, another study showed that high consumption of vegetable-source polyunsaturated fats was associated with cognitive impairment. A high fish diet, however, very much like a high monounsaturated fat diet, improved elderly cognition. The beneficial effect of monounsaturated fat and the omega-3 polyunsaturates found in seafood (Chapter 2, "Omega-3 Polyunsaturated Fat") on brain function may be in part due to incorporation of these fatty acids into brain cells, making them healthier and less prone to oxidization or natural cell-death. These fatty acids also reduce the risk of repeated "mini-strokes," which can slowly destroy a substantial part of the brain's cortex, causing senility that may mimic Alzheimer's disease.

Does this suggest that we should all increase our dietary fat? Obviously, it depends on the fat. People die of coronary heart disease five times more often than they die of stroke. Such a one-sided, five-to-one trade-off is a losing proposition. On the other hand, increasing monounsaturated fat and omega-3 polyunsaturated fat from seafoods, while decreasing saturated fats (to less than 7 percent energy intake), and trans fatty acids (preferably none), lowers the risk of both coronary artery disease and stroke—a win/win situation. A recent fourteen-year follow-up study of more than eighty thousand female nurses in the United States showed that replacement of 5 percent of energy from saturated fats with energy from unsaturated fats (monounsaturated fat or nonhydrogenated polyunsaturated fat) would reduce the risk of coronary artery disease by 42 percent. Replacement of 2 percent of energy from trans fatty acids (margarine, shortenings, and cooking fats), would reduce the risk even more—by 53 percent.

Olive Oil: The Oil for All People

Olive oil is not just a liquid form of monounsaturated fat. It is also a rich source of many antioxidants and phenolic compounds that enhance the healthfulness of the oil. For this reason, extra virgin olive oil (first pressing) is always preferable and more healthful. Virgin olive oil (second pressing) does not have as much flavor, color, and antioxidants or other phenolic compounds as the extra virgin oil, but it is still a wonderful and healthy oil.

Extra light, light, or plain olive oil is the oil extracted from what is left after the second pressing. In this third pressing, the manufacturers often use steam pressure or other techniques to remove the oil. This olive oil is mostly stripped of its personality, antioxidants, and anti-carcinogenic phenolic compounds, but it is still superior to all other vegetable oils such as corn oil, soybean oil, and safflower oil, all of which have only a small amount of monounsaturated fat. Here, strangely, "light" refers to color and taste, not the percent of fatty acids or their composition. The advantage of using light olive oil is that because it lacks taste and aroma, it is very much like other cooking oils. Thus, people who object to the taste of olive oil, can use extra light olive oil for a wide range of baking and cooking purposes, including muffins or cookies. The only problem with olive oil is that at high heat it smokes more quickly than vegetable oils such as canola or corn oil. Thus, for sautéing or searing food at high temperatures, especially indoors, canola oil (which has about 57 percent monounsaturated fat) can be substituted. Canola oil, however, lacks the antioxidants present in virgin or extra virgin olive oil. Although hazelnut oil has the highest concentration of monounsaturated fat (about 78 percent) and very low levels of saturated fat (about 7 percent), it is too expensive and impractical for everyday cooking. But no matter which olive oil, from the most exotic to the ordinary, it is the oil for all people and all occasions.

Olive oil, of course, contains fat, and each gram of fat contains approximately ten calories. Nowhere is this small, and sometimes forgotten, fact more important than in people with weight problems (34 percent of the U.S. population). Fat cells cannot differentiate, select, or reject calories from corn oil, butter, or olive oil. Each one gram of fat is still ten calories to a fat cell, no matter where it comes from. If those calories are not burned, they will be stored in fat cells, adding to body weight. Thus, in obese persons, any dietary program must also focus on reducing total energy intake (calories) from all sources—especially fats and carbohydrates. The idea is to replace all other fats (cream, butter, vegetable oils, margarine, or shortening) with olive oil. Adding olive oil to a rich, fat-laden Western diet serves absolutely no purpose, and by contributing to obesity, may even be harmful. Clearly, a teaspoon of olive oil in the salad dressing cannot redeem or counteract an unhealthy load of saturated fats and trans fatty acids in a steak and fries dinner, not to mention the fat-laden dessert.

Regrettably, many foods served at Italian or French restaurants in the United States (and other developed countries) have extremely high TRF (Twenty Risk Factor) scores. These pseudo-Mediterranean foods have no resemblance to, and share none of the benefits of, a genuine Mediterranean diet (Chapter 3).

Table 6
The Health Impact of Monounsaturated Fats

- REDUCE LDL CHOLESTEROL, BUT RAISE HDL LEVELS
- REDUCE OXIDIZATION OF LDL CHOLESTEROL AND VARIOUS CELLS IN HUMAN BODY
- REDUCE THE RISK OF HEART ATTACK AND STROKE
- REDUCE THE RISK OF CANCERS SUCH AS BREAST, COLON, OR PROSTATE
- IMPROVE INSULIN RESISTANCE IN DIABETICS

Dietary fat is not cardio-toxic. In fact, you need a sufficient amount of fat to maintain the integrity of your blood vessels and significantly reduce your risk of a heart attack or stroke. The key is to replace all oils and fats in your diet with monounsaturates (olive oil, hazelnut oil, or even canola oil). But don't look at a piece of red meat, cheese, pizza, or fried chicken as a poison dart that will go straight through your heart.

You can buy 7 percent or 10 percent fat ground meat and mix it with a tablespoon of olive oil to prevent it from getting too dry on the grill. This not only improves the taste (regrettably, fat is a major taste enhancer), but makes your hamburger more healthful. Similarly, you can sauté your fish, chicken, or vegetables in olive oil (or canola oil) instead of butter, shortening, or corn oil. If you are a diabetic, or have low HDL cholesterol, increasing monounsaturated fat should be an essential part of your dietary changes.

Omega-6 Polyunsaturated Fat:
Not the Advertised "Healthy Alternative"

Vegetable Oils and Fats: Omega-6 Polyunsaturated Fat

Over the past hundred years, human consumption of vegetable oils and fats, the primary sources of omega-6 polyunsaturated fat, has increased progressively.[4] Since the cholesterol-lowering crusade began over three decades ago, vegetable oils and margarine have become synonymous with the "good fat"—the "right stuff" to replace dietary saturated fat. The edible oil and margarine industry has exploited this misinformation and grown into a multibillion dollar industry. The world, developed and developing, is now awash with "100 percent natural and 100 percent cholesterol-free" margarines, shortenings, cooking fats, and various cooking oils.

The rise of vegetable oils and fats has clearly been one of the most successful (and perhaps regrettable) dietary manipulative campaigns ever. At present, the most charitable judgment on vegetable fats is that they may have been relatively harmless, but mounting evidence suggests that high consumption of vegetable fats, in particular hard margarine and cooking fat, may be just as harmful as the butter they replaced.[5]

Partially hydrogenated omega-6 polyunsaturated fats such as margarines, shortenings, and cooking fats contain a number of trans fatty acids with their own unique undesirable profile (Chapter 2, "Trans Fatty Acids"). Some hard margarines and shortenings may have as much as 30 percent saturated fatty acids to go along with 20 to 30 percent trans fatty acids, making them as unhealthful as, or even worse than, butter or cream.[6]

For most people with elevated blood cholesterol and normal HDL levels, liquid vegetable oils (which have high concentrations of omega-6) can be substituted for saturated fat. However, this should not exceed 4 to 5 percent of total energy intake (which is half of the present dietary recommendations). This amounts to approximately one tablespoon of vegetable oils or soft margarine per day. Unfortunately, many snacks such as chips, deep fried foods, pastries, cookies, cakes, chocolate, and doughnuts contain a good deal of hidden omega-6 polyunsaturated fat and trans fatty acids.

Although as a substitute for saturated fat, omega-6 polyunsaturated fat reduces LDL cholesterol by about 5 to 10 percent, there is more to

Table 7
Side Effects of Vegetable Oils/Fat (Omega-6 PUFA)

- REDUCE HDL CHOLESTEROL
- MAY INCREASE BLOOD PRESSURE
- INCREASE OXIDIZATION OF LDL CHOLESTEROL AND ENDOTHELIAL DYSFUNCTION
- PROMOTE BLOOD CLOTTING
- MAY INCREASE THE RISK OF GALLSTONE FORMATION
- CAN SUPPRESS THE FUNCTION OF T-LYMPHOCYTES AND DECREASE IMMUNE RESPONSE
- MAY BE CARCINOGENIC IN SOME ANIMALS

cardiovascular health than a small variation in LDL cholesterol. No amount of misleading or exaggerated claims by margarine manufacturers alters this simple fact. Moreover, the concern over increased susceptibility to oxidization of LDL, VLDL, and lipoprotein(a) particles containing omega-6 polyunsaturated fat, may offset the slight cholesterol-lowering effect of these fats.

Is switching from butter to hard, stick margarines and shortenings jumping from the frying pan into the fire? The answer is probably "yes." Although liquid, nonhydrogenated vegetable oils such as corn and soybean oil in small amounts are reasonably safe, a better switch, as suggested, is to use olive oil, canola oil, or hazelnut oil for all occasions. But if you are one of the people who has to butter up his toast or potatoes, then you can use a small amount of soft, tub margarine with low concentrations of, or preferably no, trans fatty acids (such as Benecol, Brummel & Brown Spread, Smart Balance, Take Control, and others). Mayonnaise, stick margarines, shortenings, or cooking fats have the convenience of long shelf life, but have no healthful virtue. You should avoid them whenever possible (TRF scores of various oils and fats can be found in Chapter 3).

Trans Fatty Acids: No Redeeming Value?

In the 1930s a process was developed to make liquid oils more solid. Partial hydrogenation of liquid fats (by adding hydrogen atoms to them) made these oils not only solid at room temperature, but also less likely to become rancid. It also increased their shelf life.[7]

Over the past two decades, a large body of evidence in humans and various animal species has provided compelling data showing that trans fatty acids are not as safe as was once thought. In a long-term study of over ninety thousand women in the United States, those with the highest intake of trans fatty acids (from partially hydrogenated vegetable fats) had a 35 percent higher risk of coronary artery disease than women who consumed none or very little of these fats. Other studies in both men and women have shown a similar association.

Pregnant women or nursing mothers who frequently eat pastries, cakes, pies, cookies, chocolate, doughnuts, croissants, french fries, or other deep-fried foods expose their fetuses or infants to high levels of trans fatty acids. It is conceivable that such exposures may contribute to the high prevalence of early coronary lesion in children and adolescents in the United States (Part II, (17)).

What Are the Major Side Effects of Trans Fatty Acids?

Trans fatty acids have virtually no benefit. And, as summarized in Table 9, they have many major side effects. Because they raise the LDL and lower the HDL, the cholesterol/HDL ratio goes up. Two independent groups of investigators have calculated that the shift to a higher cholesterol/HDL ratio with the rising dietary intake of trans fatty acids may increase the risk of death from coronary artery disease by 6 to 8 percent. Such an increase translates into approximately thirty thousand premature coronary deaths each year in the United States (6 to 8 percent of nearly 500,000 deaths annually). In addition, trans fatty acids are highly oxidizable and enhance oxidization of LDL particles in the arterial wall, which further contributes to the coronary quartet (Chapter 1).

Table 8
Trans Fatty Acid Content of Selected Foods

FOOD	% TFA RANGE	GRAMS TFA PER SERVING
BEEF*	4 (2 TO 5)	0.20 (3 1/2 OZ)
BENECOL SPREAD	TRACE	TRACE
BUTTER*	4 (2 TO 7)	0.4 (1/2 OZ)
CHICKEN	1 (0.5 TO 1.5)	0.04 (3 1/2 OZ)
COOKIES	18 (4 TO 36)	1.5 (ONE PIECE)
COOKING OILS, SOY, ETC.	12 (1 TO 13)	1.5 (1/2 OZ)
FISH	0	0
FRENCH FRIES	21 (3 TO 34)	4 (LARGE)
HAMBURGER*	4 (3 TO 5)	0.5 (SERVING)
POTATO CHIPS	13 (0 TO 40)	1.5 (SERVING)
PORK	0.2 (0.1 TO 0.3)	0.01 (3 1/2 OZ)
SHORTENINGS	37 (34 TO 44)	5 (1/2 OZ)
SMART BALANCE	0	0
STICK MARGARINE	27 (19 TO 49)	3 (1/2 OZ)
TAKE CONTROL SPREAD	TRACE	TRACE
TUB, SOFT MARGARINE	17 (11 TO 28)	2 (1/2 OZ)
WHOLE MILK*	3 (2.5 TO 3.5)	0.20 (3 1/2 OZ)

* TFA are produced in the rumen by fermentation and absorbed from the intestine of these animals. Eventually, these TFA appear in their meat and milk.

Table 9
Undesirable Effects of Trans Fatty Acids

- INCREASE LDL CHOLESTEROL
- INCREASE OXIDIZATION OF LDL AND MANY HUMAN CELLS
- INCREASE THE RISK OF HEART ATTACK AND STROKE
- INCREASE THE RISK OF ASTHMA AND ALLERGIC RHINITIS AMONG CHILDREN
- MAY INCREASE THE RISK OF BREAST, COLON, AND PROSTATE CANCER
- LOWER HDL CHOLESTEROL LEVEL

The average consumption of trans fatty acids in the United States is about 4 to 6 grams per day, or roughly 2 to 5 percent of daily fat intake. In Europe, daily intake of trans fatty acids is lowest in Greece, Portugal, and Italy (0.6 percent of energy), and highest in Iceland (2 percent), Netherlands (1.6 percent), and Norway (1.5 percent). Lower intake of trans fatty acids in Europe is due, in part, to the edible oil industry's effort to decrease or eliminate these unnecessary and undesirable elements from various hydrogenated fats such as margarine.

A large number of Americans may consume a lot more trans fatty acids than 4 to 6 grams per day, especially those who, ironically, have switched to margarines and shortenings for health reasons. Stick margarines, on average, have more than 20 percent trans fatty acids with a range of 19 to 49 percent (Table 8). Many tub or soft margarines contain about 15 percent trans fatty acids (with a range of 11 to 28 percent). Commercial shortenings (used for baking pastries, cakes, cookies, croissants, doughnuts, or in cooking and frying) consistently have a much higher concentration of trans fatty acids, averaging more than 30 percent (with a range of 34 to 42 percent).

Trans fatty acids have no nutritional virtue, and are far worse than their parents, omega-6 polyunsaturated fats. Almost surely they would be rejected by the Unites States Food and Drug Administration for human consumption if they were presented for approval today. You should make every effort to avoid deep-fried anything, especially at fast food eateries or other restaurants where they often use previously heated cooking fats. Aside from their cardiovascular side effects, the concern over the carcinogenic potential of trans fatty acids—and their role in aggravating allergic disorders, especially asthma—is an additional reason for avoiding these undesirable fats, at home and away from home. In the TRF scoring system, the impact of trans fatty acids in foods and snacks has been computed and accounted for, providing you with a helpful guide to healthful eating.[8]

Omega-3 Polyunsaturated Fat: Is Seafood the "Right Stuff"?

Cardiovascular Benefits of Omega-3 Polyunsaturated Fat

Over the past decade, several hundred studies have examined the beneficial health impact of (seafood) omega-3 polyunsaturated fat. Seafood omega-3 polyunsaturated fats lower triglycerides by as much as 30 percent. In fact, in many people with very high triglyceride levels, fish oil is one of the most effective triglyceride-lowering "drugs," and is much safer than any of the currently available drugs (Part II, (14)).

Omega-3 polyunsaturated fats[9] have a significant anti-arrhythmia (irregularity of heart rate) effect. The results of a six-year follow-up of 45,000 male health professionals (ranging in age from forty-five to seventy) were recently reported. Each was free of cardiovascular disease at the beginning of the study. In the six-year follow-up, there were 25 percent fewer cardiac deaths among those who had eaten at least some fish each week as compared to those who had eaten no fish at all. In another study, more than twenty thousand male physicians were followed up for twelve years. Eating even a single seafood meal per week reduced the risk of sudden cardiac deaths (the vast majority due to arrhythmias) by 50 percent. The finding of this study was identical to the study from Seattle, Washington, which showed that eating just one serving of a fatty fish per week (equivalent to two to three nonfatty fish meals) reduced the risk of sudden cardiac arrest by 50 percent. With higher seafood consumption, equal to three to four seafood meals per week, the risk of cardiac arrest was lowered by 70 percent.

In a recent Italian study, more than eleven thousand men and women who had had a heart attack within the previous three months were randomly given 1 gram of fish oil (containing a relatively small amount of omega-3 polyunsaturated fat), or no fish oil. They were followed up for an average of three-and-a-half years. Participants were also given "blood thinners" (anti-clotting agents), and other drugs, and were placed on a Mediterranean diet. Even with all these protective measures, the group that received a small amount of fish oil still showed an additional 15 percent lower risk of fatal or nonfatal heart attacks or strokes.

Table 10
Fatty Acid Composition of Seafood*
(*Grams/3.5 oz*)

FISH	FAT	SFA	MUFA	OMEGA-3 PUFA	CHOLES-TEROL
BASS, STRIPED	2.3	0.5	0.7	0.8	80
BASS, FRESHWATER	2	0.4	0.7	0.8	60
BLUEFISH	4.5	1	2	1	59
CATFISH	3	0.8	0.9	0.5	58
COD	0.7	0.1	0.1	0.3	43
FLOUNDER	1	0.2	0.3	0.4	46
HADDOCK	0.7	0.1	0.1	0.2	58
HALIBUT	2.3	0.3	0.7	0.4	32
HERRING	9	2	3.8	1.8	60
MACKEREL	13	3.3	4	2.7	70
PERCH	1	0.2	0.2	0.4	76
PIKE	1.2	0.3	0.3	0.4	86
POLLOCK	1	0.2	0.2	0.5	71
ROCKFISH	1.5	0.4	0.5	0.4	44
SABLEFISH	15	3.5	8	1.7	50
SALMON, CHINOOK	10.5	2.5	4.5	1.7	66
SALMON, COHO	6	1.3	2.2	1.5	45
SEA BASS	2	0.5	0.4	0.4	42
SHARK	1.9	0.3	0.4	0.5	44
SNAPPER	1.4	0.3	0.3	0.3	38
SOLE	1.2	0.3	0.4	0.2	50
SWORDFISH	4	1.1	1.6	0.3	39
TROUT, RAINBOW	3.4	0.7	1.2	0.6	60
TUNA	6.6	1.7	2.2	1.7	60
WHITEFISH	5.8	1	2	1.6	60

* The composition may vary depending on the habitat and the natural diet of the fish.
SFA = Saturated Fatty Acids; MUFA = Monounsaturated Fatty Acids; Omega-3 PUFA = Omega-3 Polyunsaturated Fatty Acids

Table 11
Fatty Acid Composition of Shellfish*
(Grams/3.5 oz)

SHELLFISH	FAT	SFA	MUFA	OMEGA-3 PUFA	CHOLES-TEROL
CLAMS	1.2	0.2	0.2	0.4	36
CRAB	1.1	0.2	0.3	0.6	60
LOBSTER	1	0.2	0.2	0.3	90
MUSSELS	2	0.2	0.2	0.4	67
OYSTERS	2.6	0.7	0.5	0.9	72
SCALLOPS	0.9	0.3	0.2	0.3	35
SHRIMP	1.7	0.4	0.5	0.5	157
SQUID	1.8	0.7	0.4	0.6	280

* The composition may vary depending on the habitat and the natural diet of the fish.
SFA = Saturated Fatty Acids; MUFA = Monounsaturated Fatty Acids; Omega-3 PUFA = Omega-3 Polyunsaturated Fatty Acids

The longest follow-up data relevant to omega-3 polyunsaturated fat were recently reported by the investigators of the Chicago Western Electric Study Group. In this study, 1,822 men, forty to fifty-five years old and free of cardiovascular disease at entry into the study, were followed up for thirty years. The risk of sudden or nonsudden deaths from heart attack was 44 percent lower among those who, on average, ate more than 8 ounces of fish per week, compared to those who did not eat any. Although studies dealing with the impact of omega-3 polyunsaturated fat on women's health are not as extensive as those for men, the results of available studies show a nearly identical response.

These and other studies, along with a large number of animal investigations, have clearly documented that consumption of omega-3 polyunsaturated fat from seafood reduces the vulnerability of heart muscle to serious arrhythmias and cardiac arrest. Since more than half of all coronary deaths are due to cardiac arrhythmias (such as ventricular tachycardia) and cardiac arrest, omega-3 polyunsaturated fat from seafood provides one of the most effective measures against coronary death. In fact, at present, no single drug or combination of currently available anti-arrhythmia drugs can match the life-saving benefits and safety of eating three to four seafood meals per week.[10]

Other benefits of omega-3 polyunsaturated fat are summarized in Table 12.

Table 12
Benefits of Seafood Omega-3 PUFA

CARDIO-VASCULAR BENEFITS	• LOWER TRIGLYCERIDES BY AS MUCH AS 30 PERCENT • HAVE ANTI-ARRHYTHMIA EFFECT: REDUCE THE RATE OF SUDDEN CARDIAC DEATH BY 50-70 PERCENT • LOWER LIPOPROTEIN(A) BY 10-20 PERCENT • HAVE ANTI-CLOTTING EFFECT • REDUCE THE RISK OF INFLAMMATION WITHIN CORONARY PLAQUES • INCREASE HDL AND DECREASE LDL CHOLESTEROL • DECREASE THE NUMBER OF SMALL, DENSE LDL PARTICLES
OTHER BENEFITS	• ANTI-INFLAMMATORY EFFECT IN CERTAIN FORMS OF ARTHRITIS AND COLITIS • ANTI-DIABETES EFFECT • ANTI-OBESITY EFFECT • ANTI-DEPRESSANT EFFECT • ANTI-CARCINOGENIC EFFECT

Eating three to four seafood meals per week is one of the most important dietary changes you should make. The reason is twofold. First, by increasing your intake of omega-3 fatty acids, you can dramatically reduce your risk of a cardiovascular event and heart rate irregularities. Second, each seafood meal replaces another meal with much higher calories, saturated fats, or trans fatty acids.

Since omega-3 polyunsaturated fat is the principal cardio-protective nutrient in seafood, you should choose fish or shellfish with the highest (not the lowest) fat content. Tables 10 and 11 provide you with a guide for choosing among many different types of seafood. In this instance, the fattier the fish, the better (nearly 40 percent of the fat in seafood is omega-3 polyunsaturated fat).

Most shellfish contain high concentrations of poorly absorbable cholesterol look-alikes, which, much like their plant counterparts "phytosterols," reduce the absorption of dietary cholesterol. Thus, the absorbed cholesterol from clams, shrimp, or crab legs is actually much lower than 50 percent, making a shellfish meal (without butter or margarine, please) a guilt-free and enjoyable experience.

The use of olive oil, canola oil, or hazelnut oil (monounsaturated fats) is a reasonable alternative to margarine, butter, creams, or cooking fats in preparing your seafood. Grilling, barbecuing, baking, broiling, and poaching are other healthful alternatives when cooking seafood or shellfish. Eating several servings of vegetables with a shellfish dinner will also lower cholesterol absorption further (because of their phytosterol compounds), making the meal even more healthful (Chapter 2, "Fruits, Vegetables, Herbs, and Nuts").

The two unforgivable "sins" with seafood are: (1) buying stale fish (more than two or three days old, especially if not kept in the coldest part of the refrigerator), and (2) overcooking it (which releases unpleasant fishy odors and "kills" the seafood's texture, flavor, delicacy, and unique personality). Although most frozen or canned seafood loses a good deal of its taste and texture, its nutritional value will remain unchanged. However, frozen fried seafood is no better than deep-frying fresh fish yourself in cooking fat: it defeats the purpose of eating seafood. Fried fish sticks or deep-fried fish sandwiches from fast food eateries fall in the same category.

Carbohydrates and Proteins: Fads vs. Facts

In general, dietary carbohydrates (simple or complex)[11] should constitute no more than 50 to 55 percent of daily calories. This allows for about 30 to 35 percent of your calories to come from dietary fats and 10 to 15 percent from proteins. It also allows plenty of fuel for your brain, heart, and muscles. Low- or very low-carbohydrate diets force the body to use fat stores for fuel. This fat-for-fuel conversion, along with lower calorie intake (because of reduced dietary carbohydrates), has proved to be an effective approach to weight loss (Part II, (1)), especially if continued for more than several weeks.

Excessive dietary carbohydrates can contribute to obesity, elevated blood glucose and insulin resistance even among nondiabetics (Part II, (12)), elevated triglycerides, and an increase in the number of small, dense LDL cholesterol particles which are highly coronary-unfriendly (Part II, (15)). The change from large LDL particles to small particles with long-term, high carbohydrate intake is coronary-unfriendly even if carbohydrates lower the LDL cholesterol by 5 to 10 percent. Indeed, consuming excessive dietary carbohydrates (especially simple ones) is a thoroughly unhealthy practice.

Dietary extremists on both sides argue frivolously about the benefits or evils of very high or very low carbohydrate intake. On one side, the proponents of cholesterol-free and very low-fat diets extol the virtue of high dietary carbohydrate intake (in excess of 65 percent of calories). On the other side, "carbo busters" denounce and blame dietary carbohydrates for everything from tooth decay to early aging, chronic fatigue syndrome, cholesterol disorders, and a variety of other ailments. Fortunately, both camps are wrong.

Dietary Proteins

In general, dietary proteins do not play a significant role in the process of coronary artery disease. However, maternal protein malnutrition, which often results in low birth weight (Part II, (2)), is a major risk factor for future development of coronary artery disease and diabetes. On the other hand, excessive protein intake may increase blood levels of homocysteine, another major risk factor for coronary artery disease (Part II, (8)), or contribute to poor kidney function—especially among the elderly, diabetics, or those with preexisting kidney disorders. But adequate intake of high quality proteins such as those in seafood, eggs, poultry, and other lean meats provides a variety of essential amino acids for growth, development, and normal function of nearly all humans cells.

Although elite athletes and bodybuilders need slightly more protein than an average person, this need can almost always be met by an increase in dietary protein. Despite commercial hype and celebrity testimonials, there is scant evidence to show that protein powders or supplements have any advantage over dietary sources of protein for athletes. Elite athletes need more complex carbohydrates to enhance their performance by providing adequate amounts of glucose to their muscles. Since glucose also has a protein-sparing effect, these athletes can actually benefit more by increasing dietary carbohydrates to about 55 to 60 percent of daily energy intake than by taking protein supplements.

Dietary proteins do not have any cardiovascular or cancer-related side effects. Unlike dietary fat or carbohydrates, proteins do not contribute to obesity (Part II, (1)), and thus high quality proteins such as seafood, poultry (without skin and not fried), legumes, and low fat dairy products provide a large number of choices for enjoyable eating. Since the rate of protein absorption is relatively slow, overeating at one meal loaded with dietary proteins may be a wasteful effort. This should be kept in mind by athletes or body builders who can more effectively utilize dietary proteins by spreading their intake over three or four meals instead of eating huge steaks at dinner.

There is no scientific evidence, moreover, to support the usefulness of high protein supplements, whether for weight loss, body building, enhancing "immune-power," or anything else. Long-term use of very high-protein diets, especially those with very high-fat content, are counterproductive for individuals with cardiovascular disorders, kidney disease, or diabetes.

Regular consumption of soy protein (about one ounce per day, equivalent to about 40 percent of daily protein requirement of an adult) lowers LDL cholesterol levels by 7 to 10 percent. But recent studies have shown that the active ingredients in soy protein are various isoflavones (plant chemicals), and not the protein itself. Thus soy protein, soy milk, tofu, and other soy products do not offer any advantage over proteins derived from lean meats, low fat dairy products, seafood, or poultry.

Supplemental Vitamins and Minerals: Which Ones and How Much?

Inside each living cell, hundreds of ultrafast biological actions take place at any given time, some lasting no more than milliseconds. These programmed but hectic biological exchanges produce supercharged chemical compounds that are called "free radicals," or "oxygen free radicals," or simply "oxidants."

Sometimes, free radicals can cause havoc within a cell, interfere with its normal function, or actually destroy it. An example is the impact of ultraviolet light that sunbathers are exposed to. In addition to causing physical damage, ultraviolet light triggers the release of free radicals inside the top layers of the skin, which in turn cause a self-perpetuating tissue damage, even long after sun exposure has stopped.

Most cells readily defend themselves against the onslaught of oxidant charge: otherwise life would not exist. The brave defenders that fight off and neutralize the oxidants are appropriately called antioxidants. Some antioxidants are made within our own body, but many come from outside sources such as foods or supplements. These two groups of antioxidants work in tandem and often in tiers, much like the deployment of military defensive forces; when one defensive line is exhausted or depleted, the other takes over.[12]

Vitamin E

In the past ten years a large body of experimental studies in various animals, and clinical studies in humans, have provided compelling evidence that vitamin E has a major role in preventing heart attack, stroke, and other vascular diseases.[13]

The United States Female Nurses Study and the United States Male Health Professionals Study have shown that among those who had taken supplemental doses of vitamin E (exceeding 200 IU per day), coronary artery disease rates were reduced by approximately 40 percent. This impressive cardio-protection equals the response to any of the present day cholesterol-lowering drugs, at a fraction of the cost.

In a recent study a group of men, forty to fifty years of age with coronary artery disease, were followed up for several years. Coronary plaques of subjects who took vitamin E supplements deteriorated at a much lower rate than people who did not take supplements. In fact, vitamin E had an additive effect when combined with cholesterol-lowering drugs, so that those who received the combination had a more significant regression in their coronary artery disease.

In a study of European countries with different coronary mortality rates (ranging from 66 per 100,000 population in Catalonia, Spain, to 470 in eastern Finland), blood levels of vitamin E were the most significant determinants of coronary heart disease. In this sixteen-country study, vitamin E levels predicted coronary events more accurately than high cholesterol, high blood pressure, or smoking.

Two recent short-term studies among people with coronary artery disease showed that vitamin E did not alter the course of their disease in the first three to four years. However, it is important to remember that these studies were short-term, and the impact of vitamin E in reducing the risk of new coronary plaques and future heart attacks should not be measured in three to four years. Furthermore, in someone with established coronary artery disease, multiple risk factors have been present for years. Vitamin E cannot be expected to negate the ongoing impact of every risk factor.

Although long-term use of vitamin E at doses of 400-1000 IU per day is safe and devoid of any significant side effects, not everyone needs supplements. For most people, the sensible approach is to increase daily consumption of fruits and vegetables rather than popping a handful of pills. Most of the cardiovascular or anti-carcinogenic benefits of vitamin E, however, require supplementation with 400-800 IU per day.

One main reason for the higher efficacy of alpha-tocopherol is that in humans and many mammals, vitamin E has a special "transfer agent," a protein that carries it from the intestine to and from the liver for distribution to various organs. The ability of other forms of vitamin E to hitch a ride on this transfer protein is 50 to 70 percent less than alpha-tocopherol. This reduced transportability makes these other compounds less effective. No matter how potent an antioxidant is in a test tube, it is of no value if it cannot be transported within the bloodstream and to target organs.

Since the biological potency (but not antioxidant potency) of all vitamin E preparations are standardized by using international units (IU) instead of milligrams, one should not worry too much about the natural versus the synthetic varieties. For those with severe cholesterol disorders or high triglyceride levels, and in diabetics, the high antioxidant potency of synthetic alpha-tocopherol is actually a desirable feature. For all other indications, either the natural form or a mix of both natural and synthetic forms are reasonable alternatives. Either way, except in cases of Alzheimer's disease, there is no valid scientific study to suggest that doses exceeding 400-1000 IU per day are necessarily better.

Vitamin C

Vitamin C is perhaps the most abused vitamin. Among the 40 percent of adults in this country who take nutritional supplements, more than 90 percent take vitamin C, either alone or as a component of multivitamins, but frequently both.

Vitamin C can prevent (and cure) scurvy. That said, a long list of other benefits attributed to vitamin C are vastly exaggerated and should be viewed with a healthy dose of skepticism. For example, although taking 1000-2000 mg of vitamin C (approximately ten to twenty times the recommended daily allowance) can shorten the course of a common cold by anywhere from twelve hours to one day, this trivial benefit can hardly justify taking such large doses on a daily basis. The absorption of vitamin C from a 200 mg dose is almost complete (100 percent of the oral dose). However, as the intake of vitamin C increases beyond 200 mg per day, its absorption from the intestine decreases sharply, so that a large portion of higher doses is essentially wasted in the stool. For example, of a 2500 mg dose, only 10 to 12 percent (about 250 to 300 mg) will be absorbed. Also, as the blood level of vitamin C goes up, its excretion and elimination in the urine increases considerably.[14]

Although vitamin C is a potent antioxidant in the bloodstream, the eyes, adrenal glands, and the stomach, because it is a water soluble (not fat soluble) vitamin, it cannot get into, or ride on, LDL particles. As such, it does not play any role in protecting LDL particles against oxidization once they have entered the wall of the coronary artery. But since a small amount of LDL (about 1 to 5 percent) is oxidized during its transit through the bloodstream, vitamin C, soluble in blood plasma (which is water based), may help reduce its oxidization.

Vitamin C plays additional roles in reducing the risk of coronary artery disease. As a co-antioxidant, it can help restore antioxidant potency of exhausted vitamin E. Recent studies have also shown that vitamin C reduces the oxidization of nitric oxide—a potent dilator and protector of coronary arteries. This role of vitamin C in preserving or promoting the function of nitric oxide may have a potentially beneficial impact for people with coronary artery disease or hypertension. For example, a recent study showed that a 500 mg daily dose of vitamin C lowered the systolic blood pressure by 10 points (Part II, (3)).

In diabetics or people with abdominal obesity, a larger fraction (about 5 to 10 percent) of LDL particles may be oxidized in the bloodstream. Undoubtedly this increases the risk of various cardiovascular diseases among diabetics (Part II, (12)). Supplemental vitamin C in doses of 200-500 mg per day may help reduce this oxidant burden and should be encouraged in all diabetics.

For achieving optimal benefits from supplemental vitamin C with minimal or no side effects, you should not exceed 500 mg per day. Clearly no smoker should assume that taking 500 or 1000 mg of vitamin C daily can protect him or her against all harmful effects of smoking. Nevertheless, in those who are unable to stop smoking, supplemental vitamin C may have some relevance. In people who have diabetes, elevated blood cholesterol, abdominal obesity, or other coronary risk factors, and in those with chronic gastritis or pernicious anemia (which predisposes a person to a higher risk of stomach cancer), taking vitamin C at a dose of 200-500 mg per day is a reasonable addition to a diet high in fruits and vegetables.

Beta-carotene and the Heart

Carotenoids are made up of a group of more than 1,200 compounds that are, more or less, close to vitamin A. Beta-carotene is the most touted and perhaps one of the least useful commercially available carotenoids.

At least at current doses of 25-100 mg per day, beta-carotene has no significant cardiovascular benefit. Based on its biological activity, there is no plausible reason why larger doses would prove cardio-protective. Although other carotenoids such as lutein, zeaxathine, and lycopene have no significant cardio-protective role, they have a vast number of other benefits (Chapter 2, "Fruits, Vegetables, Herbs, and Nuts").

The B Vitamins[15]

In spite of the nuisance or side effects associated with niacin (vitamin B-3), it is still the best drug for raising the HDL cholesterol, lowering lipoprotein(a), and reducing the number of small, coronary-unfriendly LDL particles. The minimum effective dose of niacin is about 1000-1500 mg per day.

At high doses, niacin has a number of undesirable side effects that can force up to 50 percent of people to stop taking it. It can cause flushing of the face and chest and a sunburn sensation that may last from minutes to an hour or so after each dose. It can also produce a generalized rash and itching. All these skin side effects can be prevented by taking one regular aspirin (325 mg) or ibuprofen (200 mg). However, frequent doses of aspirin or ibuprofen increase the risk of gastrointestinal side effects, including bleeding.

Niacin can also cause heartburn, nausea, elevation of blood sugar levels, and abnormalities of liver tests. Liver test abnormalities are often innocent findings, and are due to overproduction and leakage of certain markers (enzymes) into the bloodstream. Rarely, niacin can cause a drug-induced hepatitis. Nearly all niacin side effects can be avoided if it is used judiciously and under a physician's supervision. Starting doses of niacin should not exceed 125-250 mg at mealtime with the understanding that the dose can be increased slightly every week or two, so as to allow for adaptation to higher doses. As the dose of niacin is increased, the side effects gradually subside and go away. But if the drug is stopped for even a day or two, some of the side effects may return when it is restarted. This points out the importance of daily compliance and not skipping here and there.

More than thirty different formulations of niacin are commercially available, some of which are not absorbed adequately when taken by mouth. While certain brands may claim to produce no flushing, they may also go through the intestine unabsorbed and be essentially useless. That is, some "no flush" products may contain niacinamide or nicotinamide, which have some niacin-like effects, but completely lack any effect on blood cholesterol or triglycerides.

Delayed-release, sustained-action, long-acting, or similar products are somewhat more likely to cause liver injury than the short-acting varieties, but they may also cause less flushing or stomach irritation. You can take one brand (Niaspan) once at night instead of two or three times per day. Unfortunately, as with all other brands at high doses (more than 1500 mg), a large number of people may experience flushing and upper abdominal symptoms with Niaspan also. In addition, the cost is several times higher than other brands.

At present, some pharmaceutical companies are in the process of developing niacin-like drugs that are better tolerated and have fewer side effects. Some of these drugs should be available within the next few years, and may prove to be extremely useful for raising HDL cholesterol or lowering elevated levels of lipoprotein(a).

Recent data from a fourteen-year follow-up study of more that eighty thousand nurses in the United States showed that for every additional 100 mcg (each microgram = 1/1000 of a milligram) of folic acid (vitamin B-9) in their diet, the risk of a heart attack fell by about 6 percent. When researchers compared 940 female nurses who had suffered a heart attack during the study to those who had not, women whose dietary folic acid intake was the highest had a third fewer heart attacks. In the same study, the role of vitamin B-6 was very similar to that of folic acid: every additional 1 mg of vitamin B-6 provided a 6 percent protection. Another study showed that among men and women who had coronary artery disease, 10 percent had low blood levels of vitamin B-6 as compared to only 2 percent of those who did not have coronary artery disease.[16]

In some individuals, elevated homocysteine levels (Part II, (8)) may be lowered 15 to 20 percent by using as low as 400 mcg of folic acid (0.4 mg) along with 1000 mcg of vitamin B-12 (1 mg) daily. However, more than 35 percent require much higher doses of folic acid—at least 1 to 2 mg twice a day—to effectively bring down homocysteine levels to below eight. The relatively small reduction in homocysteine levels with low-dose folic acid, and the large percentage of nonresponders, suggest that all individuals with elevated blood homocysteine levels should be treated with higher doses, at least initially.[17]

Large doses of vitamin B-6 (pyridoxine) can cause sensory nerve damage. For this reason, doses exceeding 200 to 300 mg per day should not be used. Since many individuals with elevated blood homocysteine levels do not show a good response to vitamin B-6 alone, it should always be used as co-therapy with folic acid and vitamin B-12.

What about multivitamins? In healthy young adults who eat enough fruits and vegetables, there is no evidence that multivitamin pills serve any purpose. Yet, approximately 40 percent of the population of the United States, many of whom are young individuals, take multivitamins or other supplements. Three pharmaceutical companies control 80 percent of the multivitamin industry in this country. On May 20, 1999, in an out-of-court settlement with the U.S. Justice Department anti-trust division, F. Hoffman La Roche & Company of Switzerland and BASF AG of Germany agreed to pay $725 million in fines for "price-fixing conspiracy." The third company, Rhone-Poulenc of France, was not fined because its officials had cooperated with the Justice Department in the investigation. Most multivitamin pills lack high enough concentrations of vitamin E, B-6, folic acid, or B-12 to have a significant cardio-protective effect. However, as noted earlier, appropriate doses of individual vitamins or minerals tailor-made to an individual's needs may be more meaningful.

There is no evidence to suggest that taking one or two multivitamin pills daily has any side effect (other than the cost). The question is, do they provide any benefit? Folic acid (400 mcg) present in some multivitamins can reduce the risk of hydrocephalus and spina bifida in babies when it is taken by women before conception and during the course of pregnancy. Doses of 400-800 mcg per day may have a significant impact in reducing the risk of colon cancer and, by lowering blood homocysteine level, the risk of coronary artery disease. On the other hand, for those with moderate to severe elevation of homocysteine, or for people with a history of colon polyps which are precursors to colon cancer, the amount of folic acid in multivitamins is quite inadequate. For some, doses of 2000-4000 mcg of folic acid may be required to lower their homocysteine levels (Part II, (8)).

For older persons, or for those with chronic digestive diseases, and for pregnant or nursing women, taking one or two multivitamin pills daily should actually be strongly encouraged. But multivitamins should never be used as a substitute for plenty of fruits and vegetables.

Cardiovascular and Health Impact of Minerals

Several minerals, including selenium, chromium, calcium, magnesium, iron, sodium, and potassium have significant impacts on the cardiovascular system.

Selenium

At present there are insufficient data to support the use of selenium to prevent or treat coronary artery disease.[18] But it is perhaps one of the most effective dietary anti-carcinogens (especially against prostate, colon, and breast cancers), and any cardio-protective benefit is a bonus. At 200-400 mcg (0.2-0.4 mg) per day, selenium supplements are safe. At these doses, blood selenium levels will still be below 1000 nanogram per millimeter of whole blood, the safe level set by the Environmental Protection Agency. Higher intakes may be associated with diarrhea, irritability, hair loss, and nail changes. Seafoods, kidney, and liver (and to a lesser extent, other meats and grains) are good sources of selenium. Fruits and vegetables generally contain little selenium, especially if grown in areas with poor soil selenium content.

Chromium[19]

A recent U.S. Department of Agriculture study showed that taking chromium supplements of 200-1000 mcg per day substantially improves blood sugar control in type 2 diabetics (those who do not require insulin). Higher doses showed proportionately better improvements, approaching the results obtained with oral anti-diabetes medications. The average dietary intake of chromium in the U.S. population is about 50 mcg per day. In another study, even adding 100 mcg of chromium picolinate—the most common form of over-the-counter chromium—to a daily diet significantly improved blood sugar control.

Some studies have suggested that extra chromium can reduce blood levels of LDL cholesterol and triglycerides by as much as 10 percent while raising the level of the good HDL cholesterol by 5 percent. These beneficial cholesterol actions of chromium, combined with improved sugar metabolism, undoubtedly contribute to better cardiovascular health.

A recent study suggested that chromium supplementation (200-400 mcg per day) can help overweight people lose body fat and improve their lean-to-fat ratio. This is an important distinction when compared to other weight loss medications which nearly always cause loss of lean muscle tissues as well as body fat.

Thus because chromium can decrease insulin resistance and improve the metabolism of carbohydrates, it is a reasonable and safe supplement, especially for sedentary or obese individuals and diabetics. For all of these

uses, 200 mcg (0.2 mg) twice a day should be sufficient. Foods containing high levels of chromium include: processed cheeses (such as
American or cheddar), wheat germ, brewer's yeast, organ meats (liver and
kidney), and seafood. Since vitamin C interferes with the absorption of
chromium, the two should not be taken together, especially with vitamin
C doses exceeding 100 to 200 mg.

Iron

Numerous studies over the past decade have strongly suggested that
excessive body iron increases the risk of heart attacks, while iron depletion
has a cardio-protective role. It is thought that iron, especially at high concentrations in the bloodstream, may act like an oxidant, promoting the oxidization of LDL cholesterol, and increase tissue damage within the heart
muscle. However, the presence of several tiers of antioxidants may nullify
the oxidant impact of high blood iron levels. Iron released from breakage
of red blood cells (within the bloodstream) has also been shown to promote
platelet's potential to clump and cause intra-vascular thrombosis (blood
clot). The consensus of recent studies is that excessive body iron does not
play a role in the initiation of a coronary quartet, but does increase the risk
of a heart attack and other cardiovascular events.

Although excessive body iron can increase the risk of a heart attack,
iron deficiency is not exactly harmless. It is associated with a host of
drawbacks including anemia, tiredness, and the reduced capacity of the
heart and other muscles to perform at optimum levels.

Nearly one out of four hundred persons in the United States has a
genetic disorder that predisposes him or her to absorb a very high percentage of dietary or supplemental iron. This condition is called
"hemochromatosis," and it causes severe heart, liver, pancreas, and brain
damage due to iron overload. Recent studies have shown that in people
with hemochromatosis, even in its mild form, the risk of heart attack is
increased more than twofold. The combination of high body iron with
smoking and high blood pressure is even more cardiotoxic, vastly increasing the risk of a heart attack. Clearly, inadvertent or routine use of iron
supplements for "energy," "pep," "stress," or other falsely advertised
reasons—especially when combined with vitamin C, which increases iron
absorption—is quite harmful for these individuals.

The majority of people with a family history of premature heart attacks (before the age of fifty-five) have several identifiable coronary risk factors. Excessive body iron may be one of the "unknown" risk factors among individuals who do not have one or more major coronary risk factors.

Supplemental iron, invariably present in "multivitamins with minerals," is totally unnecessary for men and post-menopausal women who do not have severe iron deficiency. More importantly, iron products do not boost or provide energy, and cannot help tiredness or fatigue in someone who is not iron-deficient. Since the potential harmful effect of iron supplements is even larger among people with elevated blood cholesterol or homocysteine, and in hypertensives and smokers (because of iron's oxidant effect), you should avoid iron pills unless there is a clear-cut case of iron-deficiency anemia.

Women in their childbearing years who lose some blood with their monthly menstrual flow might benefit from small amounts of iron added to their daily diet. For all others who wish to take multivitamin or mineral supplements, they should choose one without iron.

Dietary sources of iron include red meats, poultry, seafood, eggs, vegetables, and fortified cereals. Absorption of iron from various meats (red or white) is far more efficient than from vegetables, fruits or cereal, because they contain different kinds of iron, with different degrees of bioavailability.

Calcium

Calcium is essential for the proper function of many cells, including muscle cells of the heart and arteries throughout the body. Calcium's impact on coronary arteries, however, is relatively minor.[20] Although calcium lowers the blood pressure, this effect is also small. Data from twenty-two randomized studies showed that calcium supplementation decreases systolic blood pressure by an average of only two points. Unfortunately, for most hypertensives, this is a trivial drop.

Since there may well be a threshold of calcium intake below which the blood pressure may rise, calcium supplementation may still be useful in some hypertensive individuals. For example, some hypertensives tend to eat less dairy products (a rich source of calcium), either on their own or on the advice of a health provider to "cut down fat and cholesterol."

Pregnant women are also at risk for developing hypertension. Recent studies have shown that calcium supplementation reduces pregnancy-induced hypertension by 70 percent, and toxemia of pregnancy—a serious disease—by nearly 60 percent. Certainly, in this group of individuals, extra calcium can be beneficial in helping to keep the mother and fetus healthy.

Chelation Therapy: Faith, Hope, and Hoax

Advertisers promote chelation therapy as an effective method to remove calcium and other mineral deposits from the arterial wall, thereby "reversing the process of atherosclerosis." Unfortunately, chelation therapy is no more than a modern-day snake oil. Chelation therapy involves intravenous infusion of a compound called EDTA, usually in combination with vitamins and minerals, once or twice a week for four to six months. This is not an inexpensive, harmless treatment. The total cost may amount to thousands of dollars, and hardly any insurance policy in the United States covers it. Recent studies have clearly established that chelation therapy with EDTA is a useless practice and cannot reduce the size of coronary artery plaques, improve blood circulation, or even remove much of anything from the atherosclerotic arteries.

The reason for EDTA's ineffectiveness is that it cannot penetrate the plaque core; even if it could, it cannot dissolve, separate, and take out the calcium from the pile of debris in the plaque. Calcium, iron, copper, fibrous tissues, overgrown muscle cells, plenty of oxidized cholesterol, and other deposits within coronary artery plaques have all contributed to a tough and haphazard, cement-like structure that would not permit EDTA to penetrate it. Even if (and here we are stretching the limits of our assumptions) some of these deposits could be removed by EDTA, the plaques will not shrink or disappear, and the underlying processes that caused hardening of the arteries in the first place will continue during and after chelation therapy. In brief, chelation therapy is a hoax and may even sidetrack people from seeking proper care for their serious disease, not to mention the hazard to your pocketbook.

Calcium supplementation (1000-2000 mg) is reasonably safe and inexpensive, provided it is not abused. To avoid kidney stones, all calcium supplementation should be taken with meals. Most kidney stones are made up of a mixture of calcium and oxalate. When supplemental calcium is taken with meals, a small portion of it binds with oxalate, making a non-absorbable mix which is then eliminated in the stools. This way, very little oxalate will be absorbed to be excreted later on in the urine. On a daily basis, approximately 200-300 mg of calcium are used up to bind oxalate in the intestine and dispose of it. Thus, anything in excess of this amount will be utilized for other body needs, including bone formation and prevention of osteoporosis, without increasing the risk of kidney stones.

Bioavailability of different calcium products may vary depending on their formulation by as much as 200-300 percent. Calcium citrate seems to be more efficiently absorbed than calcium carbonate. On average, about 30-50 percent of an oral dose of calcium is absorbed through the intestine. This fractional absorption of calcium decreases further with high doses. For this reason, dividing the dose between breakfast and dinner should improve the absorption efficiency of calcium products compared to a single daily dose. Calcium from dairy products and fortified orange juice is more bioavailable than other types of calcium such as Oscal, oyster shell pills, Tums, or Rolaids.

Good dietary sources of calcium and phosphorous are:

- All low fat dairy products that contain more calcium than phosphorous (processed cheeses contain too much saturated fat and salt; as a result, they are not good sources of calcium)

- Leafy and green vegetables such as kale, spinach, and broccoli

- Calcium-fortified foods and beverages (including orange juice)

- Drinking water, surprisingly, contains some calcium and phosphorous. However, home water filters or water purifiers remove a substantial amount not only of calcium and phosphorous but other minerals as well. Most bottled waters have practically no calcium, phosphorous, fluoride, or other minerals.

Excessive vitamin D intake may have the undesirable effect of contributing to coronary artery disease by enhancing calcium deposits in the arterial wall. Instead, regular exercises and exposure to sun, especially among older persons, stimulate vitamin D synthesis by the skin, which is then carried to bones but will not accumulate in the arterial wall. Older persons wear hats and cover themselves before going outside to minimize the risk of skin cancers. Regrettably, this is often taken to the extreme. Far too many people die of coronary artery disease and osteoporosis complications, while very few die of nonmelanoma skin cancers. (Most skin cancers are "basal cell" or "squamous cell," and are curable by surgical removal.) For these elderly persons, even thirty to sixty minutes of exposure to early morning or late afternoon sun (arms, legs, abdomen, or back) may provide sufficient vitamin D without increasing their risk of skin cancers.

Magnesium

Magnesium is the second most abundant mineral in all human tissues except in bones (potassium is first). Magnesium has numerous functions, but within the cardiovascular system, its main role is to relax the arteries and prevent irritability and irregular beating of the heart. Intravenous infusion of magnesium in people who suffer an acute heart attack may significantly reduce the risk of life-threatening cardiac arrhythmias.

To examine the relation of blood magnesium levels to coronary artery disease, nearly fourteen thousand middle-aged adults from four communities in the United States (who were free of cardiovascular diseases at the beginning of the study) were followed up for four to seven years. Women with the highest blood magnesium levels had about 50 percent less risk of developing coronary artery disease compared to women with the lowest blood levels. Among men, those with the highest blood magnesium levels had 27 percent less risk than men with the lowest blood levels. Mortality from coronary artery disease is significantly lower among men and women who live in hard water areas (containing higher calcium and magnesium levels) than among those living in soft water areas (Chapter 2, "Beverages").

It is unclear how or why magnesium deficiency contributes to coronary artery disease. In animal studies, magnesium deficiency can cause swelling and distortion of endothelial cells (lining the inner wall of the arteries), thereby allowing LDL cholesterol and white blood cells to cross through this barrier. Still, the number of studies examining the role of dietary and blood magnesium levels in human coronary artery disease is too limited to draw a valid conclusion.

Since kidneys have a dominant role in sparing or eliminating magnesium, daily variations in dietary magnesium do not play a critical role, unless the intake is quite deficient. In general, magnesium supplementation is unnecessary and, at best, of doubtful benefit. But in people with chronic recurrent diarrhea, vomiting, profuse sweating (during sustained rigorous exercises or outdoor activities on hot days), short-term supplementation may be helpful. Rich dietary sources of magnesium include whole seeds such as nuts, legumes, and various grains. Unfortunately, processing removes more than 80 percent of the magnesium in cereal grains. Green vegetables are also rich in magnesium, but fruits (except bananas), meats, dairy products, and seafood are poor sources.

Potassium

The role of potassium in cardiovascular health, like calcium, is to regulate heart rhythm, smooth muscle tone in the arterial system, and lower blood pressure. Under normal circumstances, dietary potassium deficiency does not occur. However, a good deal of potassium can be lost through the kidneys (especially when diuretics are used on a regular basis), the gastrointestinal tract (in people with protracted vomiting, diarrhea, or laxative abuse), or by profuse sweating. Excessive potassium loss can cause tiredness, weakness, poor appetite, nausea, listlessness, or irrational behavior. It can also cause severe (and, rarely, fatal) irregularities of the heart rhythm.

Three recent studies showed that higher potassium intake is associated with a modest drop in systolic (by three points) and diastolic (by two points) blood pressure. African Americans and older persons are especially responsive to increased potassium intake.

Because potassium is abundant in all living cells, it can be found in a wide variety of foods. Rich sources of potassium include: most fruits (such as figs, oranges, bananas, and cantaloupe), fruit juices, and vegetables (including root vegetables such as potatoes, carrots, and radishes), and various meats, red or white. The average daily intake of potassium in the United States is about 3500 mg per day, but for African Americans it is half the average, a factor that may be relevant to rampant hypertension among this segment of the population.

One of the easiest ways to increase your dietary potassium and at the same time reduce sodium intake is to use salt-substitutes. Many salt-substitutes contain mainly potassium chloride instead of sodium chloride. There are also different "light" or "lite" salts that, depending on the manufacturer, may contain various combinations of sodium chloride, potassium chloride, or magnesium chloride. The net result is that they all have less table salt (sodium chloride) than regular salt. These are all perfectly safe and reasonable alternatives to regular salt.

Potassium supplements are available by prescription, but they are not without side effects, especially in the pill form. Many are not readily dissolved and may cause irritation of the esophagus and the stomach, causing indigestion and, in rare instances, ulcers. But for those who are on diuretics for various indications, taking potassium supplements under supervision is reasonably safe.

Salt: Sodium Chloride

Salt is the most intensively studied mineral in medicine, yet it is still the most controversial. It seems as if almost everyone, medically trained or not, feels obligated to deliver a stern lecture on the evils of salt intake as soon as they spot a "sinner" looking at a salt shaker.

The evangelical proponents of salt restriction have manipulated public opinion, and many health providers, into believing that dietary salt intake should be restricted for everyone (the currently recommended allowance is about 10 grams per day). On the other side, the salt lobby has stubbornly resisted a sensible response to the compelling new scientific data showing that the present high level of salt consumption is unnecessary and may be harmful. The anti-salt evangelists have countered by accusing the salt lobby of collusion with the soft drink industry: in tandem they conspire with food processors to maintain the high salt content of processed foods that increase thirst, thus contributing to greater intake of soft drinks. Here is another case in which science, facts, fiction, emotions, and commercial interests all clash in a whirlpool of controversy. As these battles go on, consumers are left confused by the conflicting messages from all sides.

Salt restriction is helpful to some, harmful to a few, and of very little value to most people. Recently, researchers have discovered two versions of a gene called the "anti-angiotensinogen gene" which determine the salt-responsiveness of an individual. Those who have inherited the AA version of the gene (one copy of the gene from each parent) are sensitive to fluctuations in salt intake, whereas people with the GG version are not salt-responsive. Among African Americans, 65 to 80 percent have the AA version, and as a result their hypertension responds much better to decreased dietary salt intake. In contrast, only 10 to 15 percent of white Americans and 35 to 50 percent of Hispanics have the AA gene. Approximately 85 to 90 percent of white Americans do not respond to dietary salt restriction.

Although the test for the salt-responsiveness genes is not widely available, it should be considered before long-term, severe salt restriction (to below 4 grams per day) is recommended for white Americans with hypertension who do not have severe heart, kidney, or liver failure. On the other hand, because up to 80 percent of African Americans have the AA gene, salt restriction even for those with mild hypertension is a rational intervention.

A rigorous analysis of twenty-three recent studies of mostly white people showed that even with a drastic reduction in salt intake, on average there was only a 6-point drop in systolic blood pressure and a 3-point drop in diastolic. Clearly, for someone who has a blood pressure of 180/105 (systolic over diastolic), this rather small response will only lower the blood pressure to 174/102, numbers which are just as dangerous, and still in need of vigorous anti-hypertensive treatment.

A large number of people who develop a stroke or heart attack do not necessarily have very high blood pressure. Most have "borderline" hypertension (i.e., systolic blood pressure of about 140-150, or diastolic of 90-95). In the past, many physicians did not prescribe medications at these levels, relying instead on lifestyle changes and salt restriction, but often without much success. Even with the availability of a vast number of safe and effective anti-hypertensive medications over the past several years, moderate salt restriction (to below 6 grams per day) is still a necessary component of hypertension treatment. Although the goal is to lower the systolic pressure to less than 140 and diastolic pressure to less than 85, ideally, the systolic pressure should be closer to 110-120, and the diastolic closer to 70-80.

Salt restriction is not without harmful side effects. A significant decrease in salt intake to below 4000 mg per day may be associated with higher blood triglycerides, lower HDL cholesterol, and increased vascular tone (stiffness of the arteries) which, paradoxically, can raise the blood pressure. This is of particular importance in white hypertensive persons younger than forty-five to fifty years of age, for whom the potentially adverse metabolic effects of salt restriction may be compounded further by increasing the blood pressure rather than lowering it.

The average salt intake of an adult in the United States, Great Britain, and other developed countries is relatively high at about 10000 to 12000 mg per day, about half of which is sodium and the rest of which is chloride. Most of this dietary salt (70 to 80 percent) comes from processed foods; only 20 to 30 percent is from salt added to foods during cooking or at the table. Thus, any effort at reducing salt intake even modestly should be directed at these salty processed foods such as cold cuts, sausages, bacon, canned soups, pickled products, vegetable juices, chips, pretzels, and fast foods.

High dietary salt intake results in high urinary output of sodium, the major route by which the body eliminates sodium. But along with sodium, calcium is also dragged out through the kidneys, a process that may contribute to osteoporosis, particularly in post-menopausal women and in older men as well. In fact, a modest reduction (not restriction) of dietary salt may have the same effect on bone mineral density as an increase in calcium intake of nearly 900 mg per day. This is an important consideration, especially among young girls whose calcium intake is habitually low and who tend to eat a lot of salty processed foods including fast foods, french fries, pizzas, chips, pretzels, and other salt-laden snacks.

Numerous studies have shown that long-term compliance with a modest salt reduction is feasible. There is good evidence that when individuals choose to cut down their salt intake, their taste preference changes rather quickly. This is because salt taste receptors on the tongue become more sensitive, and salt-reduced foods give them the same taste as salty ones. In fact, after several weeks on a lower salt diet, most people prefer less salty foods, which helps them stay with their salt-reduced diet.

On the basis of the available information, the following recommendations provide a rational guideline for dietary salt intake:

Older persons, African Americans, and obese persons of any age who have high blood pressure tend to be salt-responsive and therefore should lower their salt intake to less than 4000 mg per day (sodium intake of less than 2000 mg). This is equivalent to slightly less than one teaspoon of salt for the entire day. To achieve this level of salt intake, nearly all salt-laden processed foods should be avoided. Using salt substitutes or sodium-reduced salt products for cooking or in the salt shaker is another way of cutting down salt intake. Salt substitutes (sodium-free or reduced-sodium salts) have the added advantage of providing potassium which helps lower the blood pressure.

All other persons with high blood pressure, and post-menopausal women with or without risk factors for osteoporosis, should cut back their salt intake to less than 6000 mg per day. This can be achieved by cutting down on salty processed foods. Here, too, the use of salt substitutes should be encouraged.

For those without hypertension, avoiding salty processed foods whenever possible is a rational way of cutting back on salt intake to less than 8000 mg per day (less than two teaspoons for all foods and drinks).

Food processors should voluntarily cut back the amount of sodium (salt) they add to their products. This makes good public health sense, and with today's advanced food technology it is practical enough to make good business sense as well.

Cafeterias at schools and military bases are notorious for serving salt-laden fatty meals to children as well as young adults. These young people often adapt to a salty diet, and follow the same kind of eating behavior for years to come. It is scandalous that health messages have bounced off the walls of these institutions, and that no one has taken the initiative to change these practices. Fast food restaurants are where children and adolescents eat most of their salt-laden foods. At restaurant chains such as Burger King, Pizza Hut, or Taco Bell, some entrees contain more than 1500 mg of sodium (or 3000 mg of salt). By the time other side dishes are added in, the total sodium content of the entire meal may exceed 2000 mg (or 4000 mg of salt). Unfortunately, these eateries are unlikely to "clean up their acts," at least not in the foreseeable future.

Fruits, Vegetables, Herbs, and Nuts: Proven Cardio-protection

Fruits and vegetables are irreplaceable in human nutrition. They contain, among other things, minute quantities of a vast number of compounds which contribute to balanced nutrition. Multivitamin pills and other supplements offer only a limited number of compounds, often at unbalanced quantities and qualities.

Numerous studies have shown an inverse relation between cardiovascular diseases and the consumption of fruits, vegetables, herbs, and nuts. These cardio-protective benefits have been observed across many populations—among both those with high, and those with low rates of cardiovascular diseases.

Of course all fruits, vegetables, herbs, and nuts do not have similar cardio-protective or anti-cancer benefits. In fact, even among populations with relatively high consumption of these foods, there are profound differences in the types and quantities they consume. Regional and seasonal availability of different fruits and vegetables also implies that although the dietary fiber content of different populations may be similar, the source of the fiber and other ingredients in the diets may be vastly different (Table 13). These differences play a far more significant role than dietary fiber in the rates of cardiovascular diseases and cancers among various populations (Tables 14 and 15).

In addition to providing a vast number of healthful ingredients, consumption of fruits, vegetables, herbs, and nuts may also lead to reductions in the intake of saturated fat, trans fatty acids, and excess calories. The shift in dietary fat to more monounsaturates, primarily derived from olive oil, or more omega-3 fatty acids from seafood, also provides additional health benefits in populations that consume large amounts of fruits and vegetables.

Recent studies suggest that consumption of blueberries and dark, purple grape juice decreases the oxidization of LDL cholesterol by 30 percent, as well as improving the ability of the arteries to relax and dilate, both of which decrease the risk of coronary artery disease. In laboratory experiments (U.S. Department of Agriculture and Tufts University), researchers gave some rats daily doses of blueberry extracts (equivalent to one cup of blueberries for humans). These animals showed considerable

Table 13
Ranking of Fruits and Vegetables with High Concentrations of Carotenoids

RANKING	BETA-CAROTENE	LUTEIN	LYCOPENE
1	APRICOTS	KALE	TOMATO CATSUP
2	CARROTS	SPINACH	TOMATO PASTE
3	SWEET POTATOES	MUSTARD GREENS	TOMATO SAUCE
4	COLLARDS	DILL	TOMATO JUICE
5	KALE	CELERY	RAW TOMATOES
6	SPINACH	BROCCOLI	WATERMELON
7	PARSLEY	ROMAINE LETTUCE	GUAVA, RAW
8	SWISS CHARD	GREEN PEAS	GUAVA, JUICE
9	MUSTARD GREENS	GREEN PEPPERS	PINK GRAPEFRUIT
10	CHICORY	PUMPKIN	APRICOTS

improvement in age-related loss of balance and lack of coordination when compared with rats who were not given the extract. Strawberry and spinach extracts showed similar benefits but to a lesser extent.

In a recent study from Finland (which has one of the highest rates of coronary artery disease in the world), people who ate apples and onions frequently (both rich sources of antioxidant compounds) had a nearly 30 percent reduction in the rate of heart attacks or death from coronary events. Two recent Harvard University studies also showed that high consumption (more than five servings per day) of vegetables and fruits reduced the five-year risk of coronary events by 30 percent.

Undoubtedly, various nutrients in fruits, vegetables, herbs, and nuts such as potassium, antioxidants, vitamins, flavonoid compounds, and blood "thinners" may account for a substantial part of these benefits. However, the role of other healthy eating habits and healthy lifestyles, such as regular exercises, not smoking, and better control of other coronary risk factors are all relevant.

The main reason you should eat a variety of deeply colored fruits (which should be eaten with their skins), vegetables, and herbs is because their healthful nutrients, including vitamins, antioxidants, flavonoids, and other plant chemicals, vary from one fruit, vegetable, or herb to the next. Also, some of these compounds may be more, or less, digestible depending on the source.

As a rule, eating too much of a single nutrient, even if it is a fruit or vegetable, is too unbalanced to provide a fighting tool against cardiovascular diseases. What is in tomatoes is not the same as what is in spinach or broccoli, and what berries contain is distinctly different from the contents of apples, melons, or oranges. Although dark-colored fruits (such as berries, black grapes, plums, nectarines, and peaches), and vegetables (such as spinach, broccoli, outer leaves of lettuce, watercress, parsley, and herbs) are the most helpful, you should not dismiss other fruits or vegetables because of their lighter color.

A recent study from Johns Hopkins University showed that a diet rich in fruits and vegetables without the use of vitamin supplements resulted in sufficient blood antioxidant levels to reduce oxidization of LDL cholesterol. This and other studies have clearly established that habitual intake of several servings of fruits, vegetables, herbs, and nuts does indeed provide a genuine and effective increase in the concentration of antioxidants in the blood (Figure 5). The problem is that many children and adolescents do not learn to eat sufficient amounts of these foods, and maintain their poor dietary habits into adulthood. Although, ideally, prevention of cardiovascular diseases and cancers requires an early start and almost a lifetime of healthy dietary and lifestyle practices, it is never too late to start.

In the United States and most developed countries, fresh fruits and vegetables are available year round. Certainly fresh frozen fruits or vegetables are just as nutritious, if not as tasty, as their fresh counterparts. Canned fruits in juices (but not in heavy syrup) are another alternative in winter months, but because of higher salt content, you should avoid canned vegetables and choose the fresh frozen (or preferably fresh) variety. Dried fruits such as raisins, apricots, peaches, figs, black cherries, and various berries are wonderful for snacking (as opposed to cookies, candies, and chips). Even a few chocolate-covered almonds or raisins are far better than Almond Joys, Trix, Baby Ruths, or Reese's Peanut Butter Cups.

Incredibly, some people take a handful of multivitamins or other "nutritional" supplements on a daily basis with the explanation, "I don't eat enough fruits or vegetables." This is a terribly unbalanced and illogical alternative to eating all kinds of the real thing: fruits and vegetables containing a vast number of healthful nutrients that can never be put in a pill or capsule.

Table 14
Biological Potencies of Some Compounds in Vegetables and Fruits

COMPOUND	SOURCE	ANTI-OXIDANT	CARDIO-PROTECTION	ANTI-CANCER
CAROTENOIDS:				
BETA-CAROTENE	YELLOW FRUITS AND VEGETABLES	++	0	0
ZEAXANTHIN	FRUITS, DARK LEAFY VEGETABLES	+++	++	+++
LUTEIN	GREEN LEAFY VEGETABLES	++	++	++
LYCOPENE	TOMATO AND TOMATO PRODUCTS	+++	++	++++
ALPHA TOCOPHEROL	GREEN LEAFY VEGETABLES	++++	++++	+
FLAVONOIDS	BERRIES, APPLES, ONIONS, TEA	++++	+++	++++

+ to ++++ = Low to High Level of Effectiveness
0 = No Effect

Table 15
The Impact of Different Nutrients on Human Cancers

CANCER	VITAMIN C&E	FOLIC ACID	LYCOPENE	SELENIUM	FRUITS AND VEGETABLES
BREAST	0+	++++	0	+	++
OVARY	0	+	0	+	++
PROSTATE	++	+	++++	++++	++
LUNGS	0	0	++	+++	0+
MOUTH AND ESOPHAGUS	++	+	0+	0	++
STOMACH	++	+	0	0+	++
COLON AND RECTUM	+	++++	+	++++	+++

+ to ++++ = Low to Very High Protection
0 = No Protection
0+ = Minimal Protection

Figure 5
Rise in Blood Antioxidant Activity After Two Weeks of Eating 10 Servings of Fruits and Vegetables Every Day

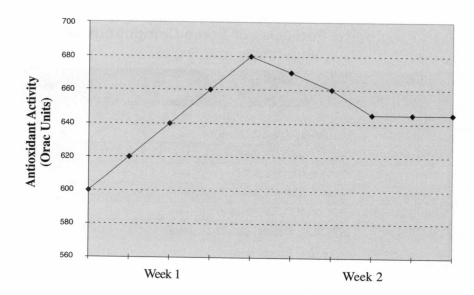

A reminder: you should rinse all fruits, vegetables, and herbs—whether domestic or imported—thoroughly before eating. Many outbreaks of food-borne illnesses from imported raspberries, domestic alfalfa sprouts, and other produce have occurred in the past several years. These outbreaks are obviously exceptions rather than the rule, and efforts are underway to correct the problem at the source of contamination. Still, people whose immune system is not normal (including diabetics, those with chronic liver or kidney disorders, those who have been on long-term cortisone and immune suppressant drugs, and people with a transplanted organ, AIDS, or other immune-deficiency disorders) might be better off avoiding imported berries and domestic alfalfa sprouts altogether. This is because washing alone may be inadequate to lower the contaminants significantly and make it safe to eat them raw. This cautionary note should not be generalized to all domestic or imported fruits and vegetables since various state and federal agencies in the United States have helped to make the produce available here the safest in the world.

Garlic: No Magic Bullet

Hardly a week goes by without a headline or a sound bite praising one fruit or vegetable for all its potent, life-saving virtues. These claims are almost always exaggerated, out of context, and, in some instances, quite nonsensical. Nevertheless, a number of fruits and vegetables may contain distinct ingredients with cardio-protective or anti-carcinogenic effects.

For instance, promoters of garlic tout it as an effective cholesterol-lowering, "natural" alternative to drugs. Unfortunately, most of the studies reporting positive results (5 to 7 percent cholesterol lowering) with garlic are flawed because, among other study design problems, they have ignored the role of simultaneous dietary changes. In other words, the observed cholesterol-lowering is primarily due to changes in dietary practices, and not garlic pills.

The findings of four diet-controlled, double-blind studies (from the United States, Great Britain, and Germany) using garlic powder pills (Kwai) or steam-distilled garlic oil capsules were recently published. All of these controlled studies showed that garlic had no effect on any blood lipids; LDL, HDL, or triglyceride levels were no different in those who took garlic preparations compared with those who took placebos. Even if we assume that much higher doses of garlic (fresh, powder, or oil) could lower blood cholesterol levels, the effect is no more than 5 to 7 percent, too meager to have any relevance to cardiovascular health.

Garlic contains a large amount of a certain sulfide compound called "allinin," which is odorless. But allinin is quickly converted to allicin by garlic's own enzyme (called "allinase") upon crushing or dicing a garlic clove. Allicin is the major active ingredient of garlic and is also responsible for the unmistakable odor of garlic and garlic breath. Aged garlic preparations are far less odorous than fresh garlic, garlic extracts, or some garlic pills because they have much smaller amounts of allicin. Still, the cholesterol-lowering effect of various garlic preparations is simply too small, too impractical, and too odorous for most people.

Garlic reduces the clumping of blood platelets, and by doing so, it reduces the risk of clot formation, a component of heart attacks. This particular benefit of one or two cloves of garlic per day is almost equal to taking one low-dose aspirin tablet daily. Since not all garlic products have a similar anti-platelet effect, the choice of one over other garlic products is important. For example, fresh garlic and freeze-dried garlic powder are similar in potency, whereas steam-distilled oils are 35 percent as effective, and oil macerates about 10 percent as effective. Aged garlic preparations have no such anti-clotting effects.

Garlic products are not exactly harmless; in some individuals, especially those with irritable bowel or esophageal acid reflux, garlic preparations can aggravate symptoms of belching, heartburn, gaseousness, and bloating. Garlic can also cause allergic reactions including contact dermatitis. A strong garlic breath or garlic body odor also has an anti-social and repellent effect that should be considered before starting an odorous garlic regimen.

A small amount of garlic adds a distinct flavor and taste to most meals, and you should enjoy it for that reason. As a bonus, garlic is also a rich source of many nutrients, antioxidants, and anti-clotting compounds which can provide some minor cardio-protection. No amount of packaging, gimmickry, or advertising makes garlic supplements more effective than a bit of fresh or powdered garlic added to foods. For those who hope to lower their cholesterol or to prevent a cardiovascular event there are, fortunately, other safe and effective means of reaching their goal. Relying on garlic for this purpose is an illusion based on folklore and perpetuated by anecdotal testimonials of well-paid celebrities. A high blood cholesterol level and coronary artery disease are not trivial matters, and you should never trivialize them by taking one or two garlic pills daily.

Onions

Like garlic, onion is also extremely versatile and a rich source of many nutrients. For example, it has a high concentration of quercetin, a flavonoid with very potent antioxidant effects. A recent European study suggests that people who consume onions frequently (or apples and tea, which also contain high levels of flavonoids) have significantly lower rates of cardiovascular disease, especially heart attacks.[21]

Onion has far less sulfides than garlic, and therefore fewer volatile compounds that come out with breathing. This makes onion more user-friendly and avoids the stale garlic odor that remains in the breath for twelve to twenty-four hours. However, if you have certain digestive disorders such as acid reflux or irritable bowel syndrome, you may not be able to tolerate too much onion, especially uncooked.

Fortunately, makers of nutritional supplements have left onion alone, so that one can enjoy the real thing without the distraction of pills and capsules or the gaseous and misleading testimonial of actors and television personalities. Since healthful ingredients of onion and garlic are mostly heat resistant, both raw and cooked versions provide the same benefits.

Tomatoes

Tomato is a rich source of an antioxidant called "lycopene," as well as other nutrients. Because lycopene (like vitamin E) is a fat-soluble antioxidant, it is carried by various lipoproteins into the arterial wall, where it backs up vitamin E to fight the oxidization of LDL cholesterol. The available studies, however, suggest that the cardio-protective role of lycopene is relatively small.

Since lycopene (like vitamins A, D, E, and K) is fat soluble, it requires some fat to facilitate its absorption. Thus, drinking tomato juice with your breakfast of cereal and skim milk is not the same as drinking the same glass of juice with lunch or dinner, or with a breakfast that contains some fat such as 1 percent or 2 percent milk. Also, heating releases more lycopene from tomato and tomato products, and because lycopene is relatively heat stable, it is not destroyed by cooking. In fact, since tomato sauces or pastes are used in foods with some fat (preferably olive oil), they are excellent sources of lycopene—even better than tomato juice or a tomato itself. For those who are concerned about (or have) prostate cancer, lycopene supplement of 10 to 25 mg once or twice a day is, in addition to a diet containing a good amount of tomato products, both reasonable and safe.

Cruciferous Vegetables

Broccoli, broccoli sprouts, cauliflower, cabbage, and brussels sprouts not only reduce the risk of cardiovascular diseases, but significantly lower the rates of many cancers, especially esophagus, stomach, colon, pancreas, prostate, and ovaries. Aside from a vast number of antioxidants, cruciferous vegetables also provide a good deal of dietary fiber that can prevent blood sugar surges in diabetics or obese persons.

Since cruciferous vegetables are available year-round in the United States (and to varying degrees in other countries), every effort should be made to eat several servings per week. Unfortunately, these vegetables are not very popular, and overcooking them—a rather common mistake—can give them an unpleasant odor, color, or texture. Adding salt, pepper, olive oil, a touch of lemon juice, or other herbs and spices during a short three to five minute steaming (in the microwave or on the stove top) should make them more appealing to a larger number of people.

Green, Leafy Vegetables

Dark, green, leafy vegetables are rich sources of many vitamins including A, C, and E, trace minerals, as well as a vast number of flavonoids. Numerous studies have shown that, much like cruciferous vegetables, green leafy vegetables are both cardio-protective and anti-carcinogenic.

Among all vegetables, kale, spinach, and watercress have the highest concentrations of antioxidants. (As mentioned, their fruit counterparts with the highest concentrations of antioxidants are blueberries, blackberries, raspberries, strawberries, and concord grapes.)

Eating green, leafy vegetables on a regular basis provides you with a number of cardio-protective antioxidants. It is also one of the most effective dietary means to reduce your risk of many cancers. Using kale, spinach, and watercress (instead of lettuce), and a few broccoli florets, provides a healthful and tasty alternative to regular salads. Some physicians warn their patients who are on "blood thinners" (anti-coagulants like Coumadin) to cut down on or avoid green leafy vegetables, but this is simply recycled pseudoscience. Their concern is that vitamin K in these products may counteract the effect of anti-coagulants. For this to happen, however, you need to eat several pounds of kale or spinach every day—which is unlikely to happen. Furthermore, these green, leafy vegetables also contain vitamin E and tiny amounts of aspirin-like substances that would negate the impact of any vitamin K they might also have.

Herbs and Spices

Is there any food whose personality, character, and delectability cannot be enhanced or brought to life by herbs and spices? Happily, herbs and spices also contain a vast number of vitamins, trace minerals, antioxidants, and other compounds that are cardio-protective, anti-carcinogenic, or have other health benefits. Some herbs and spices also contain low levels of salicylates (close relatives of aspirin), which enhance their cardio-protectivity.

Among those with high concentrations of salicylates are oregano, mint, rosemary, paprika, pepper, curry, and cumin.

A recent joint study by Swedish and Greek investigators showed that extracts of thyme and sage reduced oxidization of fats in various cells to the same extent as vitamin E. This and other studies suggest that frequent use of herbs may also provide many health benefits beyond pleasurable eating.

Unlike fruits and vegetables, herbs and spices cannot be consumed in large quantities. This limits their overall contribution to a cardio-protective or healthful diet. Nevertheless, because of higher concentration of health-promoting compounds in herbs and spices, even at a low level of consumption they can still make your foods delicious and, at the same time, healthful.

Grapefruit

Grapefruit has been touted to have cardio-protective, anti-cancer, and weight control benefits along with a number of other equally exaggerated health claims. Although grapefruit is a rich source of vitamin C, potassium, and some antioxidants, it is not a wondrous fruit. If grapefruit has any anti-obesity effect (which is highly improbable), it is due to its filling effect, the same as with any other fruit, vegetable, or even plain drinking water. Grapefruit does not possess any magical or mysterious ingredient that enables it to do all that it is alleged to do.

Grapefruit and its juice, however, have a unique action on the intestinal lining that is different from all other fruits. Grapefruit juice deactivates a special enzyme in the wall of the intestine called "cytochrome P3A4." Cytochrome P3A4 is responsible for the partial breakdown of many drugs taken by mouth, making them less available for absorption. When a particular drug is taken along with grapefruit or grapefruit juice, the actual dose of the drug available for absorption is decreased by a third compared to taking the same drug with water or other juices. For most drugs, this is not a major problem. In fact, for some drugs it improves their bioavailability and, therefore, efficacy. But for many cardiac medications—especially calcium channel blockers, digoxin, and all cholesterol-lowering statins except Pravachol and Lescol (Part II, (16))—it could pose a problem if you switch from one drug to another, creating a situation where the absorption of these drugs could fluctuate from dose to dose. For some drugs such as "blood thinners" (anti-coagulants such as Coumadin), heart medications, or diabetes drugs, these fluctuations may prove problematic.

Grapefruit provides no significant advantage over other citrus fruits. Moreover, to repeat, it has no known cardio-protective, anti-cancer, or anti-obesity benefits. Because of the peculiarities noted above, you should avoid grapefruit or grapefruit juice for at least two hours before or after taking various heart, blood pressure, diabetes, anti-coagulants, or anti-AIDS drugs, and all oral chemotherapy (anti-cancer) agents.

Some recent studies suggest that a daily glass of grapefruit juice might increase the risk of kidney stones by more than 40 percent. It is unclear how grapefruit juice contributes to kidney stones, but one possibility is that an ingredient in grapefruit combines with dietary oxalate, a main component of most kidney stones, and makes it form a sediment when it is excreted by the kidneys.

Except for some of the above precautions and reservations, grapefruit and its juice should be enjoyed for what they are, no more and no less.

Oranges and Orange Juice

Oranges and their juice are rich sources of various antioxidants as well as vitamin C, folic acid, and potassium. In one recent study, Canadian researchers gave a group of volunteers three glasses of orange juice daily (more than 1.5 pints) for several weeks. On average, HDL cholesterol levels rose by about 20 percent with no change in LDL cholesterol. Lower intakes did not have a significant HDL-raising benefit. Since three glasses of orange juice add an additional 80 grams of carbohydrates (or about 320 calories) to the diet, this is an impractical way of raising HDL levels for diabetics or obese individuals. Still, even one or two glasses of orange juice with pulp and fortified with calcium is far superior to soda or apple juice, especially for teenagers and older persons.

Cranberries and Cranberry Juice

Although cranberries are a rich source of antioxidants, because of their tartness they are used sparingly. As such, they have no significant cardio-protective benefit.

Taste and Distaste for Fruits and Vegetables

Nearly everyone knows that eating plenty of fruits and vegetables is good and healthful. So why is it that in the United States and many developed countries so few eat adequate servings?

Recent data suggest that genetic makeup has something to do with distaste for certain fruits and vegetables. Nearly a third of the population of the United States is genetically very sensitive to certain tastes such as bitter and tart—tastes which, in most fruits and vegetables, are due to flavonoid compounds. These individuals are called "supertasters." Without retraining their taste buds or making a conscious effort, they shy away from broccoli, other cruciferous vegetables, and certain tart fruits such as various berries—all of which are the best plant sources for a vast number of healthful flavonoids. The rest of the population is made up of "normal tasters" and "nontasters." This latter group can eat anything and everything.

By and large, nontasters are thinner, more physically active, and have higher levels of good HDL cholesterol and lower levels of bad LDL cholesterol and homocysteine. Those who are genetically blessed and are among the nontasters should enjoy their good fortune. Normal tasters can adapt to eating more fruits and vegetables containing flavonoids. Unfortunately, supertasters (like former president George Bush, who made "I hate broccoli!" one of his lasting legacies) have a hard time with their fruit and vegetable selections. They often eat few vegetables other than perhaps the occasional salad.

Besides genetic factors, cultural and culinary experiences in childhood and adolescence also undoubtedly influence "likes and dislikes." Many supertasters can accept a few vegetables or fruits without a lot of fussing. Even switching from orange juice in the morning or from soda with meals to mixed vegetable juices such as V-8 (and others) is a step in the right direction. They should also make the effort to eat at least two or three servings of fresh, seasonal fruits daily, something they usually seem to be willing to do, especially since fruits do not require cooking or preparing to make them more palatable. Multivitamin pills can never be a substitute for the "real thing," so almost everyone should aim for several servings of fruits and vegetables daily.

Nuts

Most nuts provide a vast number of healthful nutrients including proteins, monounsaturated or omega-3 polyunsaturated fats, various vitamins, antioxidants, trace metals, calories, added dietary fiber, and excellent taste. Several studies have shown that frequent consumption of various nuts is associated with a 20 to 25 percent lower risk of developing coronary artery disease. Whether this benefit is directly attributable to nuts or the fact that people who eat nuts regularly also have other healthy behaviors or lifestyles is not clear.

Eating an ounce (30 grams) of nuts several times a week reduces the risk of coronary artery disease and sudden cardiac death. In a study of 22,071 male physicians in the United States followed up for eleven years, the risk of sudden cardiac death decreased in a linear fashion with increasing nut consumption. This association seemed genuine and persisted even after adjustments for lifestyles and other coronary risk factors or dietary practices. Although only Persian and English walnut have modest amounts of omega-3 polyunsaturated fatty acids, this alone cannot explain the benefits, especially the significant reduction in sudden cardiac death. Many nuts contain a high concentration of magnesium which is known to reduce heart rhythm irregularities, providing another plausible explanation for their healthful benefits.

English or Persian walnuts, almonds, filberts (hazelnuts), macadamias, pecans, and pistachios are rich sources of monounsaturates with little saturated fat, and provide delicious and healthy snacks for people of all ages. Peanuts, however, have a relatively high concentration of saturated fat (18 percent in peanut oil), and contain small amounts of longer-chain saturated fats (arachidic acid with 20 carbons, and behemic acid with 22 carbons), both of which are highly coronary-unfriendly, at least in monkeys. Brazil nuts, pine nuts, and pumpkin, sesame, or sunflower seeds also have high concentrations of saturated fats and omega-6 polyunsaturated fat which make them less desirable than other nuts.

Except for Brazil nuts, pine nuts, cashews, and peanuts, you can enjoy all other nuts as a component of a heart-friendly diet. The main drawback of nuts is that they are all energy-dense and provide far more calories per 100 gm weight than fruits. For example, 100 gm (3.5 oz) of dry roasted sunflower seeds provides more than 600 calories. On the other hand, with the exception of avocados, all fresh fruits are fat-free and contain fewer than 100 calories per each 100 gm serving. In fact many fruits and nearly all vegetables contain less than 50 calories per each 100 gm serving. Still, a handful of tasty almonds, filberts, pistachios, or walnuts is superior to a piece of cake, pastry, doughnut, chocolate bar, or a scoop of ice cream.

Whole Grains

Whole grains are important sources of many nutrients including fiber, starch, proteins, trace minerals, vitamins, plant chemicals, and antioxidants. All of these provide a balanced blend of ingredients that have proved in numerous studies to be cardio-protective, and reduce the risk of developing hypertension, diabetes, or stomach and colon cancers. Unfortunately, most other healthful nutrients (except for the starch and protein) are removed in the milling process, making the resulting grain products (white breads, rice, pastas, and most cereals) no more than ghosts of the real things. These stripped grain products are devoid of any significant cardio-protective or anti-carcinogenic benefits (Chapter 2, "Dietary Fiber").

Several recent studies in both men and women have shown that long-term use of whole grains on a regular basis can reduce the risk of coronary artery disease by about 30 percent. Although some of this benefit may be attributable to healthier dietary and lifestyle behavior of people who eat whole grain products, the ingredients in whole grains contribute to their cardio-protective benefit.

Of course, eating whole wheat grains should not be confused with overdosing on wheat bran or bran cereals. For many people, a portion of the bran is often fermented in the colon producing a good deal of gas, bloating, or cramps. This is especially true among those who have diverticulosis or an irritable bowel. On the other hand, oat products and whole wheat or multigrain breads (whole wheat cereals or pastas, and wild rice) are all healthful alternatives.

Herbal Supplements: A Marketing Hoax?

Herbal and "nutritional" supplements have become increasingly popular in the United States. The allure of "natural" products is, in part, rooted in the belief that natural products are benevolent, safe, and—with the help of a good deal of misleading advertising—also "effective" against a wide variety of diseases.

The central theme perceived by consumers is that natural products are inherently better or healthier than synthetic ones. The truth is that just because herbal products are "natural," it does not follow that they are safe, healthful, or harmonious with human nature. Poisonous mushrooms, snake bites, pneumonia, malaria, cancers, hurricanes, and earthquakes are all natural, but hardly good for you. A large segment of adult populations in many European countries, and now in the United States, take various herbal supplements, either for their perceived health benefits or for therapeutic purposes. This is even more common among people with chronic diseases.

In most instances, herbal products are no more than very weak chemical compounds or drugs that lack the scrutiny of the Food and Drug Administration. How can it be that these untested, unproven, often contaminated, and ineffective "natural" drugs flourish in a technologically advanced and well-informed society?

Since there is no standard for many herbal products, both their ingredients and whatever biological activity they might have vary from manufacturer to manufacturer and indeed from batch to batch. Soil conditions, storage, handling, manufacturing, and shelf life of the finished product affect their potency. The potency of different brands of a given herbal supplement may vary by 5,000- to 10,000-fold. While a particular herbal supplement may claim to have, for example, 500 mg of this or that herb, it may actually contain only 5 to 10 mg. Sometimes stores sell one botanical product as something else. Or manufacturers select and mix the wrong part of the plant or herb with the proper parts. Not infrequently, the product is inadvertently contaminated with toxic or nontoxic materials. In brief: there are few (and often no) checks and balances, so that you can never be sure that a given herbal supplement is safe or even genuine.

In the United States, herbal supplements with claims of cardioprotection include ginseng, ginkgo biloba, garlic products, hawthorn, and evening primrose.

Ginseng

Ginseng is perhaps the most heavily hyped and controversial supplement. It has achieved the status of an all-healing, cure-all, born-again, miracle supplement. Ginseng comes from the roots of some plants grown in the Far East (Korea, China, and Japan), Canada, the United States, and Brazil. And therein lies the problem.

Almost all fruits, vegetables, herbs, or spices are more or less similar all over the world. But the ginseng in Korea is not the same as that found in Russia, Brazil, or the United States. More than fifty different plants are called ginseng, but with the exception of a few, they have nothing in common with the genuine Asian or American ginseng. Moreover, in spite of claims of purity (nearly always false) by ginseng manufactures and retailers, there is no standardization of the product, or guarantee of its purity.

One has the assurance that 500 mg of aspirin manufactured by different companies is the same in London, Stockholm, or Seoul, Santa Fe, Seattle, and almost anywhere else in the world. By contrast, 100 mg of ginseng means different things, with different ingredients, to different manufactures, in different regions of a country—not to mention different countries.

More than 25 percent of the products sold under the name ginseng have no detectable ginseng. Another 60 percent contain very little (far less than half) of what is advertised or printed on the bottle. Some types of ginseng, like the Brazilian or the Russian (Siberian) varieties, are not even true ginseng, but they are still sold as such.

In the United States, about 90 percent of the ginseng crop is grown in Wisconsin by over fifteen hundred ginseng growers. Although ginseng is supposed to be cultivated without any pesticides, Wisconsin's Department of Agriculture recently uncovered widespread and illegal use of the pesticides Lindane and PCMB by ginseng growers.

Exaggerated claims for what ginseng can do have no boundaries. Depending on the zeal of the promoter and the gullibility of the target audience, ginseng "can do anything." These claims include: the ability to improve cardiovascular health, lower cholesterol and blood pressure, protect against cancers, reduce stress, increase sexual potency, and improve physical performance for athletes. All of them are trivial or nonexistent.

Because Oriental ginseng is expensive, there is often a tendency to cut and dilute it with all sorts of fillers. The more greedy and unscrupulous merchants do not even bother to put any ginseng at all in their products, but have no qualms about labeling and promoting their nonginseng product as a "pure" and "potent" ginseng.

In people with chronic heart failure who are taking digitalis, Siberian "ginseng" can raise digitalis blood levels to toxic and even fatal levels. For this reason, if you have any cardiovascular disease for which your doctor has prescribed digoxin or other digitalis derivatives, you should not take any ginseng product since often the label does not identify the source of ginseng in the bottle.

Ginkgo Biloba

Unlike ginseng, which comes from the plant's roots, ginkgo biloba is extracted from dried leaves of ginkgo trees. People have taken ginkgo preparations since 2800 B.C., but it has become very popular only recently, so that it is currently one of the best-selling herbal medicines in Europe. Ginkgo is among the few herbs for which standardized extracts are available.

A number of European studies have suggested that the regular use of ginkgo biloba over two to four months might improve cognitive functions, memory, and stress tolerance. Since ginkgo has a slight anti-platelet effect, it might also have some relevance to reducing the risk of heart attack or stroke. Because of this anti-platelet activity, it may enhance the effect of aspirin or other anti-clotting drugs slightly, but it does not contribute to bleeding tendencies.

Ginkgosan

Ginkgosan is a combination of ginkgo biloba (60 mg) and ginseng (100 mg). At the dose of two tablets per day, ginkgosan may synergistically enhance the effects of both agents. The combination may also have a mild blood pressure-lowering effect.

The "benefits" of ginseng or ginkgo biloba lack scientific studies to show the claimed benefits, and for most users, provide no more than a placebo effect. Since it is almost impossible to obtain genuine ginseng or ginkgosan at a reasonable price, the meager benefits of most commercially available products do not justify the trouble and expense. Although at one to three pills per day they have no major side effect, it is highly unlikely that you will see or feel a sustainable health benefit from either ginseng or ginkgo biloba.

Hawthorn

The flowers, fruits, and leaves of hawthorn were popular at the turn of the twentieth century for palliating various cardiovascular ailments, at a time when we had no safe or effective drugs. Hawthorn has been shown to increase blood flow through coronary arteries and improve the heart's performance in people with mild heart failure. It has also shown a very mild anti-hypertensive effect. These effects, however, are minor at best, and pale in comparison with today's highly effective and safe cardiovascular drugs.

In the United States alone, nearly one million people die of cardiovascular diseases each year. In the dawn of the twenty-first century, you should not rely on hawthorn to treat such deadly diseases. At the commonly used dosage, hawthorn is relatively free of major side effects, but it has very little clinical usefulness. On occasions, hawthorn can cause digitalis toxicity in people with chronic heart failure who take digoxin (or Lanoxin), very much like the effects of Siberian ginseng.

Evening Primrose

The seeds of this native North American weed contain about 14 percent oil. A small portion of this oil, amounting to less than 2 percent overall, is made up of gamma-linolenic acid, a plant omega-3 fatty acid with some cardiovascular benefits.

Exaggerated claims for primrose oil include its ability to help with weight loss, lowering cholesterol, hypertension, and rheumatism, as well as relieving menstrual cramps and premenstrual syndrome. Because of its gamma-linolenic oil content, some claim evening primrose has cardio-protective benefits. But to obtain this questionable cardiovascular benefit you would need to take ten or more capsules per day (costing a few dollars daily). Then there is the problem of adulterated products that include impurities, and dilution with other oils by unscrupulous manufacturers. Another important concern is that a portion of the oil in evening primrose may be oxidized during its shelf life in the capsules. These oxidized fatty acids may potentially cause liver damage and could possibly be carcinogenic.

The trivial and unproven benefit of evening primrose oil certainly cannot justify spending $50 to $100 a month on this supplement. At lower doses, it is practically useless. Several pieces of Persian or English walnut provide more plant omega-3 fatty acids than two capsules of primrose oil, and they are not only more delicious but far safer, with the same number of calories.

In general, herbal supplements have no magical, hidden cardiovascular benefits that are measurable or reproducible. More importantly, cardio-vascular diseases are not simple cosmetic disorders that can be trivialized and treated with nineteenth-century remedies. In developed countries, the average life span has gone up from forty-seven to seventy-seven years since the mid-nineteenth century, almost entirely due to advances in med-icine, public health, and food technology. Most herbal remedies did little then and can do no more today. Subsequent chapters provide you with evidence-based, practical recommendations that will reduce your risk of cardiovascular events while avoiding the trappings of herbal remedies.

Dietary Fiber: No Need for Supplements

The term "dietary fiber" refers to certain components of plants that are not broken down or digested in the human small intestine. Horses, cattle, and all herbivores have the necessary enzymes such as cellulase and hemicellulase to digest plant fiber. Humans lack these enzymes. Thus, a grazing cow does quite well on green pasture, whereas humans would starve to death eating grass or tree leaves.

When, why, and how humans lost these enzymes is a question that dates back at least two million years to our distant ancestor Homo erectus, who began walking, making various hunting tools, and displaying the behavior of a hunter-gatherer. Certainly the modern human over the past ten thousand years has been mainly carnivorous, even though we still eat plenty of fruits, vegetables, and seeds. Although humans cannot digest or absorb plant fiber (it is mostly eliminated in the stool), many other ingredients in fruits and vegetables are readily processed and absorbed from the intestine.

Clearly, the hollow argument of some fanatic vegans that "humans are born to be herbivores" is not based on fact but on emotions and personal belief systems. Even today, many monkeys and other primates in the wild are not purely vegetarian. They hunt for animal proteins in ways that vary from eating ants and other insects to cannibalism. In addition, there are well over five hundred species of carnivorous plants.

There is a vast difference between a high fiber diet and a diet that contains plenty of fruits and vegetables. Certain nutrients such as bran cereals contain very high concentrations of dietary fiber, whereas fruits and vegetables have between 1 to 10 percent dietary fiber (Tables 16-A and 16-B). The physical form of dietary fiber (for example, coarse grains compared to finely milled flour products) can also alter the impact of dietary fiber.

In a recent study, researchers studied 34,500 post-menopausal women for an average of nine years. Women with the highest intake of whole grains (an average of three servings per day), had a 30 percent lower risk of developing coronary artery disease when compared to women with the lowest intake (less than three servings per week). Although dietary fiber accounted for some of the benefit, most of the benefit was attributable to various antioxidants, plant chemicals, folic acid, and other (as yet unidentified) ingredients in whole grains. In addition, people who eat whole grains are usually more health conscious, and have other healthy habits and lifestyles (such as being physically active and weighing less).

One characteristic of all plant fibers is their ability to hold water and swell. Fibers that have a high water holding capacity are soluble fibers and those with very low capacity are insoluble. Some examples of soluble fiber include psyllium (such as metamucil and bran bud), pectins, and gums from plants, fruits, and some vegetables. Most plant fibers are a mix of soluble and insoluble. Oat bran, for example, has approximately 16 grams of fiber in each 100 grams, of which 40 percent is soluble. More importantly, oat bran contains 10 percent beta-glucan, a highly soluble viscous compound that is responsible for oat bran's cholesterol-lowering effect. In contrast, wheat bran has nearly 42 grams of fiber in each 100 grams, most of which is insoluble. Wheat bran has only 2 percent beta-glucan, which explains why wheat bran products do not lower blood cholesterol levels.

Beta-glucan binds with bile in the intestine and helps to eliminate it. Since the liver makes bile from cholesterol, the more bile is eliminated, the more cholesterol is taken out of blood circulation by the liver to form new bile. This bile-eliminating and, therefore, cholesterol-lowering effect of soluble fiber depends on the dose. An effective dose of oat bran, for example, is approximately three to five servings per day to lower cholesterol by 5 to 7 percent. Higher doses of oat bran, phyllium, guar gum, pectin, or other soluble fibers—along with other dietary modifications—can reduce blood cholesterol level by an average of 7 to 10 percent. Higher doses, however, amounting to 50-60 grams per day, are almost always associated with many unpleasant gastrointestinal side effects, including excessive gas, bloating, fullness, diarrhea, and abdominal pain. In rare occasions, they may even cause intestinal obstruction, especially in older persons.

Since the average diet of an American male contains less than 15 grams of fiber per day (for women it is less than 12 grams), increasing this 300 to 400 percent and maintaining it indefinitely is neither practical nor justifiable for most people. Fiber pills, regardless of their promotional claims, are even more problematic and should be avoided by most people, particularly older persons or those with a history of digestive problems. On occasions these fiber pills can swell up and cause small bowel obstruction, especially among individuals with abdominal adhesions from previous surgeries.

There are a large number of well-promoted and highly touted fiber products on the market, all geared towards cholesterol-reduction. Some of these are terribly costly (as much as $6 to $8 a day). For others, to achieve a 5 to 7 percent cholesterol reduction, as many as twelve tablets should be taken daily for almost a lifetime! This is a rather impractical, expensive, and wasteful use of resources for such meager cholesterol-lowering results. In spite of much deceptive advertising, these products, even if they do lower blood cholesterol by 5 to 10 percent, have no relevance to cardiovascular health. This is particularly true at low doses which are utterly ineffective but give consumers a false sense of security, perhaps influencing them not to seek proper medical care. Moreover, since women require even more fiber for a cholesterol-lowering response than men, taking lower doses of these commercially touted and highly expensive fiber supplements is even more inappropriate.

In general, you should try to eat several servings of fruits and vegetables (fresh, canned, frozen, or dried) along with legumes or nuts (excluding Brazil nuts, peanuts, pine nuts, and pumpkin or sunflower seeds), and frequent use of cereals containing soluble fiber such as oat and barley. This is certainly far superior to taking any kind of fiber supplement, be it pills, capsules, powder, or granules.

People often assume that they have enough fiber in their diet because they eat an occasional serving of salad or fruit. As seen in Table 16, ingredients of a typical garden salad have very little fiber. If one medium-sized cucumber has 1 gram of fiber, how much fiber can there be in two or three slices? Or in two or three small wedges of a tomato? Similarly, most of the commonly eaten summer fruits (such as cantaloupe or melons) do not have much fiber.

Some simple ways you can increase dietary fiber include switching to rye or dark bread from white bread, to oat-based cereals or whole wheat from Frosted Flakes or Rice Krispies, and to baked potato with skin from french fries. Fresh or dried figs, prunes, apricots, peaches, and various berries, beans, peas, corn, and carrots are all healthful alternatives to pills and powders. Another easy way is to eat fruits (such as oranges, apples, and prunes) instead of drinking their juices, which are practically devoid of any fiber. To avoid the digestive side effects such as gas and bloating, you should increase your dietary fiber slowly to reach desirable levels of more than 20 gm per day.

Table 16-A
Total Fiber Content of Fruits and Vegetables
(Per 100 gm)

FRUITS	GRAMS	FRUITS	GRAMS
APPLES, WITH SKIN	2.2	NECTARINES	1.6
APPLES, W/O SKIN	1.8	OLIVES, GREEN	2.8
APPLESAUCE	1.5	OLIVES, BLACK	3
APRICOTS, DRIED	8	ORANGES	2.5
APRICOTS, FRESH	2	ORANGE JUICE	0.2
AVOCADOS	2	PEACHES, DRIED	1.6
BANANAS	2	PEARS, DRIED	8
BLACKBERRIES	7	PEARS	2.6
BLUEBERRIES	2.2	PINEAPPLES	1.2
CANTALOUPE OR HONEYDEW	1	PINEAPPLES, CANNED	1.3
CHERRIES	1.5	PLUMS, FRESH	2
FIGS, DRIED	9.2	PLUMS, DRIED	7
FRUIT COCKTAIL	1.5	PRUNES, STEWED	6
GRAPEFRUIT	1	RAISINS	5
GRAPES, SEEDLESS	1	RASPBERRIES	5
KIWI FRUIT	3.4	STRAWBERRIES	2.6
MANGOES	1.5	WATERMELONS	0.4

Table 16-B
Total Fiber Content of Vegetables and Breads
(Per 100 gm)

VEGETABLES	GRAMS	VEGETABLES	GRAMS
ARTICHOKES	5.2	LETTUCE, ICEBERG	1
ASPARAGUS, GREENWHITE	2	LETTUCE, ROMAINE	1.7
BEANS, BLACK, KIDNEY	7	MUSHROOMS	1.3
BEANS, LIMA	7	ONIONS	1.6
BEETS	1.7	PEAS, SWEET	2.6
BROCCOLI	2.8	PEAS, BLACK-EYED	9.6
BRUSSELS SPROUTS	4.3	PEPPERS, SWEET	1.6
CABBAGE	1	POPCORN	4
CABBAGE, RED	2	POTATOES, WITH SKIN	4
CARROTS	3.2	POTATOES, W/O SKIN	1.5
CAULIFLOWER	2.4	SPINACH, RAW	2.2
CELERY	1.6	SQUASH	2
CORN, SWEET	3.7	SWEET POTATOES	3
CUCUMBERS, WITH SKIN	1	TOMATOES, RAW	1.3
CUCUMBERS, W/O SKIN	0.5	TURNIPS, GREEN	2.4
EGGPLANT	2.5	WATERCRESS	2.3
KALE	2	ZUCCHINI	2

Table 16-C
Total Fiber Content of Nuts, Seeds, and Breads
(Per 100 gm)

NUTS AND SEEDS	GRAMS
ALMONDS, ROASTED	11.2
CASHEWS, ROASTED	6
CHICKPEAS, CANNED	5.8
FILBERTS (HAZELNUTS), ROASTED	6.9
MIXED NUTS, ROASTED	8
PEANUTS, ROASTED	8
PEANUT BUTTER, CHUNKY	6.8
PEANUT BUTTER, CREAMY	6
PECANS, ROASTED	6.5
PISTACHIOS, ROASTED	10.8
SUNFLOWER SEEDS, ROASTED	6.8
WALNUTS, ROASTED	5
BREADS	GRAMS
CORNBREAD	2.4
CRACKED WHEAT	5.3
FRENCH	2.7
ITALIAN	3.1
MIXED GRAIN	7.1
OATMEAL BREAD	3.9
PITA, WHITE	1.6
PITA, WHOLE WHEAT	7.6
PUMPERNICKEL	5.9
RYE	6.2
WHEAT	4.3
WHITE	2.3
WHOLE WHEAT	6.9

Beverages: Tea, Cocoa, Coffee, Alcohol, Water, Soft Drinks, and Fruit Juices

Tea

Next to water, people drink tea more than any beverage in the world, particularly in Asia and Europe. Black tea is the fermentation by-product of green tea leaves. Much like wine making, it is the tea master's expertise and creativity in combination with the soil condition, region of the world, weather, rain, and other growing conditions, that account for the tea's taste, flavor, aroma, and other characteristics.

Tea is a rich source of many antioxidants. Within thirty to fifty minutes after drinking a cup of brewed tea, blood levels of tea's antioxidants rise by 40 to 50 percent and may last for up to eighty minutes. Green tea, but not black tea, has certain polyphenolic compounds that can block the action of an enzyme called "urokinase" in some cancer cells.

Black tea contains various antioxidants including quercetin and catechins that can reduce the risk of coronary artery disease and stroke significantly. A substantial portion of these antioxidants are readily absorbed from the intestine and go to work soon after arrival in the bloodstream.

Tea also lowers the blood level of homocysteine, a protein compound that is highly damaging to the cardiovascular system (Part II, (9)). Recent data from the Boston Area Health Study showed that among men and women with no previous history of coronary artery disease, those who habitually drank more than one cup of tea per day had 45 percent less risk of developing a heart attack compared to those who didn't drink tea. In another study from the Netherlands, the risk of suffering a stroke during a fifteen-year follow-up was 70 percent less in men who drank an average of four-and-a-half cups of tea per day compared to those who drank less than two-and-a-half cups.

The cardiovascular and anti-cancer benefits of tea (green or black) are substantially reduced if milk is added to the tea, a practice all too common in England, Canada, Australia, and New Zealand. This is because some ingredients in milk (such as lactalbumin, fatty acids, and calcium) may bind to tea's antioxidants and phenolic compounds at high temperatures, and reduce their absorption from the digestive tract. In other words, these compounds become less bio-available when milk is added to a cup of hot tea. However, the same reaction would not occur when tea without milk is drunk after a meal which contains milk or other dairy products. This is because gastric acidity and lower temperature of the stomach content (98-99 degrees as compared to more than 200 degrees in a cup of hot tea) prevents this kind of binding and, as a result, food does not interfere with the absorption of tea's ingredients.

The evidence to date strongly suggests that drinking a few cups of tea daily is a healthful practice that can indeed reduce your risk of heart attack, stroke, and perhaps certain cancers such as esophagus, stomach, or bladder. Since tea has other ingredients that act like diuretics, it may reduce the risk of bladder cancer by increasing the volume of the urine and diluting any carcinogens in the bladder (see "Water," this chapter). Tea can also reduce the risk of forming kidney stones by diluting the urine. Since coffee has no cardio-protective or anti-cancer benefits, it would seem prudent to consider tea as an alternative to drinking coffee. Although iced tea is still preferable to carbonated beverages, it is too diluted to contain a significant amount of phenolic compounds or other antioxidants when compared to a cup of brewed hot tea.

To ensure that the qualities of tea are fully extracted from tea leaves, you should boil water in excess of 210 degrees. This will also allow the tea's phenolic antioxidants to seep through. Although microwave-heated water may look as if it is boiling, the water temperature is not as hot as kettle- or pot-boiled water. This is because in the microwave the bubbles rise from the outer layers of water while the center is not fully heated, so that when you pour the water over a tea bag, the temperature is usually much less than 210 degrees. The result is a cup of tea with not much personality or healthfulness. A slight foaming over the surface of the cup indicates that the water was not adequately hot. Brewing the tea in the old-fashioned way is still the best way to have a healthful and enjoyable cup of tea.

The practice of adding milk to tea not only turns a delightful cup of brew into an unappealing and muddy-looking drink, but strips it of its cardio-protective and anti-carcinogenic properties. A better alternative is to add a teaspoon of dark honey to each cup of tea. Dark honey (more so than light honey) is a rich source of antioxidants and anti-carcinogenic phenolic compounds that can further enhance the flavor and healthfulness of your tea.

Cocoa

Cocoa (and hence chocolate) is a paradox. Despite its relatively high sugar and saturated fat content, chocolate is a rich source of antioxidants. These antioxidants not only prevent the fat in chocolate from turning rancid and reduce the need for adding preservatives to extend the chocolate's shelf life, but they can also reduce oxidization of LDL cholesterol.

A cup of hot chocolate, for example, contains approximately 150 mg of phenolic compounds, and a piece of milk chocolate bar (1.5 oz or 41 gm) provides almost 200 mg. For comparison, a standard 5 oz (140 ml) glass of red wine contains approximately 210 mg of phenolic compounds.

Chocolate is also a rich source of many vitamins, including A and B vitamins, as well as a number of minerals such as calcium, phosphorous, potassium, copper, and iron. Moreover, it contains phenylethylamine, which stimulates the brain and produces euphoria and pleasure. In addition, good, dark chocolate (unlike the cheap varieties) does not contain added shortening or a big dose of butter, and nearly one-third of its fat content is stearic acid, a saturated fat that behaves like monounsaturates.

Contrary to a common misconception, an occasional piece of chocolate or a cup of hot chocolate, instead of being among the evil foods and drinks, offers pleasure to many, and perhaps some minor cardio-protection to a few. Alas, if you are a chocolate lover you cannot assume that overdosing with the tasty morsels is entirely safe. Over time, unfortunately, the cholesterol-raising potential of excessive, daily chocolate intake may prove more harmful than the sum of its antioxidants or pleasurable benefits.

Coffee

Moderate amounts of coffee (less than five to six cups per day) have no desirable or undesirable cardiovascular effects. On the other hand, high consumption (more than eight cups per day) of either regular or decaffeinated coffee can raise the blood level of LDL cholesterol and, as a result, increase the risk of coronary artery disease. The cholesterol-raising compound in coffee is not caffeine, but a special oily substance in the ground coffee that seeps out during brewing. The active compounds of this oily substance are mainly cafestol and kahweol, which are usually filtered out by paper coffee filters, and to a lesser extent by metal filters. Because relatively high levels of these compounds are present in boiled coffee (Scandinavian style), as well as unfiltered and espresso coffee, drinking more than six to eight cups of these brews on a regular basis may increase the LDL cholesterol by as much as 10 percent.

Large amounts of coffee (in excess of six to eight cups per day) can also increase the blood level of homocysteine, a particularly harmful protein compound that damages coronary arteries (Part II, (9)). At present, it is unclear whether cafestol, kahweol, or other compounds in coffee are responsible for this harmful effect.

Heavy coffee drinkers are often heavy smokers, a common problem especially among Europeans and Latin Americans. For these people, smoking plays a far more important role in increasing the risk of cardio-vascular diseases than drinking a few cups of coffee daily.

Excessive coffee drinking may cause some irregularity of the heart rhythm (usually fast beating or extra beats). It may also cause palpitation (skipped beats), as well as jitteriness, sleeplessness, indigestion, heart-burn, or diarrhea in some susceptible individuals. Caffeine, not other ingredients in coffee, accounts for most of these side effects. Some stud-ies suggest that regular coffee (but not decaffeinated) has a mild anti-depressant effect. This mood-elevating property may explain why coffee drinkers experience irritability, mood swings, fatigue, and headaches when they stop drinking coffee.

Aside from the pleasure, taste, and slight physical and emotional lift, coffee (unlike tea) lacks any cardio-protective, anti-cancer, or other sig-nificant health benefits. Of course not everything we do has to have a par-ticular positive health impact. Wearing makeup, shaving, ironing our clothes, or a variety of other things we do are not directly (or even indi-rectly) relevant to our physical health. We do these things because we like them, they give us pleasure, and they enhance our quality of life. Drinking a few cups of coffee is a harmless and often pleasurable habit. For this rea-son, if you enjoy a few cups of coffee each day, there is no compelling rea-son to change. However, switching to tea is a healthful alternative.

Alcohol

Alcohol, very much like tea or coffee, is not a nutrient, yet many con-sume it around the world. In the past decade, over one hundred long-term studies have consistently shown that a small amount of alcohol (less than two drinks per day) is associated with 30 to 50 percent reduction in the risk of developing coronary artery disease. Mortality data from twenty-one developed and relatively affluent countries have also shown cardio-protective benefits from all alcoholic beverages, not just red wine. To date, the weight of the evidence supporting the cardio-protective effect of light drinking is so strong that it can no longer be considered controversial.

How Do Alcoholic Beverages Help the Heart?

Alcoholic beverages (wine, beer, or cocktails) reduce cardiovascular mortality in three distinct ways:

(1) Alcohol, and not other ingredients of alcoholic beverages, raises blood levels of HDL cholesterol by approximately 7 to 10 percent, depending on the individual's initial HDL level. In people with low levels, it is much harder to raise their HDL with alcohol (or with exercises) than in those with higher HDL levels. This is an unfortunate "catch 22," because people with low HDL cholesterol need to have their levels raised far more than individuals who have high levels. The rise in HDL cholesterol level accounts for approximately 50 percent of alcohol's cardio-protective benefit.

(2) Alcohol reduces the tendency of blood to clot, and therefore significantly decreases the risk of coronary thrombosis. This anti-coagulant effect is especially helpful when alcohol is consumed with meals, as many French and Mediterraneans do. This is because following a meal, the blood's tendency to clot inside the arteries increases for several hours, raising the risk of a heart attack or stroke. The post-meal anti-coagulant effect is, of course, not relevant to the practice of "happy hour" or random drinking, common among many Americans and populations of other affluent countries. Nearly all anti-clotting effects of alcoholic beverages are related to their alcohol content and not other compounds. Thus, various alcoholic drinks serve the same purpose. The anti-clotting effect of alcoholic beverages accounts for approximately 30 percent of their cardio-protective benefits.

(3) Some, but not all, alcoholic beverages contain certain flavonoid antioxidants (such as catechin and quercetin) that can potentially reduce the oxidization of both HDL and LDL cholesterol by more

than 75 percent. These antioxidants in both red and white wine seep through the grape's skin during the wine-making process, and account for approximately 10 to 20 percent of the cardio-protective benefits of alcoholic beverages.

Red or White Wine vs. Other Alcoholic Beverages

A torrent of publicity has recently surrounded the "wonders of red wine," as if it were man's last best hope. Although red wine contains a number of ingredients other than alcohol that may not be present in other beverages, their importance to cardiovascular health is greatly exaggerated. During wine making, a number of compounds in the grape's skin can seep through, giving different wines their distinct color, aroma, flavor, and other characteristics. The grape's skin also contains a variety of oxidants (substances that cause oxidization), as well as antioxidants and phenolic compounds. The same compounds, however, are also present in grape juice, grapes, and raisins, provided they are chewed well to crush the skin.

The concentration of various compounds in wine may vary from batch to batch because of geographic location of the vineyards, soil characteristics, vintage, and variety. In addition, the multitude of chemicals and proprietary compounds that are used in the process, filtering techniques, and aging, all can influence and change concentrations of these compounds in the wine. Even decorking the wine and letting it sit for a while at room temperature can alter many of these ingredients, some of which may become oxidized and lose their cardiovascular benefit.

Aside from concentration and potency, the absorption of a wine's various compounds from the intestinal tract varies. Equally relevant is the fact that the result of laboratory studies performed in test tubes cannot be extrapolated to humans, even if we were able to digest and absorb all of these compounds.

A recent study demonstrated that in people who drank white (chardonnay) wine, oxidization of LDL cholesterol was reduced by 30 percent. In contrast, those who drank red (cabernet) wine showed only a 15 percent reduction in their LDL oxidization. Furthermore, the blood's tendency to clot decreased by 29 percent among the white wine drinkers compared with 12 percent among the red wine drinkers. The reason for the better efficiency of white wine in reducing clot formation and LDL oxidization is that the phenolic compounds and antioxidants may be absorbed more readily from white wine than from red wine.

The review of data from twenty-two recent studies in which the types of alcoholic beverages consumed were identified offers highly diverse and inconsistent conclusions regarding various alcoholic beverages. Fortunately, or perhaps unfortunately, these conclusions suit everyone's taste. These data show that depending on the design of the study, the type of beverage used, and the population and the gender of the study population, red wine, white wine, beer, and liquor, each come out on top. For example, in a study from California, white wine appeared to be more cardio-protective than red wine, red wine was more protective than beer, and beer was more protective than liquor. In the Female Nurses Study, beer was associated with the lowest risk of coronary artery disease, while in the Male Health Professionals Study, liquor was the most cardio-protective alcoholic beverage. And in France, red wine won the honors.

Red wine may still possess some hidden virtues beyond its alcohol content or its antioxidants. Red wines, especially young wines, have tannins that give the wine its astringent taste. In aged wines, tannin often settles at the bottom of the bottle. Recent studies in rats have shown that after the anti-clotting effect of alcohol wears off in a few hours, there is a rebound effect in the clotting tendency, a condition referred to as a "hypercoagulable state." This increased tendency to form clots within the arteries may increase the vulnerability to a heart attack or stroke. When rats were given tannin along with alcohol, it prevented the rebound phenomenon. Rats given red wine also showed far less clotting rebound than animals given other forms of alcohol. Whether this phenomenon occurs in humans is not clear, but if it exists its impact is relatively minor, especially with one or two glasses of wine.

Red wine (and the skin or juices of all dark grapes) contains a special antioxidant called "resveratrol," which can significantly reduce oxidization of LDL cholesterol in a test tube. Unfortunately, its blood concentrations even after drinking more than two to three glasses are still ten- to one-hundredfold lower than necessary to protect LDL cholesterol against oxidization. However, even at blood concentrations reached with two or three glasses, resveratrol significantly reduces the sticking of the white cells to the endothelial surface of the arteries, and thereby prevents their trespassing into the arterial wall. This novel action of resveratrol may indeed have significant cardio-protective benefits during the post-meal period, assuming that the wine or the purple grape juice (12 to 16 oz) is drunk with meals.

Low doses of alcohol (two drinks or less per day) also reduces the risk of a stroke by 50 percent. But among heavy drinkers, the risk is increased threefold.

Since over 80 percent of cardio-protection from alcoholic beverages is due to alcohol itself, there is not a lot of room for the other ingredients of various beverages to be relevant, especially with one or two drinks per day. For all practical purposes, there are no significant cardio-protective differences among various alcoholic beverages.

Is There a "French Paradox"?

For centuries the French diet has contained relatively high levels of fat. Yet, except for the Japanese who are unique in their own right, certain regions of France have had the lowest rates of coronary artery disease of all developed nations. This apparent "paradox" is attributed, erroneously, to the traditional French habit of drinking red wine. Such misleading oversimplification ignores a host of other cardio-protective factors that lower the risk of coronary artery disease among the French. For example:

- Although the French (from the regions of France with low rates of coronary artery disease) have a diet that is relatively high in fat, a large portion of the fat is made up of monounsaturates, especially olive oil. And unlike other developed countries, they eat very little partially hydrogenated polyunsatuates or trans fatty acids in the form of margarine or shortenings. Most of their poultry or red meats come from free-range and grazing animals whose flesh has less saturated fat and more monounsaturates than feed-lot fed animals. In addition, meats and eggs from free-range animals contain some omega-3 polyunsaturated fats, absent in cage-fed poultry or feed-lot fed cattle.

- The French eat a lot of seafood, which results in higher blood levels of omega-3 polyunsaturated fat, with all of the benefits this brings.

- The French eat a lot more fruits and vegetables (in fact several times more) than their northern European counterparts who have much higher rates of coronary artery disease.

- The French eat 58 percent of their total 24-hour calories by 2 P.M., compared to 38 percent of Americans. They are also physically more active before and after meals. This distinct lifestyle, combined with other factors, has contributed to much lower rates of abdominal obesity in many regions of France.

- The French drink wine with their meals, not at "happy hour" as is prevalent in the United States, Great Britain, and other developed countries. Given this meal-related alcohol consumption, it is quite likely that even if the French drank beer or liquor with their meals, they would still have the same results. This is because alcohol from any source taken with meals reduces the risk of coronary artery disease during the vulnerable post-meal hours.

- In many regions of France the population has remained homogeneous for centuries, transferring to its offspring some, if not all, of its cardio-protective genes. Some of these genes are responsible for normal cholesterol patterns, low homocysteine levels, reduced risk of hypertension, less abdominal obesity, and less diabetes.

For all of the above reasons, the "French paradox" is not a paradox at all. It is a readily explainable phenomenon that does not justify the exuberance of the red wine aficionados or the news media.

Light drinking can make insulin's action more efficient and therefore the breakdown or metabolism of carbohydrates becomes much easier. Thus in diabetics, especially those who are treated with oral medications, one or two drinks with the evening meal might help control diabetes more efficiently.

Contrary to a common misconception, sautéing with wine or beer does not result in total evaporation of alcohol content or denaturing of alcohol's other ingredients. In fact, as much as 70 to 80 percent of alcohol may be retained in such foods. However, the amount of alcoholic beverages used for this sort of gourmet cooking is so small and infrequent that it has virtually no health impact.

Alcohol's Side Effects

Alcohol is a nonspecific drug with a narrow safety margin. Beyond one or two drinks per day, alcohol has no medically beneficial virtue and is associated with a vast number of side effects, some of which are serious or even fatal. Nearly all cardio-protection of alcohol is achieved with the first drink. After the second drink, it is all downhill. Some negative effects of alcohol include:

- Light drinking increases the level of apoprotein A-1, a protein complex that is a component of HDL particles and is responsible for HDL's cardio-protective action. But as the drinking increases, apoprotein A-1 level decreases progressively, even if the HDL cholesterol continues to rise. Without adequate apoprotein A-1, HDL cholesterol cannot function properly. It is for this and a number of other reasons that excessive drinking, no matter what happens to HDL, increases the risk of heart attack.

- Among heavy drinkers, men are twice, and women are seven times, as likely to suffer a stroke as nondrinkers.

- Most heavy drinkers have already damaged their heart muscle. A recent study of sudden deaths in women without a history of heart problems showed that nearly 40 percent were alcohol-related. A number of studies have shown similar data in men. The culprit in almost all of these fatalities is sudden irregularities of the heart rate and eventual cardiac arrest.

- Heavy alcohol consumption is a known risk factor for premature mortality. A recent long-term study of sixteen hundred middle-aged men revealed that the risk of all-cause mortality was substantially increased in people who regularly drank six or more beers at a time. The association was even stronger with deaths from external causes (such as accidents) and heart attacks. Unfortunately, heavy drinkers are also often heavy smokers. Undoubtedly, the combined burden of excessive alcohol intake and smoking, along with poor intake of antioxidants and poor dietary and unhealthy lifestyle practices, contribute to increased cardiovascular mortality among heavy drinkers.

If you have no personal objection to alcoholic beverages, one or two drinks with dinner (or with lunch for some people) provide a vast number of cardio-protective and other healthful benefits. Most of the benefits of alcoholic beverages are due to alcohol and not to other ingredients.

This simple fact, unfortunately, means that grape juice or raisins cannot provide the same benefits as low-dose alcohol.

So what kind of alcoholic beverage is best? The answer is that, with a few minor differences, they are all essentially the same. One interesting distinction is that beverages produced by fermentation such as beer, wine, cognac, and champagne, cause a 50 to 90 percent increase in stomach acid secretion. Distilled beverages such as gin, vodka, and whisky, on the other hand, have no measurable impact on gastric acid secretion. When wine or beer are distilled, their distillates do not increase acid secretion, whereas the remaining fraction does. This suggests that fermented alcoholic beverages have one or more ingredients, as yet unidentified, that stimulate acid production. Because of this difference, if you have acid reflux or stomach problems you may be better off with distilled beverages.

Given the compelling evidence favoring low-dose alcohol intake, it does make sense to recommend one or two drinks per day, with a meal, for those at high risk of cardiovascular diseases. Coexistence of multiple risk factors for coronary artery disease, especially among men and women past the age of forty, is also an indication for low-dose alcohol therapy.

In spite of the vast benefits of low-dose alcohol therapy, it is not necessary to drink alcoholic beverages to reduce your risk of heart attack. We should not get caught up in the fashionable fantasy that alcohol is the answer to the worldwide epidemic of coronary artery disease. Alcohol can be a deadly drug when abused. Beyond the narrow indications for low doses of alcohol recommended here, William Shakespeare had it right when he wrote: "First the man takes a drink, then the drink takes a drink, then the drink takes the man!"

Table 17
Alcohol's Effects and Side Effects

BENEFITS (<2 Drinks/Day)	• INCREASES HDL CHOLESTEROL • REDUCES CLOT FORMATION • REDUCES THE RISK OF HEART ATTACK AND STROKE • REDUCES THE RISK OF MACULAR DEGENERATION • REDUCES THE RISK OF KIDNEY STONES • REDUCES INSULIN RESISTANCE • REDUCES THE RISK OF COLON CANCER
SIDE EFFECTS (>4 Drinks/Day)	• COSTS THE U.S. >$150 BILLION ANNUALLY • INCREASES THE RISK OF STROKE AND HEART ATTACK • DAMAGES THE HEART MUSCLE, PANCREAS, BRAIN, AND LIVER (A COMMON CAUSE OF LIVER CIRRHOSIS) • INCREASES THE RISK OF BREAST CANCER IN WOMEN • INCREASES THE RISK OF VIOLENT ACCIDENTS (2/3 OF ALL FATAL MOTOR VEHICLE ACCIDENTS) • INCREASES DEPRESSION • CAUSES TESTICULAR ATROPHY AND IMPOTENCE • IS ADDICTIVE AND TEARS FAMILIES APART

< = Less Than   > = More Than

Water

Over the past decade, sales of bottled water in the United States have increased by more than 400 percent. The annual per capita consumption of bottled water has risen to over thirteen gallons, while in California, it exceeds twenty gallons. In Europe and urban areas of many countries the craze is also mushrooming.

There are well over forty national and regional brands of bottled water in the United States, some of which, contrary to their misleading claims, are nothing more than bottled city water with no relation to "pure spring water." Nearly one-third of bottled water is filtered tap water to which a dash of this or that mineral is added. Some have the audacity to add oxygen to bottled water and make outlandish claims that the product improves athletic performance, as if humans were fish. Needless to say, extracting a few molecules of oxygen from water in the intestine will not make you grow gills.

Aside from successful advertising, the growth of the bottled water industry is mainly due to consumers' concern about the taste and safety of tap water, even in Western societies with relatively stringent safety standards for drinking water. Whether concerns over the safety of tap water are exaggerated or not, bottled water is here to stay. Taste and packaging aside, all bottled waters are not the same. Some bottled waters such as Lithia Springs, Monclair, and Vichy Springs, contain high levels of sodium. On the other hand, many brands contain little or no sodium. Some of these latter include: Canadian Glacier, Carolina Mountain, Deer Park, Evian, Great Bear, Mountain Valley Spring, Poland Spring, Pure Hawaiian, Sierra, Talking Rain, and Zephyrhills.

Most bottled waters, regrettably, have little or no magnesium or calcium, two minerals that reduce the risk of cardiac rhythm irregularities in dehydrated individuals. In fact, among the more than thirty brands, only Mendocino has an adequate and balanced amount of these two minerals without going overboard with sodium. Evian is a distant second to Mendocino.

Is the current craze another fading fad? Perhaps; but water, strange as it sounds, is quite cardio-protective and can significantly reduce the risk of heart attack. In a recent six-year study of more than 34,000 Seventh-Day Adventists, men who drank five or more glasses of water a day had a

51 percent lower risk of fatal heart attacks compared to those drinking less than two glasses per day. Women who drank more than five glasses of water daily had a 35 percent lower risk of fatal coronary events. Even after adjusting for other risk factors, these remarkable differences persisted. Just as important was the finding that men and women who drank more than five glasses of water a day had a 44 percent lower risk of fatal strokes.

In a Swedish study, women fifty to sixty-nine years of age, who had lived in counties with hard water (high levels of calcium and magnesium), had a 30 percent lower risk of dying from a heart attack. Among Swedish men, high-magnesium water conferred similar protection against fatal heart attacks.

Why should water lower the risk of fatal heart attacks? One plausible explanation is that water dilutes the blood, making it less viscous, and there-fore less likely to cause clot formation. Another untested explanation is that platelets in a well-hydrated bloodstream do not stick together or to the endothelial cells of coronary and cerebral arteries to initiate clot formation. A well-hydrated person also passes a lot of urine. Because certain clotting substances circulating in the bloodstream are eliminated through the kid-neys, a high urine output makes the blood even less prone to clotting. In addition, both calcium and magnesium in hard waters lower death rates from coronary artery disease and decrease the risk of fatal arrhythmias after a heart attack. These observations cast doubt on whether bottled waters are ever as healthful as regular city waters which are not heavily filtered and stripped of their mineral content. Moreover, bottled waters are also devoid of other important minerals including fluoride, iodine, and selenium.

Bottled water offers no advantage over city water in areas maintaining high standards for water purification and safety. In fact, because most city water contains healthful minerals such as magnesium, calcium, fluoride, iodine, selenium, and zinc, you are better off with city water than you are with the heavily filtered and mineral-stripped bottled waters. This is not a trivial matter, especially for athletes who exercise vigorously and might deplete their potassium and magnesium. Similarly, individuals exercising strenuously may have a higher risk of cardiac rhythm irregularities. Children, too, need calcium and fluoride for healthy teeth and bones, and therefore should be discouraged from drinking bottled waters and colas. Admittedly, the taste and smell of some city water leaves a lot to be desired. In such locales, bottled waters are certainly preferable to dehydration.

Most faucet-mounted home water filters (with solid block carbon filters) remove a very high percentage (more than 90 percent) of water-borne parasites from the tap water and provide a tasty and safe source of drinking water. However, you must change the filter frequently, at least once every two to three months. Some newer models of granular activated charcoal filters can also remove water-borne parasites, but this varies from manufacturer to manufacturer. For those whose immune systems are severely compromised, more expensive and effective under-the-sink filters should not only remove the parasitic contaminants but other micro-organisms as well.

Bottled waters in general provide some convenience and often a false sense of safety. But since the majority of bottled waters are neither pasteurized nor sterilized (they are usually filtered), they may still have some bacterial contaminants.

Soft Drinks

In general, an occasional soft drink with or without caffeine or sugar has no relevance to cardiovascular health, cancer, or any other health issue. Although drinking too many caffeinated soft drinks may trigger heart rhythm irregularities in susceptible people, there are a vast number of caffeine-free soft drinks, especially for children and those who cannot tolerate caffeine, as well as sugar-free products for "dieters."

Fruit Juices

All unsweetened fruit juices (with or without calcium fortification) are excellent alternatives to colas. But unpasteurized juices (such as apple juice) may pose a health risk due to bacterial contamination. Several recent outbreaks of E. coli infection in the United States and Canada have been traced to these unpasteurized products, even though the manufacturers had used standard procedures. (Most of these outbreaks of E. coli infection have been traced to the farm or orchard from which the produce came, and not to the factories themselves.) For this reason, only pasteurized fruit juices should be chosen, especially for those who have compromised immune systems.

Chapter 3
The Twenty Risk Factor Diet

Because the risk factors that contribute to coronary artery disease are numerous, any nutritional approach must take into account each individual risk factor, its relative importance, and how it interacts with other risk factors. Most popular diets designed to lower cholesterol or to aid quick weight loss don't do that; they often take a simplistic, and sometimes harmful, approach. Before I introduce my nutritional approach to cholesterol-lowering, let's see why current dietary programs are obsolete, ineffective, or even unsafe.

Coronary artery disease is almost always due to the interaction of multiple risk factors, and no dietary measures that focus on one or two risk factors are likely to provide a significant degree of protection for the heart. Yet, for decades, many have parroted the outdated recommendation to "cut down the fat and cholesterol" without questioning the effectiveness of such advice. Just as troubling are the growing concerns about the safety of some of the current diet fads.

Low-fat, Low-cholesterol Diets: Ineffective and Possibly Harmful

Low-fat, low-cholesterol diets began over thirty years ago, when the medical community assumed that coronary artery disease was a direct consequence of an elevated blood cholesterol level. Today, we know that this was a flawed assumption. The other flawed assumption was that a low-fat, low-cholesterol diet would significantly lower blood cholesterol and, by doing so, would lower the risk of coronary artery disease. Regrettably, these diets did not live up to their high expectations. Among the general population, approximately 30 percent respond to low-fat, low-cholesterol diets, and drop their harmful LDL cholesterol by an average of 7 to 10 percent. Unfortunately, this modest reduction in LDL cholesterol is unlikely to have a significant cardiovascular impact, especially in those who have already developed coronary artery disease. Moreover, the

70 percent of persons who do not respond to dietary cholesterol and saturated fat benefit even less from low-fat, low-cholesterol diets.

Low-fat, low-cholesterol diets may lower LDL cholesterol by 7 to 10 percent, but they also lower beneficial HDL cholesterol by the same percentage, offsetting their minor benefits. Since a low-fat, low-cholesterol diet is almost always supplemented by a high carbohydrate intake, this further lowers the HDL cholesterol, raises triglycerides, and may convert the large LDL particles, which are relatively harmless, into small dense LDL particles, which are particularly coronary-unfriendly.

The total dietary fat is irrelevant to coronary artery disease. Eskimos obtain more than 60 percent of their energy supply from fat, but they have the lowest risk of coronary artery disease in the world. Similarly, many low-risk populations—such as Mediterraneans, many ovo-lacto-vegetarians, or the large majority of the U.S. population that does not have coronary artery disease—have a dietary fat intake that ranges from 33 percent to more than 40 percent. As seen in Figure 6, dietary fat intake among various populations is not correlated with their rates of coronary artery disease. In a recent fourteen-year follow-up of more than eighty thousand healthy American women who were between thirty-four and fifty-nine years of age at the beginning of the study, the total amount of dietary fat had no relation to coronary artery disease. The investigators, however, estimated that the replacement of 5 percent of energy from saturated fat with energy from unsaturated fats (monounsaturates or non-hydrogenated vegetable oils) would reduce the risk of coronary artery disease by 42 percent, and the replacement of 2 percent of energy from trans fatty acids (present in margarines, shortenings, cooking fats, and other foods) with energy from unsaturated fats would reduce the risk by 53 percent, without reducing the total fat intake.

The Multiple Risk Factor Intervention Trial followed up nearly thirteen thousand healthy (low-risk) men with no previous history of coronary artery disease for sixteen years. One group followed the American Heart Association phase II diet, which has less than 20 percent fat and less than 200 mg of cholesterol per day. They also took medications to lower their high blood pressure, stopped smoking, and lost some weight. During the sixteen-year follow-up, deaths from coronary artery disease in the treated group dropped by only 11 percent compared to the control group (which was not so treated). In contrast, a recent study from Lyon, France, showed that in a group of high-risk individuals (i.e., people who have already developed coronary artery disease and experienced at least one heart attack), those who followed a Mediterranean diet experienced 70 percent fewer heart attacks, 56 percent fewer overall deaths, and, surprisingly, 61 percent fewer cancers. These dramatic effects occurred even though the fat content of the diet was more than 30 percent, mostly from monounsaturates along with omega-3 polyunsaturates from seafood.

Aside from depriving people of the joy of eating and imposing unnecessary and inflexible restriction on their food choices, low-fat, low-cholesterol diets may even be harmful. In a twenty-year follow-up of 832 men who were between forty-five and sixty-five years of age at the beginning of the study, a low-fat, low-cholesterol diet increased the risk of a stroke by more than 50 percent compared to those who were not on cholesterol- and fat-restricted diets (Chapter 2, "Monounsaturated Fat"). Is this an effective, practical, or safe diet to prevent a heart attack?

Figure 6
Dietary Fat Intake Is Not a Predictor
of Coronary Artery Disease

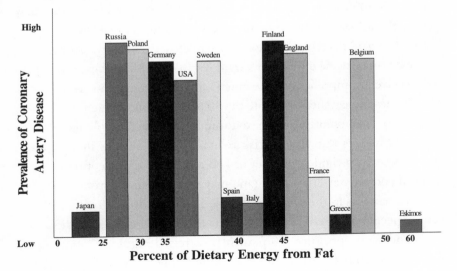

Very Low-fat, Very Low-cholesterol Diets: Helpful or Harmful?

Let's now look at some of the very low-fat, very low-cholesterol diets. Pritikin's Longevity Program contains less than 10 percent of calories from fat (less than 3 percent from saturated fat), and about 25 mg of cholesterol per day, whereas Ornish's Lifestyle Heart Trial provides 7 percent of calories from fat and no cholesterol. In addition, the Lifestyle Heart Trial forbids all oils, meats, poultry, seafood, nuts, dairies (except a small amount of skimmed milk), eggs, alcohol, tea, coffee, and chocolate (what's left?).

Unlike many studies that are based on hundreds or thousands of cases, Dean Ornish's Lifestyle Heart Trial diet evolved from the study of only twenty-two men with severe coronary artery disease, obesity, and sedentary lifestyles. Those individuals were enrolled in a supervised program of regular exercise (one died while exercising), stress management, weight reduction, smoking cessation, anti-hypertensive therapy, aspirin and various vitamins, along with repeated follow-up visits. In addition, they closely followed the strict vegan diet alluded to above.

After five years on this rigid program—impossible to follow for free-living people—the researchers reported a 50 percent lower relative risk of new coronary events compared to another small control group. They touted this 50 percent response rate as proof that a rigid vegan diet may well be the answer to the epidemic of coronary artery disease.

But does a 50 percent reduction in the relative risk of coronary events in five years support the efficacy of a rigid vegan diet? Since these individuals also received comprehensive treatment for numerous other risk factors, why do these researchers attribute the 50 percent improvement (as meager as it is) to their punitive and next-to-impossible diet? Table 64 (Part II, (15)) summarizes the average risk reduction from various interventions, and shows why a rigid vegan diet has no relevance to prevention or treatment of coronary artery disease (and may well be counterproductive).

Since patients in the Ornish Lifestyle Diet took aspirin (with a 30 percent expected risk reduction), lowered their LDL cholesterol (30 percent) and blood pressure (30 percent), exercised regularly (50 percent), lost weight (40 percent), stopped smoking (30 percent), and participated in regularly scheduled, twice-a-week stress management therapy (at least an expected 50 percent risk reduction), they should have earned a risk reduction close to 260 percent. Yet their relative risk reduction was only 50 percent. Is this a rational, safe, effective, or practical way to deal with a deadly epidemic?

A frivolous argument by some vegetarian zealots and proponents of very low-fat, no-cholesterol diets is that the human digestive tract is genetically unsuitable for carnivorous diets. The fact is that our distant ancestors, Homo erectus, made tools and chased animals for food at least two-and-a-half million years ago. Thus any genetic mutation since those days would, if anything, have favored a carnivorous diet, not the other way around. With a few exceptions, even rodents, insects, birds, and fish are also avid carnivores whenever they have the opportunity. Monkeys and other primates, as mentioned, often supplement their protein-deficient diet by devising ingenious tricks to catch ants and other insects. They also resort to occasional cannibalism. It is of interest that there are also more than five hundred species of carnivorous plants in the world.

Extremely low-fat, low-cholesterol diets (or the newer cholesterol-free versions) began some twenty years ago, at a time when there were no effective or safe cholesterol-lowering drugs. These diets were the counterparts of salt-free diets (for hypertensives and people with heart or kidney failure) and sugar-free diets (for diabetics). Fortunately, salt-free and sugar-free diets had their "fifteen minutes of fame" and faded into oblivion as effective anti-hypertensive and antidiabetes drugs became available. Very low-fat, cholesterol-free diets are punitive, accomplish very little, and may even be harmful. They have no relevance to prevention or treatment of coronary artery disease, especially on a population-wide basis.

The Ten Dietary Commandments

Now that we have dismissed the obsolete low-fat, low-cholesterol diets, let's ask the key question: What should the aims of dietary interventions be? An ideal dietary intervention should prevent, slow down, or stop the coronary quartet (Chapter 1). To achieve these goals such a diet should be consistent with most or all of the following "ten commandments." An ideal coronary-friendly diet should:

(1)   Reduce LDL cholesterol, especially the small, dense particles

(2)   Reduce triglycerides

(3)   Reduce the oxidization of LDL cholesterol

(4)   Reduce insulin resistance and blood sugar

(5)   Reduce activation of white blood cells and platelets inside the coronary artery

(6)   Reduce the blood's viscosity and tendency to clot

(7)   Increase HDL cholesterol

(8)   Increase the body's antioxidants

(9)   Increase choices, practicality, and flexibility for long-term adherence

(10) Be safe and not increase the risk of stroke, cancer, or other diseases

The Twenty Risk Factor (TRF) diet presented here addresses all of these dietary "commandments." Low-fat, low-cholesterol, and vegetarian diets do not.

The TRF diet is not based on a personal belief system, a bias for or against any particular nutrient or food group, or the author's own unsupported opinions. In sciences, and especially in medicine, no one is entitled to his own opinion unless it is supported by facts. The TRF diet is based on a modified and contemporary Mediterranean diet, analyzed and computed for use by people of all ages, with or without any risk factors for coronary artery disease. It is backed by several thousand scientific works published in the past ten years and a three thousand-year-old history of healthfulness and safety. In addition to its cardio-protective role, the TRF diet also reduces the risk of many cancers (such as colon, prostate, and breast), diabetes, hypertension, obesity, kidney stones, and osteoporosis. It provides you with endless choices without the boredom of a fixed, rigid menu. In essence, the TRF diet is designed to replace almost all other diets.

One Diet for All Coronary Risk Factors: The TRF Rating System

For more than thirty years, we have promoted the notion that dietary fat and cholesterol, by raising blood cholesterol levels, cause coronary artery disease. All existing dietary programs designed to impact the cardiovascular system are based on this flawed premise. Today, even though it is clear that an elevated LDL cholesterol is only one among twenty major coronary risk factors, we are still stuck in the quicksand of dietary saturated fat and cholesterol (Chapter 1).

Food is not the enemy. Foods have a vast number of cardio-protective and anti-carcinogenic ingredients. They also can promote health in numerous other ways. On the other hand, excessive consumption of some nutrients, such as saturated fats, trans fatty acids, or carbohydrates, can have a negative health impact. It is this dual role that has given foods a Dr. Jekyll and Mr. Hyde persona: credited for their health-promoting role and blamed for their disease-causing potential.

Eating should be pleasurable, not an exercise in algebra, food biochemistry, or bewilderment about what the various ingredients in a given food mean. Clearly, judging food solely on the basis of its fat and cholesterol content is wrong, because this narrow focus ignores the exceedingly diverse roles of different nutrients in foods. Although a small, select group of people might be willing to follow a rigid and impractical diet, such punitive dietary practices have no relevance to the general public or to preventive medicine. Fad diets that put an inordinate emphasis on a single nutrient such as broccoli, grapefruit, oat bran, or garlic, or on components such as carbohydrates, fat, and cholesterol, are unbalanced and often harmful.

Short bursts of dieting for a week or a month have no long-term benefits. Regrettably, you can't place benefits of short-term dietary or lifestyle changes in a biological bank somewhere in the human body, and then take out some of the savings or long-term dividends at will.

The Twenty Risk Factor diet (TRF diet) introduced here is the result of a decade of research in the area of food technology, nutrition, medicine, and health. Instead of focusing on one or two nutrients, the TRF diet is broad-based, taking into account all the important nutrient groups in foods. For example, in the TRF diet, the overall health impact of a piece of chicken is distinctly different from that of a piece of fish, even though they may have the same amount of fat and cholesterol content. Similarly, a tablespoon of olive oil or canola oil is quite different from a tablespoon of corn oil or margarine, even though they have the same amount of fat and calories, and no cholesterol.

For most consumers, it is annoying and impractical to be constantly on guard against certain foods and try to figure out how much of what is in them. The TRF diet eliminates all these concerns. Just as important, the TRF diet is designed to meet dietary requirements for the management of *all* twenty major coronary risk factors. Thus, there is no need for one dietary approach for those with heart disease, hypertension, or diabetes, and another for those with elevated LDL cholesterol, high homocysteine level, or obesity, and yet a different diet for the young or the elderly. Moreover, the TRF diet has drawn from a huge database of research on various cancers to provide a rational dietary approach to reduce the risk of the most common cancers dramatically, including breast, colon, and prostate. Thus, the TRF diet is the lifetime diet for all people—healthy or otherwise.

The formula for the TRF scoring system is presented for information only. Readers will not have to do the math themselves because the scores for a vast number of common foods and snacks are already computed and presented in Tables 19 to 58. The formula should be a helpful tool for other researchers, nutritionists, and government or private agencies involved in public health and nutrition policies.

Table 18
TRF Scoring System*

NUTRIENT	AMOUNT	SCORE
S = SALT	EACH 5,000 MG	+1
CH = CHOLESTEROL	EACH 100 MG	+1
OMEGA-6 PUFA	EACH 5 GM	+1
TFA = TRANS FATTY ACIDS	EACH 1 GM	+2
SFA = SATURATED FATTY ACIDS	EACH 1 GM	+2
VF & N = VEGETABLES, FRUITS, AND NUTS	EACH 2 SERVINGS	-1
MUFA = MONOUNSATURATED FATTY ACIDS	EACH 2 GM	-1
OMEGA-3 PUFA (PLANT-DERIVED)	EACH 2 GM	-1
OMEGA-3 PUFA (MARINE-DERIVED)	EACH 1 GM	-3

TRF Rating System

- Dietary carbohydrates and proteins are neutral (score 0) in the TRF system
- PUFA = Polyunsaturated fatty acids
- VF & N = vegetables, fruits, and nuts; also represents their antioxidants, flavonoids, and other cardio-protective ingredients

* The TRF score of a given food or snack is the sum of all its nine ingredients. This single score provides an instantaneous understanding of the total nutritional impact of a given food, instead of an isolated or unbalanced focus on cholesterol or saturated fat. The lower the TRF score of a food or snack is, the more coronary-friendly it is. The goal is to keep the total TRF scores of all foods and snacks under +30 points per day, and preferably closer to +20.

TRF Rating System

Table 19
TRF Scores of Oils and Fats
(Per 2 Tablespoons)

COCONUT {A}	+48
PALM KERNEL {A}	+44
VEGETABLE SHORTENING	+26
BUTTER {A}	+25
PALM	+23
BEEF TALLOW	+22
LAMB TALLOW	+21
STICK MARGARINE	+20
MAYONNAISE	+18
LARD	+18
SOFT MARGARINE	+16
DUCK FAT	+16
CHICKEN FAT	+15
COTTONSEED	+15
TURKEY FAT	+14
SAFFLOWER {B}	+8
SUNFLOWER {B}	+8
CORN {B}	+6
SOYBEAN	+6
PEANUT	+5
SESAME	+3
OLIVE {C}	-2
CANOLA {C}	-3
HAZELNUT {C}	-5

{A}-Coconut Oil, Palm Kernel Oil, and Butter have the highest percentage of saturated fatty acids: 86%, 81%, and 62%, respectively.
{B}-Safflower, Sunflower, and Corn Oil contain the highest percentage of Omega-6 PUFA: 77%, 69%, and 61%, respectively.
{C}-Olive, Canola, and Hazelnut Oil are rich sources of monounsaturated fatty acids and contain 72%, 56%, and 78%, respectively.

Table 20
TRF Scores of Margarine*
(Per 2 Tablespoons)

ALL FAT-FREE MARGARINES	0	FLEISHMAN EXTRA LIGHT	+7
IMPERIAL DIET, IMITATION	+8	PARKAY LIGHT	+11
BENECOL SPREAD	+1	FLEISHMAN LIGHT	+9
IMPERIAL SOFT	+14	PARKAY LIGHT CORN SPREAD	+9
BLUE BONNET	+19	FLEISHMAN MOVE OVER BUTTER	+15
IMPERIAL WHIPPED	+14	PARKAY SOFT	+15
BLUE BONNET, LIGHT SPREAD	+10	FLEISHMAN SOFT	+13
MAZOLA	+18	PROMISE, EXTRA LIGHT	+5
BLUE BONNET, SOFT	+14	FLEISHMAN TODAY'S CHOICE	+6
ABOVE, DIET 100% CORN OIL IMITATION	+5	PROMISE, SOFT	+14
BRUMMEL & BROWN SPREAD**	+4	FLEISHMAN UNSALTED	+18
MAZOLA, UNSALTED	+18	PROMISE, STICK	+20
CHIFFON	+17	LAND O'LAKES	+21
MRS. FILBERT'S GOLDEN	+19	PROMISE, ULTRA	+2
CHIFFON, SOFT	+11	*ABOVE*, COUNTRY MORNING LIGHT	+14
MRS. FILBERT'S 100% CORN OIL	+14	RICHFOOD, STICK	+18
CHIFFON, WHIPPED	+11	LAND O'LAKES SOFT	+19
MRS. FILBERT'S SOFT GOLDEN	+15	RICHFOOD 100% CORN OIL	+18
EMPRESS, STICK	+17	I CAN'T BELIEVE IT'S NOT BUTTER	+17
MRS. FILBERT'S WHIPPED MARGARINE	+15	SMART BALANCE, SOFT **	+8
EMPRESS, STICK	+20	*ABOVE*, LIGHT	+10
MRS. FILBERT'S WHIPPED SPREAD	+11	TAKE CONTROL SPREAD	+1
FLEISHMAN 100% CORN OIL	+18	IMPERIAL COUNTRY MORNING	+19
PARKAY	+21	WEIGHT WATCHERS EX. LIGHT, STICK	+5

* Because of variability in trans fatty acid content of different samples, a plus/minus 2 point variation in the TRF scores of these fats may occur.
** Benecol, Brummel & Brown, Smart Balance, and Take Control have no TFA.

Table 21
TRF Scores of Dairy and Egg Products
(Per 100 gm or 3.5 oz, Unless Otherwise Noted)

BUTTERMILK	+1
ABOVE (1 CUP)	+3
CANNED MILK, WHOLE, EVAPORATED*	+21
CANNED MILK, SKIM, EVAPORATED	+1
CHOCOLATE MILK, 1% FAT (1 CUP)	+3
CHOCOLATE MILK, 2% FAT	+2
ABOVE (1 CUP)*	+6
CHOCOLATE MILK, REGULAR	+5
ABOVE (1 CUP)*	+11
EVAPORATED, CONDENSED, & SWEETENED MILK*	+17
ABOVE (1 CUP)*	+43
MILK, SKIM (NO FAT)	+3
MILK, LOWFAT (2%)	+2
MILK, WHOLE (4% FAT)	+4
ABOVE (1 CUP)*	+9
MILK, CHOCOLATE SHAKE (8 OZ)*	+8
MILK, VANILLA SHAKE (8 OZ)*	+8
COCOA & CHOCOLATE POWDER IN NONFAT MILK	+2
COCOA & CHOCOLATE POWDER WITH WHOLE MILK *	+11
DRIED, NONFAT MILK EGG NOG*	+7
EGG NOG (1 CUP)*	+20
EGG, LARGE (1 WHOLE)	+4
EGG, YOLK (1 LARGE)	+4
EGG WHITES	+4
EGG, 1 HARD, SOFT COOKED, OR POACHED	+4
EGG, 1 SCRAMBLED WITH OLIVE OR CANOLA OIL	+3
EGG, 1 SCRAMBLED WITH ADDED MILK & MARGARINE*	+7

Table 21 continued on next page

Table 21 continued

EGG, 1 SUNNY SIDE UP COOKED WITH MARGARINE*	+7
EGG, 1 OMELETTE COOKED IN BUTTER OR MARGARINE*	+7
ABOVE WITH ADDED CHEESE*	+10

*AVOID

TRF Rating System

TRF Rating System

Table 22
TRF Scores of Cheeses and Other Dairy Products
(Cheese 1 oz Slice, Other Dairy Products 3 oz, Unless Otherwise Noted)

AMERICAN*	+11	MOZZARELLA	+8
AMERICAN SPREAD (2 TBS)	+7	MOZZARELLA, PART SKIM	+6
BLUE*	+10	MUENSTER*	+11
BRIE	+9	PARMESAN, HARD	+9
CAMEMBERT	+7	PARMESAN, GRATED (2 TBS)	+4
CHEDDAR*	+12	PIMENTO*	+11
CHEDDAR, SHREDDED	+23	PROVOLONE	+8
COLBY*	+11	RICOTTA (2 TBS)	+4
COTTAGE, CREAMED	+6	RICOTTA, PART SKIM (2 TBS)	+3
COTTAGE, 2%	+3	ROMANO*	+10
COTTAGE, 1%	+2	ROQUEFORD*	+12
CREAM CHEESE (2 TBS)*	+12	SWISS*	+10
CREAM CHEESE, LIGHT (2 TBS)	+5	SWISS, LOW-FAT	+5
CREAM CHEESE, SMOKED SALMON (2 TBS)	+7	ICE CREAM, REGULAR*	+13
CREAM CHEESE, OLIVE & PIMENTO (2 TBS)	+6	ICE CREAM, RICH (16% FAT)*	+19
CREAM CHEESE, FAT-FREE	0	ICE CREAM, SOFT (3% FAT)	+2
CREAM CHEESE, SOFT (2 TBS)	+7	SHERBET (2% FAT)	+3
FETA (2 TBS)	+8	YOGURT, FROZEN FAT-FREE	0
GOUDA*	+10	YOGURT, WHOLE MILK	+3
GRUYERE*	+11	ABOVE (8 OZ. CONTAINER)	+7
HAVARTI*	+13	YOGURT, LOW-FAT MILK, PLAIN	+2

* AVOID

Although all cheeses with TRF scores >+10 should be avoided, an occasional piece of cheese will not have any detrimental impact. Clearly, added slices of processed cheese to an otherwise lean sandwich, or "cheese lovers" pizza, are counterproductive.

Table 23
TRF Scores of Poultry
(Per 100 gm or Per Serving)

CHICKEN, FRIED	
BREAST WITH SKIN	+7
BREAST W/O SKIN	+3
BREAST W/O SKIN WITH BATTER	+5
BREAST W/O SKIN WITH FLOUR	+4
DRUMSTICKS WITH SKIN (2)	+7
DRUMSTICKS W/O SKIN (2)	+5
DRUMSTICKS WITH SKIN & BATTER (2)*	+10
DRUMSTICKS WITH SKIN & FLOUR (2)	+9
DRUMSTICKS W/O SKIN WITH BATTER (2)	+8
DRUMSTICKS W/O SKIN WITH FLOUR (2)	+7
LEG WITH SKIN (1)*	+10
LEG WITH SKIN WITH BATTER (1)*	+13
LEG WITH SKIN WITH FLOUR (1)*	+11
LEG W/O SKIN (1)	+5
LEG W/O SKIN WITH BATTER (1)	+8
LEG W/O SKIN WITH FLOUR (1)	+6
THIGH WITH SKIN (2)*	+10
THIGH W/O SKIN (2)	+6
CHICKEN, ROASTED	
BREAST WITH SKIN	+5
BREAST W/O SKIN	+3
DRUMSTICKS WITH SKIN (2)	+5
DRUMSTICKS W/O SKIN (2)	+3
LEG WITH SKIN (1)	+5
LEG W/O SKIN (1)	+3
THIGHS WITH SKIN (2)	+8
THIGHS W/O SKIN (2)	+5

* AVOID

Table 23 continued on next page

TRF Rating System

Table 23 continued

OTHER POULTRY	
CORNISH HEN WITH SKIN, ROASTED	+6
DUCK WITH SKIN, ROASTED *	+15
DUCK W/O SKIN, ROASTED	+6
PHEASANT WITH SKIN, ROASTED	+5
PHEASANT W/O SKIN, ROASTED	+2
TURKEY, BREAST (SLICED)	+2
DARK MEAT WITH SKIN	+6
DARK MEAT W/O SKIN	+4
WHITE MEAT WITH SKIN	+5
WHITE MEAT W/O SKIN	+3

* AVOID

Table 24
TRF Scores of Beef and Organ Meats
(Per 100 gm or 3.5 oz)

BONELESS CHUCK, TRIMMED*	+16
CHUCK ROAST, CHOICE (W/O BONE)*	+24
CHUCK STEAK, CHOICE (W/O BONE)*	+24
CHUCK, GROUND, LEAN*	+16
CHUCK, RIB ROAST*	+28
CHUCK, GROUND, LEAN	+11
CHUCK ROAST, LEAN*	+13
CHUCK STEAK, LEAN*	+13
CHOPPED SIRLOIN, EXTRA LEAN	+7
CORNED BEEF, COOKED*	+23
CORNED BEEF HASH (W/POTATO)*	+10
GROUND BEEF, LEAN (20% FAT)*	+17
GROUND BEEF, EXTRA LEAN (10% FAT)	+8
GROUND ROUND, LEAN*	+12
GROUND RUMP, EXTRA LEAN	+8
GROUND RUMP, REGULAR*	+21
LONDON BROIL, FLANK STEAK, CHOICE	+6
PORTERHOUSE STEAK, CHOICE*	+25
RIB ROAST W/O BONE, CHOICE*	+28
ROUND STEAK, LEAN	+10
RUMP ROAST, CHOICE*	+20
SIRLOIN STEAK, CHOICE*	+20
T-BONE STEAK, CHOICE*	+25
TENDERLOIN, LEAN	+6
BEEF BRAIN*	+22
BEEF HEART	+5
BEEF LIVER	+7
BEEF TONGUE*	+14

TRF Rating System

* AVOID

Table 24 continued on next page

Table 24 continued

BEEF TONGUE, LEAN	+8
CHICKEN HEART	+5
CHICKEN LIVER	+9
CHICKEN LIVER PATE (1 OZ)	+5
DUCK LIVER	+8

* AVOID

TRF Rating System

Table 25
TRF Scores of Lamb, Pork, and Veal Products
(Per 100 gm, Unless Otherwise Noted)

LAMB	
CHOP, BROILED, GRILLED	+8
ABOVE, 2 AVERAGE CHOPS*	+24
ABOVE, LEAN MEAT ONLY, 2 CHOPS	+9
CHOP, LOIN, BROILED, GRILLED	+9
ABOVE, 2 AVERAGE CHOPS*	+21
ABOVE, LEAN MEAT ONLY, 2 CHOPS	+6
LEG, ROASTED	+10
ABOVE, LEAN MEAT ONLY	+4
RIB, ROASTED*	+20
ABOVE, LEAN MEAT ONLY	+8
SHOULDER, ROASTED*	+14
ABOVE, LEAN MEAT ONLY	+7
PORK	
BACON, 3 SLICES	+4
CANADIAN BACON, 2 SLICES	+2
HAM, ROASTED	+5
ABOVE, LEAN MEAT ONLY	+5
HAM, CANNED	+3
HAM, LEG ROASTED	+4
ABOVE, LEAN MEAT ONLY	+4
HAM, LUNCH MEAT, 2 SLICES	+3
PORK CHOP, BROILED, GRILLED	+9
ABOVE, LEAN MEAT ONLY	+4
ABOVE, PAN FRIED*	+14
ABOVE, LEAN MEAT ONLY	+6
PORK, RIBS, ROASTED*	+14
ABOVE, LEAN MEAT ONLY	+8
PORK SHOULDER, ROASTED*	+14
ABOVE, LEAN MEAT ONLY	+6
SPARE RIBS, ROASTED, BROILED*	+19

* AVOID

Table 25 continued on next page

Table 25 continued

VEAL	
CUTLET, LEAN	+4
CHOP, BROILED, GRILLED	+8
ABOVE, LEAN MEAT ONLY	+4
RIB, ROASTED	+9
ABOVE, LEAN MEAT ONLY	+4
VENISON	
STEAK	+3

* AVOID

TRF Rating System

Table 26
TRF Scores of Seafoods*
(Per 100 gm or 3.5 oz)

BARRACUDA	-1	PERCH	0
BASS, FRESHWATER	-1	POLLOCK	0
BASS, SEA	0	POMPANO	+1
BASS, STRIPED	-1	ROCKFISH	-1
BLUEFISH	-2	SABLEFISH	-2
CATFISH	-2	SALMON, ATLANTIC	-1
CAVIAR	+1	SALMON, CHINOOK	-4
COD	0	SALMON, COHO	-3
CROAKER	-2	SHARK	-1
FLOUNDER	0	SNAPPER	-1
GROUPER	0	SOLE	0
HADDOCK	0	SPOT	+1
HALIBUT	-1	STURGEON	0
HERRING	-1	SARDINES	-1
MACKEREL, ATLANTIC	-5	SWORDFISH	-1
MACKEREL, KING	0	TROUT, RAINBOW (FARM-RAISED)	-1
MAHIMAHI	-2	TROUT, RAINBOW (LAKE)	-3
MONKFISH	0	TROUT, SEA	+1
MULLET	-2	TUNA, BLUEFIN	-1
OCEAN PERCH	0	TUNA, YELLOWFIN	-1
ORANGE ROUGHY	-2	WHITEFISH	-1

* TRF Scores of some fish such as tuna, salmon, or rainbow trout may be higher or lower depending on where the fish was caught (or canned). Wild fish invariably have higher concentrations of omega-3 PUFA than farm-raised fish.

Table 27
TRF Scores of Other Seafoods
(Per 100 gm)

TUNA & SALMON (CANNED IN WATER)	
BUMBLE BEE SOLID WHITE	-1
BUMBLE BEE CHUNK WHITE	-1
BUMBLE BEE PINK SALMON	-2
BUMBLE BEE RED SALMON	-2
CHICKEN OF THE SEA SOLID WHITE	-1
CHICKEN OF THE SEA CHUNK WHITE	-1
CHICKEN OF THE SEA SALMON	-2
STARKIST CHUNK LIGHT	-1
STARKIST SOLID WHITE	-2
TUNA (CANNED IN OIL)	
BUMBLE BEE SOLID WHITE	-1
BUMBLE BEE CHUNK WHITE	+1
CHICKEN OF THE SEA CHUNK LIGHT	-1
STARKIST CHUNK WHITE LUNCH	-1
STARKIST LUNCH KIT	-1
STARKIST SOLID WHITE	0
SHELLFISH	
CLAMS	0
CRABS, ALASKA KING	0
CRABS, DUNGENESS	0
CRAYFISH	0
LOBSTER	+1
MUSSELS	0
OCTOPUS	0
OYSTERS	0
SCALLOPS	0
SHRIMP	+1
SNAIL	0
SQUID	+2

Table 28
TRF Scores of Grain Products
(Per Serving as Noted)

BAGEL, PLAIN (1)	+1
BREAD CRUMBS (1 CUP)	+2
BREAD STUFFING (1 CUP)	+8
CRACKED WHEAT	+1
DINNER ROLLS (2)	+2
ENGLISH MUFFINS (1)	+1
FRENCH OR AUSTRIAN BREAD	+1
HOT DOG OR HAMBURGER ROLLS (1)	+1
HARD ROLLS (2)	+1
HOAGIE/SUBMARINE ROLLS (1)	+1
ITALIAN BREAD	0
MIXED GRAIN BREAD	0
OATMEAL BREAD	0
PITA BREAD	0
PUMPERNICKEL BREAD	0
RAISIN BREAD	0
RYE BREAD	0
WHEAT BREAD	0
WHOLE WHEAT BREAD	+1
WHITE BREAD	+1
OTHER EUROPEAN BREADS	+1
CORN GRITS (HOMINY) W/O BUTTER OR MARGARINE	0
CREAM OF WHEAT	0
OATMEAL OR ROLLED OATS	0
ALL BRAN (1 CUP)	-1
CAP'N CRUNCH (1 CUP)	+2

TRF Rating System

Table 28 continued on next page

Table 28 continued

TRF Rating System

CHEERIOS (1 CUP)	-1
CORN FLAKES (1 CUP)	0
CRISPIX (1 CUP)	0
40% BRAN FLAKES (1 CUP)	-1
FRUIT LOOPS (1 CUP)	0
GOLDEN GRAHAMS (1 CUP)	+1
GRAPE NUTS (1 CUP)	0
HONEY NUT CHEERIOS (1 CUP)	0
NATURE VALLEY GRANOLA (1/3 CUP)	+7
PRODUCT 19/ WHEATIES/ TOTAL (1 CUP)	0
RAISIN BRAN (1 CUP)	-1
RICE KRISPIES (1 CUP)	0
SHREDDED WHEAT (1 CUP)	-1

Table 29
TRF Scores of Nuts, Vegetables, and Fruits

NUTS (PER 1 OZ SERVING)	
ALMONDS, DRIED OR DRY ROASTED	-1
ALMONDS, OIL ROASTED	-1
BEECHNUTS, DRIED OR ROASTED	+1
BRAZILNUTS, DRIED OR ROASTED	+7
BUTTERNUTS, DRIED OR ROASTED	+2
CASHEW NUTS, DRIED OR ROASTED	+2
CHESTNUTS, DRIED OR ROASTED	0
COCONUT, DRY MEAT*	+17
COCONUT, DRIED, SHREDDED*	+17
COCONUT, RAW MEAT, 2" X 2" PIECE*	+26
FILBERTS, DRIED OR ROASTED	-4
GINKGO NUTS, DRIED	0
HICKORY NUTS, DRIED	+1
MACADAMIA NUTS, DRIED OR ROASTED	-3
MIXED NUTS, DRIED OR ROASTED	+1
PEANUTS, DRIED OR ROASTED	+2
PEANUT BUTTER (2 TBS)	+4
PECANS, DRIED OR ROASTED	-2
PINE NUTS, DRIED OR ROASTED	+3
PISTACHIO NUTS, DRIED OR ROASTED	-1
PUMPKIN KERNELS	+4
SESAME, ROASTED OR TOASTED	+2
SUNFLOWER KERNELS	+4
WALNUTS, DRIED OR ROASTED	+2
FRUITS & VEGETABLES (PER 2 SERVINGS)	
ALL FRUITS	+-1
MOST VEGETABLES**	-1

* AVOID   ** THE TRF SCORES FOR OLIVES AND AVOCADOS IS -2.

Table 30
TRF Scores of Frozen Entrees

BUDGET GOURMET	
BEEF CANTONESE	+6
CHEESE MANICOTTI W/MEAT SAUCE*	+22
CHICKEN MARSALA	+9
CHINESE STYLE VEGETABLES & CHICKEN	+4
FETTUCINE ALFREDO W/FOUR CHEESES*	+26
GLAZED TURKEY	+4
ITALIAN SAUSAGE LASAGNA*	+18
ITALIAN STYLE VEGETABLES & CHICKEN	+4
LINGUINI W/TOMATO SAUCE & ITALIAN SAUSAGE	+8
MACARONI AND CHEESE*	+10
MANDARIN CHICKEN	+3
ORIENTAL BEEF*	+10
ORANGE GLAZED CHICKEN BREAST	+3
PENNE PASTA W/CHUNKY TOMATOES	+8
PEPPER STEAK	+6
RIGATONI IN CREAM SAUCE W/BROCCOLI & CHICKEN	+5
SCALLOPED NOODLES AND TURKEY*	+21
SIRLOIN TIPS W/COUNTRY STYLE VEGETABLES	+11
SPAGHETTI W/CHUNKY TOMATO & MEAT SAUCE	+5
SPICY SZECHUAN STYLE VEGETABLES & CHICKEN	+5
SWEDISH MEATBALLS*	+32
THREE CHEESE LASAGNA*	+19
WIDE RIBBON PASTA W/RICOTTA & CHUNKY TOMATOES*	+15
BEEF SIRLOIN SALISBURY STEAK	+5
HERBED CHICKEN BREAST W/FETTUCINE	+7
ROAST CHICKEN BREAST W/HERB GRAVY	+4
SHRIMP MARINER	+5
SPECIAL RECIPE SIRLOIN BEEF	+6
STUFFED TURKEY BREAST	+4
YANKEE POT ROAST	+4

* AVOID

Table 31
TRF Scores of Frozen Entrees

HEALTHY CHOICE	
BEEF BROCCOLI BEIJING	+3
BEEF MACARONI	+3
BEEF PEPPER STEAK	+4
BEEF PEPPER STEAK ORIENTAL	+4
BEEF & PEPPERS CANTONESE	+5
CHICKEN CACCIATORE	+2
CHICKEN CON QUESO BURRITO	+3
CHICKEN DIJON	+3
CHICKEN FETTUCINE ALFREDO	+2
CHICKEN PARMIGIANA	+2
CHICKEN TERIYAKI	+2
COUNTRY GLAZED CHICKEN	+2
COUNTRY INN ROAST TURKEY	+3
FIESTA CHICKEN FAJITAS	+1
GARDEN POTATO CASSEROLE	+4
HONEY MUSTARD CHICKEN	+2
LEMON PEPPER FISH	+2
MACARONI & CHEESE	+6
MEATLOAF DINNER	+6
MESQUITE BEEF W/BARBECUE SAUCE	+4
MESQUITE CHICKEN BBQ	+3
MESQUITE CHICKEN DINNER	+3
PASTA SHELLS MARINARA	+3
SALISBURY STEAK	+5
SHRIMP & VEGETABLE MEDLEY	+2
SOUTHWESTERN GLAZED CHICKEN	+4
SPAGHETTI BOLOGNESE	+3
SWEET & SOUR CHICKEN DINNER	+2

TRF Rating System

Table 31 continued on next page

Table 31 continued

THREE CHEESE MANICOTTI	+1
TRADITIONAL BREAST OF TURKEY	+3
TRADITIONAL SALISBURY STEAK	+6
VEGETABLE PASTA ITALIANO	0
ZUCCHINI LASAGNA	0

TRF Rating System

Table 32
TRF Scores of Frozen Entrees

LEAN CUISINE	
ANGEL HAIR PASTA	+2
BAKED CHEESE RAVIOLI	+7
BEEF POT ROAST	+4
BROCCOLI & CHEDDAR	+3
CHEESE CANNELLONI	+8
CHEESE LASAGNA CASSEROLE	+6
CHEESE OVER BAKED POTATO	+9
CHICKEN CHOW MEIN	+3
CHICKEN ENCHILADA SUIZA	+5
CHICKEN FETTUCINE	+6
CHICKEN À L'ORANGE	+3
CHICKEN IN PEANUT SAUCE	+3
CLASSIC CHEESE LASAGNA	+7
FETTUCINE ALFREDO	+7
FIESTA CHICKEN	+3
FRENCH BREAD PIZZA	+6
FRENCH BREAD PIZZA DELUXE	+6
GLAZED CHICKEN	+4
HOMESTYLE TURKEY	+5
HONEY MUSTARD CHICKEN	+4
LASAGNA W/MEAT SAUCE	+6
MACARONI AND BEEF	+4
MACARONI AND CHEESE	+3
MACARONI & CHEESE W/ BROCCOLI	+3
MEATLOAF	+9
ORIENTAL BEEF	+6
RIGATONI	+4
SWEDISH MEATBALLS	+7
TERIYAKI STIRFRY PASTA W/CHICKEN & VEGETABLES	+2
THREE BEAN CHILI	+4
ZUCCHINI LASAGNA	+5

TRF Rating System

Table 33
TRF Scores of Frozen Entrees

STOUFFER'S	
CHEESE TORTELLINI IN ALFREDO SAUCE*	+36
CHICKEN À LA KING	+7
CHICKEN BREAST, BAKED	+8
CHICKEN BREAST, FRIED*	+11
CHICKEN CHOW MEIN W/RICE	+3
CHICKEN MONTEREY*	+11
CHICKEN PIE*	+20
CREAMED CHIPPED BEEF	+7
ESCALLOPED CHICKEN & NOODLES*	+14
FETTUCINE ALFREDO*	+31
FETTUCINE PRIMAVERA*	+23
GREEN PEPPER STEAK	+6
LASAGNA W/MEAT SAUCE	+8
MACARONI & BEEF*	+12
MACARONI & CHEESE*	+11
MEATLOAF & WHIPPED POTATOES*	+17
NOODLES ROMANOFF*	+15
POT ROAST, BEEF	+6
SALISBURY STEAK*	+11
SCALLOPED APPLES	0
SPAGHETTI W/MEAT SAUCE	+5
SPINACH SOUFFLÉ	+5
STUFFED PEPPERS	+8
SWEDISH MEATBALLS*	+14
TUNA NOODLE CASSEROLE	+5
TURKEY TETRAZZINI*	+10
VEAL PARMIGIANA	+6
VEGETABLE LASAGNA*	+11
WELSH RAREBIT CHEDDAR CHEESE SAUCE	+7

* AVOID

TRF Rating System

Table 34
TRF Scores of Frozen Entrees

WEIGHT WATCHERS	
BROCCOLI & CHEESE BAKED POTATO	+3
CHICKEN ENCHILADA SUIZA	+4
DELUXE COMBO PIZZA	+7
FETTUCINE ALFREDO	+5
GARDEN LASAGNA	+2
GRILLED SALISBURY STEAK	+5
ITALIAN CHEESE LASAGNA	+5
LASAGNA W/MEAT SAUCE	+4
MACARONI AND CHEESE	+4
STUFFED TURKEY BREAST	+5
SWEDISH MEATBALLS	+8
THREE CHEESE ROTINI	+5
TUNA NOODLE CASSEROLE	+5
ANGEL HAIR PASTA	+1
FIESTA CHICKEN	+1
HONEY MUSTARD CHICKEN & SAUCE	+1
LASAGNA FLORENTINE	+2
LEMON HERB CHICKEN PICCATA	+3
PASTA PORTOFINO	+1
RAVIOLI FLORENTINE	+1
CHICKEN BROCCOLI & CHEDDAR	+5
GRILLED CHICKEN SANDWICH	+5
HAM & CHEESE POCKET SANDWICH	+5
REUBEN POCKET SANDWICH	+4

TRF Rating System

Table 35
TRF Scores of Frozen Entrees

BANQUET	
BEEF POT PIE*	+15
CHARBROILED BEEF PATTIES	+8
CHICKEN NUGGET MEAL	+11
CHICKEN POT PIE*	+15
COUNTRY FRIED CHICKEN*	+12
FRIED CHICKEN*	+12
FRIED CHICKEN MEAL*	+20
GRAVY & SLICED TURKEY	+4
SALISBURY STEAK	+11
SALISBURY STEAK W/GRAVY	+9
SKINLESS FRIED CHICKEN*	+17
TURKEY & GRAVY	+6
TURKEY POT PIE	+17
TYSON	
CHICKEN MARSALA	+4
CHICKEN MESQUITE	+8
CHICKEN PICCATA	+4
GRILLED CHICKEN	+4
HONEY ROASTED CHICKEN	+4
ROASTED CHICKEN	+3

Table 35 continued on next page

Table 35 continued

SWANSON	
BEEF POT PIE*	+18
CHICKEN POT PIE*	+18
FISH & CHIPS*	+31
FRIED CHICKEN*	+21
HUNGRY MAN BEEF POT PIE*	+27
HUNGRY MAN CHICKEN POT PIE*	+25
HUNGRY MAN SALISBURY STEAK*	+29
HUNGRY MAN SIRLOIN BEEF TIPS*	+15
HUNGRY MAN TURKEY*	+12
HUNGRY MAN TURKEY POT PIE*	+25
HUNGRY MAN YANKEE POT ROAST	+7
SALISBURY STEAK	+12
TURKEY	+5
TURKEY POT PIE*	+18
VEAL PARMIGIANA*	+14
YANKEE POT ROAST	+9

* AVOID

TRF Rating System

Table 36
TRF Scores of Frozen Seafoods
(Per 100 gm, Unless Otherwise Noted)

GORTON'S	
BREADED FISH STICKS	+5
CRUNCHY FISH FILLETS	+8
CRUNCHY GARLIC & HERB FISH FILLETS	+8
HOT & SPICY FISH FILLETS	+9
MRS. PAUL'S	
BREADED FISH STICKS	+1
CRISPY CRUNCHY FILLETS	+4
CRISPY CRUNCHY FISH STICKS	+3
DEVILED CRABS	+5
DEVILED CRAB MINIATURES	+6
FRIED CLAMS	+2
HEALTHY TREASURES FISH FILLETS	+1
HEALTHY TREASURES FISH STICKS	+2
LIGHT FILLETS, FLOUNDER	+3
SEA PALS (FISH SHAPES)	+2
VAN DE KAMP'S	
BATTERED FISH PORTIONS	+8
BREADED BUTTERFLY SHRIMP	+5
BREADED FISH STICKS	+4
BREADED POPCORN SHRIMP	+5
CRISP & HEALTHY FISH FILLETS	+3
CRISP & HEALTHY FISH STICKS	+2
FISH FILLETS IN BATTER	+4
MINISTIX	+6

Table 37
TRF Scores of Canned Pasta Entrees and Beans
(Per 100 gm)

CAMPBELL'S	
BAKED BARBECUE BEANS	0
BAKED BEANS, BROWN SUGAR, BACON-FLAVORED	+2
BAKED BEANS, NEW ENGLAND STYLE	+2
PORK N' BEANS	+1
CHEF BOYARDEE	
BEEFARONI	+6
BEEF RAVIOLI	+5
CHEESE RAVIOLI	+1
CHEESE TORTELLINI	+2
CHOMPS-A-LOT BITESIZE LASAGNA	+2
CHOMPS-A-LOT BITESIZE BEEF RAVIOLI	+3
DINOSAURS	+1
FETTUCINE IN MEAT SAUCE	+6
LASAGNA*	+7
MEAT TORTELLINI	+3
MINI RAVIOLI IN TOMATO & MEAT SAUCE	+5
PASTA W/MINI MEATBALLS	+6
SPAGHETTI & MEATBALLS*	+7
TEENAGE MUTANT NINJA TURTLES	+2
TIC TAC TOE W/MEATBALLS*	+7
FRANCO-AMERICAN	
SPAGHETTIOS IN CHEESE SAUCE	+3
SPAGHETTIOS W/MEATBALLS*	+7
SPAGHETTIOS IN CHEESE SAUCE TEDDYOS	+3
SPAGHETTIOS W/SLICED FRANKS*	+9
GARFIELD RAVIOLI IN MEAT SAUCE*	+8

* AVOID

TRF Rating System

Table 38
TRF Scores of Boxed Pasta Entrees

RICE-A-RONI	
ANGEL HAIR PASTA W/PARMESAN CHEESE	+2
CORKSCREW PASTA W/FOUR CHEESES	+3
FETTUCINE	+3
FETTUCINE W/ALFREDO SAUCE	+4
FETTUCINE W/ROMANOFF SAUCE	+5
LINGUINI W/CHICKEN & BROCCOLI SAUCE	+3
PENNE PASTA, HERB & BUTTER	+2
RIGATONI W/WHITE CHEDDAR & BROCCOLI	+4
TENDERTHIN PASTA W/PARMESAN SAUCE	+4
HAMBURGER HELPER	
BEEF NOODLE	+1
CHEESEBURGER MACARONI	+3
ITALIAN RIGATONI	+1
LASAGNA	+1
PIZZA PASTA	+2
STROGANOFF	+2
TUNA HELPER, CHEESY NOODLES	+4
ZESTY ITALIAN	+1
LIPTON NOODLES N' SAUCE	
BEEF NOODLE	+1
CHEESEBURGER MACARONI	+3
ITALIAN RIGATONI	+1
LASAGNA	+1
PIZZA PASTA	+2
STROGANOFF	+2
TUNA HELPER, CHEESY NOODLES	+4
ZESTY ITALIAN	+1

Table 38 continued on next page

Table 38 continued

LIPTON PASTA N' SAUCE	
CHEDDAR BROCCOLI	+4
CREAMY GARLIC	+3
ROTINI PRIMAVERA	+4
LIPTON GOLDEN SAUTÉ	
ANGEL HAIR W/CHICKEN N' BROCCOLI	+1
PENNE PASTA, HERB W/GARLIC	+3
RICE & VERMICELLI W/CHICKEN FLAVOR	+3
KRAFT MACARONI & CHEESE	
DINOMAC	+2
ORIGINAL	+3
SUPER MARIO	+4

TRF Rating System

Table 39
TRF Scores of Processed Foods
(Per Slice)

BUTTERBALL	
ROASTED CHICKEN	+1
ROASTED TURKEY	+1
ROASTED TURKEY BREAST	+1
HEALTHY CHOICE	
BAKED COOKED HAM	+1
BOLOGNA, TURKEY	+1
SMOKED TURKEY BREAST	+1
TURKEY	+1
HEBREW NATIONAL	
BEEF BOLOGNA*	+6
BEEF SALAMI*	+6
LOUIS RICH	
BOLOGNA*	+6
COOKED TURKEY SALAMI	+2
ROASTED TURKEY BREAST	+1
SALAMI	+4
SMOKED TURKEY	+1
TURKEY BOLOGNA	+5
TURKEY PASTRAMI	+1
WHITE TURKEY	+1

* AVOID

Table 39 continued on next page

Table 39 continued

OSCAR MAYER	
BEEF BOLOGNA*	+8
BOLOGNA*	+8
BOLOGNA (THIN SLICED)	+4
CORNED BEEF (THIN SLICED)	+1
HARD SALAMI	+2
HEALTHY FAVORITES	+4
LIGHT BEEF BOLOGNA	+1
OVEN ROASTED CHICKEN	+1
OVEN ROASTED TURKEY	+1
PASTRAMI	+2
OSCAR MAYER LUNCHABLES (PER PACKAGE)	
BOLOGNA W/AMERICAN CHEESE*	+28
CHICKEN W/AMERICAN CHEESE*	+20
LEAN CHICKEN W/MONTEREY JACK*	+20
LEAN HAM W/AMERICAN CHEESE*	+20
LEAN HAM W/SWISS CHEESE W/O DESSERT*	+18
LEAN TURKEY W/CHEDDAR CHEESE & REESE'S CUP*	+20
LEAN TURKEY W/CHEDDAR CHEESE & TRAIL MIX*	+26

* AVOID

TRF Rating System

Table 40
TRF Scores of Soups
(Per Can)

CAMPBELL'S	
BEAN WITH BACON	+4
BEEF BROTH	+1
BEEF NOODLE	+3
BEEF W/VEGETABLES & BARLEY	+3
CHICKEN ALPHABET	+3
CHICKEN BROTH	+2
CHICKEN GUMBO	+2
CREAMY CHICKEN MUSHROOM*	+6
CREAMY CHICKEN NOODLE*	+6
CHICKEN NOODLE O'S	+3
CHICKEN N' DUMPLINGS	+3
CHICKEN NOODLE	+3
CREAM OF CHICKEN*	+7
CHICKEN VEGETABLE	+2
CHICKEN WITH RICE	+3
CHILI BEEF	+5
CREAM OF CELERY*	+6
CREAM OF CHICKEN & BROCCOLI*	+6
CREAM OF MUSHROOM*	+6
CREAM OF POTATO	+4
CONSOMMÉ BEEF	+1
CHUNKY BEEF	+5
CHUNKY BEEF NOODLE*	+6
CHUNKY CHICKEN BROCCOLI & CHEESE*	+10
CHUNKY CORN CHOWDER*	+12
CHUNKY CHICKEN NOODLE	+5
CHUNKY CHICKEN NOODLE W/MUSHROOMS*	+6
CHUNKY CHICKEN W/RICE	+3

Table 40 continued on next page

Table 40 continued

CAMPBELL'S	
CHUNKY MEDITERRANEAN VEGETABLE	+5
CHUNKY NEW ENGLAND CLAM CHOWDER*	+12
CHUNKY OLD FASHIONED BEAN N' HAM*	+7
CHUNKY PEPPERSTEAK	+3
CHUNKY SIRLOIN BURGER*	+7
CHUNKY VEGETABLES	+3
GOLDEN MUSHROOM	+3
MINESTRONE	+3
OLD FASHIONED VEGETABLE	+2
SCOTCH BROTH	+3
TEDDY BEAR	+2
TOMATO	+3
TOMATO BISQUE	+4
TURKEY NOODLE	+3
TURKEY VEGETABLE	+3
VEGETABLE BEEF	+3

* AVOID

TRF Rating System

Table 41
TRF Scores of Soups
(Per ½ Can)

HEALTHY REQUEST		CONDENSED SOUPS	
CHICKEN BROTH	+1	BLACK BEAN	+3
CHICKEN NOODLE	+3	BROCCOLI CHEESE	+5
CHICKEN W/RICE	+3	CHEDDAR CHEESE*	+9
CREAM OF BROCCOLI	+2	CHICKEN WON TON	+1
CREAM OF CELERY	+2	CREAM OF ASPARAGUS*	+6
CREAM OF CHICKEN	+3	CREAM OF BROCCOLI	+5
CREAM OF MUSHROOM	+3	CREAM OF SHRIMP*	+6
HEARTY CHICKEN NOODLE	+3	FRENCH ONION	+1
HEARTY CHICKEN RICE	+3	GOLDEN CORN	+3
HEARTY CHICKEN VEGETABLE	+3	GREEN PEA	+3
HEARTY MINESTRONE	+3	MANHATTAN CLAM CHOWDER	+2
HEARTY VEGETABLE BEEF	+3	NACHO CHEESE*	+8
NEW ENGLAND CLAM CHOWDER	+3	NEW ENGLAND CLAM CHOWDER	+2
SPLIT PEA W/HAM	+3	PEPPER POT	+3
TOMATO	+2	SPLIT PEA W/HAM & BACON	+5
TOMATO VEGETABLE W/PASTA	+3		
VEGETABLE BEEF	+2		
VEGETABLE WITH BEEF STOCK	+3		

* AVOID

Table 42
TRF Scores for Sauces
(Per ½ Cup = 120 ml)

CLASSICO	
FOUR CHEESE	+3
MUSHROOM & RIPE OLIVES	+2
ONION & GARLIC	+2
SPICY RED PEPPER	+2
SWEET PEPPERS & ONIONS	+2
TOMATO & BASIL	+3
HEALTHY CHOICE	
CHUNKY GARLIC & ONIONS	+1
CHUNKY MUSHROOM	+1
EXTRA CHUNKY MUSHROOMS	+1
FLAVORED W/MEAT	+1
GARLIC & HERBS	+1
TRADITIONAL	+1
ZESTY ITALIAN	+1
NEWMAN'S OWN	
SOCKAROONI	+1
VENETIAN W/MUSHROOM	+1
PREGO	
DICED ONION & GARLIC	+2
FLAVORED W/MEAT	+3
FRESH MUSHROOM	+3
GARDEN COMBINATION	+2
LOW SODIUM	+2
MUSHROOM & DICED ONION	+3
MUSHROOM & DICED TOMATO	+2

TRF Rating System

Table 42 continued on next page

Table 42 continued

PREGO (continued)	
MUSHROOM & GREEN PEPPER	+3
SAUSAGE & GREEN PEPPER	+5
THREE CHEESE	+2
TOMATO & BASIL	+2
TOMATO, ONION, & GARLIC	+3
TRADITIONAL	+4
ZESTY BASIL	+4
ZESTY GARLIC & CHEESE	+4
ZESTY MUSHROOM W/CHEESE	+3
RAGU	
CHUNKY GARDENSTYLE	+2
CHUNKY GARDEN SUPER MUSHROOM	+2
CHUNKY MUSHROOMS & GREEN PEPPERS	+3
CHUNKY SUPER VEGETABLE PRIMAVERA	+2
HOMESTYLE FLAVORED W/MEAT	+3
HOMESTYLE W/MUSHROOM	+2
HOMESTYLE TOMATO & HERB	+2
LIGHT GARDEN HARVEST	+1
LIGHT TOMATO & HERB	+1
OLD WORLD STYLE TRADITIONAL	+2
OLD WORLD STYLE W/MEAT	+3
THICK & HEARTY MUSHROOM	+2
THICK & HEARTY W/MEAT	+2
THICK & HEARTY TOMATO & HERB	+2

Table 42 continued on next page

Table 42 continued

OTHER SAUCES	
BÉARNAISE*	+8
HOLLANDAISE	+3
MARINARA (TOMATO BASED)	0
SPAGHETTI WITH MEAT	+1
SPAGHETTI WITH MEATBALLS	+1
TARTAR	+4

* AVOID

TRF Rating System

Table 43
TRF Scores of Salad Dressings
(Per 2 Tablespoons)

KRAFT	
BACON & TOMATO*	+5
BLUE CHEESE*	+6
CATALINA	+4
CAESAR RANCH	+4
CLASSIC CAESAR*	+5
COLESLAW	+4
CREAMY ITALIAN*	+6
CREAMY PARMESAN ROMANO	+5
CREAMY ROASTED GARLIC	+4
CUCUMBER RANCH*	+5
DELICIOUSLY RIGHT ITALIAN	+2
DELICIOUSLY RIGHT RANCH	+4
DELICIOUSLY RIGHT THOUSAND ISLAND	+2
DELICIOUSLY RIGHT CATALINA	+2
FRENCH	+4
GREEK VINAIGRETTE	+3
HONEY DIJON*	+5
ITALIAN, OLIVE OIL	+4
PEPPERCORN RANCH*	+5
RANCH*	+5
RANCH SOUR CREAM & ONION*	+5
SALSA ZESTY GARDEN	+2
TANGY TOMATO BACON	+3
THOUSAND ISLAND	+4
ZESTY ITALIAN	+4

Table 43 continued on next page

Table 43 continued

KEN'S	
CAESAR LITE	+2
CREAMY PARMESAN LITE	+3
RASPBERRY WALNUT VINAIGRETTE	+2
RED WINE VINEGAR & OLIVE OIL	-1
STEAK HOUSE BLUE CHEESE*	+6
STEAK HOUSE BASIL VINAIGRETTE	+4
STEAK HOUSE SWEET VIDALIA ONION	+3
THOUSAND ISLAND*	+5
NEWMAN'S OWN	
OLIVE OIL & VINEGAR*	+5
WISHBONE	
CHUNKY CHEESE*	+7
CLASSIC CAESAR	+3
ITALIAN	+2
RANCH*	+6
RED WINE VINAIGRETTE	+1
ROBUSTO ITALIAN	+2
RUSSIAN	+3
ALL FAT-FREE VARIETIES	0

* AVOID

TRF Rating System

Table 44
TRF Scores of Cakes
(Per One Slice or ⅟₁₆ of Cake)

ANGEL FOOD	0
CARAMEL, NO ICING (MADE W/VEG. SHORTENING)*	+5
CARAMEL, NO ICING (MADE W/ BUTTER)*	+7
CARAMEL, W/ICING (MADE W/VEG. SHORTENING)*	+6
CARAMEL W/ICING (MADE W/BUTTER)*	+8
CARROT W/CREAM CHEESE FROSTING*	+8
CHOCOLATE, NO ICING (MADE W/VEG. SHORTENING)*	+8
CHOCOLATE, NO ICING (MADE W/BUTTER)*	+10
CHEESECAKE*	+18
CHOCOLATE W/ICING (MADE W/VEG. SHORTENING)*	+9
CHOCOLATE W/ICING (MADE W/BUTTER)*	+11
COFFEECAKE, NO ICING (MADE W/VEG. SHORTENING)	+2
COFFEECAKE W/CHOCOLATE ICING	+4
FRUITCAKE (MADE W/VEG. SHORTENING)	+1
FRUITCAKE (MADE W/BUTTER)	+1
GINGERBREAD (MADE W/VEG. SHORTENING)*	+6
GINGERBREAD (MADE W/BUTTER)*	+9
MARBLE	+4
PLAIN (MADE W/VEG. SHORTENING)	+4
PLAIN (MADE W/BUTTER)*	+5
PLAIN, CHOC. ICING (MADE W/VEG. SHORTENING)*	+6
PLAIN, CHOC. ICING (MADE W/BUTTER)*	+7
POUND CAKE (MADE W/VEG. SHORTENING)*	+5
POUND CAKE (MADE W/BUTTER)*	+8
SPONGE CAKE	+1
CARAMEL ICING (2 TBS)	+2
CHOCOLATE ICING (2 TBS)	+4
COCONUT ICING (2 TBS)	+4
CHOCOLATE FUDGE ICING (2 TBS)	+4
CHOCOLATE SYRUP*	+14

* AVOID

Table 45
TRF Scores of Candies, Cookies, and Pastries
(Per 1 oz)

BUTTERSCOTCH	+1	YOGURT COVERED RAISINS	+1
CARAMEL, PLAIN	+3	OTHER CANDIES W/O MILK, FAT, OR CHOCOLATE	0
CARAMEL W/CHOCOLATE	+3	BROWNIES (1.5) W/NUTS	+5
CARAMEL W/NUTS	+2	BROWNIES (1.5) W/BUTTER*	+6
CHOCOLATE, BITTERSWEET*	+12	CHOCOLATE CHIP COOKIES W/SHORTENING*	+6
CHOCOLATE, SEMISWEET*	+8	CHOCOLATE CHIP COOKIES W/BUTTER*	+7
CHOCOLATE, MILK, PLAIN*	+8	COCONUT BAR (3 PIECES)*	+6
CHOCOLATE, MILK, W/ALMONDS*	+6	DANISH (1), SMALL (PLAIN)*	+6
CHOCOLATE, MILK, W/PEANUTS*	+6	DANISH (1), SMALL W/FRUIT*	+7
CHOCOLATE COATED ALMONDS	+2	DOUGHNUT (1), PLAIN*	+6
CHOCOLATE COVERED RAISINS	+4	DOUGHNUT (1), CHOCOLATE COVERED*	+9
CHOCOLATE FUDGE	+2	DOUGHNUT (1), W/CUSTARD INSIDE*	+12
CHOCOLATE FUDGE W/NUTS	+2	FIG BARS (3)	+1
CHOCOLATE FUDGE W/WALNUTS	+1	GINGERSNAPS (3)	+1
COCONUT CENTER FUDGE	+3	GRANOLA BARS (QUAKER CHEWY-1 BAR)*	+10
PEANUT BAR	+3	OATMEAL COOKIES (3) W/RAISINS	+2
PEANUT BRITTLE	+1	RAISIN COOKIES (3)	+1
YOGURT COVERED NUTS	+1	SUGAR WAFERS (3)	+2

* AVOID

TRF Rating System

Table 46
TRF Scores of Pies
(Per One Regular Slice or ⅛ of Pie)

APPLE*	+6	PEACH	+4
ABOVE, ONE SMALL SLICE	+2	*ABOVE*, ONE SMALL SLICE	+2
BANANA CUSTARD*	+6	PECAN	+2
ABOVE, ONE SMALL SLICE	+2	*ABOVE*, ONE SMALL SLICE	+1
BLACKBERRY*	+6	PINEAPPLE	+5
ABOVE, ONE SMALL SLICE	+2	*ABOVE*, ONE SMALL SLICE	+2
BLUEBERRY*	+6	PUMPKIN*	+7
ABOVE, ONE SMALL SLICE	+2	*ABOVE*, ONE SMALL SLICE	+2
CHERRY*	+6	RAISIN	+4
ABOVE, ONE SMALL SLICE	+2	*ABOVE*, ONE SMALL SLICE	+1
CHOCOLATE CHIFFON*	+7	STRAWBERRY	+3
ABOVE, ONE SMALL SLICE	+2	*ABOVE*, ONE SMALL SLICE	+1
CHOCOLATE MERINGUE*	+8	SWEET POTATO*	+7
ABOVE, ONE SMALL SLICE	+3	*ABOVE*, ONE SMALL SLICE	+2
COCONUT CUSTARD*	+10	WALNUT	+2
ABOVE, ONE SMALL SLICE	+3	*ABOVE*, ONE SMALL SLICE	+1
CUSTARD*	+7	APPLE PIE FILLING (1/2 CUP)	+2
ABOVE, ONE SMALL SLICE	+2	CHERRY PIE FILLING (1/2 CUP)	0
LEMON CHIFFON	+4	APPLESAUCE PIE FILLING (1/2 CUP)	0
ABOVE, ONE SMALL SLICE	+2	CRANBERRY (1/2 CUP)	0
LEMON MERINGUE	+5	MINCEMEAT (1/2 CUP)	0
ABOVE, ONE SMALL SLICE	+2	LIBBY'S PUMPKIN (1/2 CUP)	0

* AVOID

Table 47
TRF Scores of Cookies and Snacks
(Per Serving as Noted)

KELLOGG'S (PER 1)	
CHOCOLATE FUDGE TART	+1
FROSTED POP TARTS	+2
LOWFAT GRANOLA BAR	+2
NUTRI-GRAIN BAR	+2
POP TARTS	+2
RICE KRISPIE BAR	+2
NABISCO (PER 2)	
APPLE NEWTONS	0
CHEWY CHIPS AHOY	+3
CHUNKY CHIPS AHOY*	+11
FIG NEWTONS	0
MINI-OREO (10)	+5
MYSTIC MINT	+4
OREO	+4
OREO DOUBLESTUFF*	+8
OREO WHITE FUDGE*	+6
PURE CHOCOLATE MALLOWS*	+6
PURE CHOCOLATE MARSHMALLOWS*	+11
PURE CHOCOLATE PINWHEELS*	+10
REAL CHOCOLATE CHIPS AHOY	+3
NATURE VALLEY	
GRANOLA BAR (1)	+2
LOW-FAT CHEWY GRANOLA BAR (1)	0

* AVOID

Table 47 continued on next page

TRF Rating System

Table 47 continued

PEPPERIDGE FARM (PER 2)	
BROWN CHOCOLATE NUT	+3
BRUSSELS	+4
CARROT WALNUT	+2
FRUIT COOKIES	+4
GENEVA	+4
MILANO	+4
OLD-FASHIONED CHOCOLATE CHIP	+4
SOFT CHOCOLATE CHUNK*	+6
WHOLESOME CHOICE	+2
QUAKER (PER 1)	
CARAMEL CHEWY BAR	+2
CHOCOLATE CHIP BAR	+3
PEANUT BUTTER BAR	+3
TRAIL MIX BAR	+3

* AVOID

Table 48
TRF Scores of Various Snacks
(Per 100 gm, Unless Otherwise Noted)

ARCHWAY COOKIES (PER COOKIE)	
APPLE & RAISIN	+2
CHOCOLATE CHIP & TOFFEE	+3
DATE FILLED OATMEAL	+2
DUTCH COCOA	+3
FROSTY LEMON	+2
FAT-FREE OATMEAL RAISIN	0
FAT-FREE FRUIT BAR	0
FAT-FREE GRANOLA	0
GOLDEN OATMEAL	+2
OATMEAL	+2
OLD-FASHIONED MOLASSES	+2
ROCKY ROAD	+3
AUSTIN (PER 1 PACKET)	
CHEESE ON CHEESE*	+7
CHEESE ON PEANUT BUTTER*	+6
TOASTY PEANUT BUTTER*	+6
WHEAT & CHEDDAR*	+7
BETTY CROCKER (PER 1)	
FRUIT DINOSAURS (PER POUCH)	+2
FRUIT GUSHERS	0
FRUIT ROLL-UPS	0
FRUIT SHARKS (PER POUCH)	+2
GIANT (PER POUCH)	
BEAUTY & THE BEAST	+3
FRUIT DINOSAURS	+2
FRUIT SHARKS	+2

TRF Rating System

Table 48 continued on next page

Table 48 continued

HEALTH VALLEY	
BAKERS (BLUEBERRY, APPLE)	0
DATE ALMOND	0
FAT-FREE APRICOT FRUIT CAKE	0
GRANOLA/OATBRAN	0
OATBRAN MUFFIN	0
RAISIN FRUIT	0
RASPBERRY	0
RASPBERRY, STRAWBERRY	0
WHEAT FREE	0
KEEBLER	
APPLE CINNAMON GRAHAM (4)	+2
CHIPS DELUXE (1)	+3
CHOCOLATE GRAHAM (4)	+2
CINNAMON CRISP GRAHAM (4)	+2
COCONUT CHOCOLATE DROP (1)	+5
ELFIN DELIGHTS (1)	+1
E.L. FUDGE (1)	+2
FUDGE CARAMEL (1)	+4
FUDGE STICKS (1)	+4
FUDGE STRIPES (1)	+4
PB FUDGEBUTTERS (1)	+2
ZESTRA SALTINES (4)	+1
KELLOGG'S	
LOW-FAT GRANOLA BAR (1)	+2
NUTRI-GRAIN BARS (1)	+3
RICE KRISPIE BAR/CHOCOLATE CHIP (1)	+3

Table 48 continued on next page

TRF Rating System

Table 48 continued

KRAFT	
CHEEZ N' BREADSTICKS (1)*	+9
CHEEZ N' CRACKERS *	+10
CHEEZ N' PRETZELS*	+9
CHEEZ WHIZ (1 OZ)*	+9
CHEEZ WHIZ LIGHT (1 OZ)	+5
KUDOS (PER 1)	
CHOCOLATE CHIP SNACK BAR	+4
CHOCOLATE CHUNK SNACK BAR	+4
HONEY NUT BAR	+4
NABISCO	
BROWN EDGE WAFERS (5)	+3
BUGS BUNNY GRAHAM SNACKS (5)	+2
CHOCOLATE GRAHAM SNACKS (5)	+2
FAMOUS CHOCOLATE WAFERS (5)	+5
FAT-FREE PREMIUM SALTINES (5)	0
HONEY MAID GRAHAMS (5)	+2
ABOVE, CINNAMON (5)	+2
LOWFAT GARDEN CRISP CRACKER (5)	+
MINI OREOS (10)	+5
MULTIGRAIN SALTINES (5)	+2
NUTTER BUTTERS (2)	+5
OREOS (2)	+4
OREO DOUBLESTUFF (2)	+8
ORIGINAL PREMIUM SALTINES (5)	+2
REAL CHEDDAR CHEESE NIPS (5)	+1
SOCIABLES (5)	+1
TEDDY GRAHAM SNACKS (5)	+2

* AVOID

Table 49
TRF Scores of Various Snacks
(Per 100 gm, Unless Otherwise Noted)

NATURE VALLEY		SUNSHINE	
LOW-FAT GRANOLA BAR	+2	CINNAMON GRAHAMS (5)*	+13
OATS N' HONEY	+4	FUDGE DIPPED GRAHAMS (5)*	+31
VARIETY	+4	GINGER SNAPS (5)	+3
PEPPERIDGE FARM		HONEY GRAHAMS (5)*	+7
GOLDFISH (1/2 OZ)	+1	KRISPY MILD CHEDDARS (5)	+1
GOLDFISH SNACK MIX (1/2 CUP)	+3	KRISPY SALTINES (5)	+1
SESAME SNACK STICKS (5)	+3	OATMEAL CHOCOLATE COOKIES (2)*	+6
THREE CHEESE SNACK STICKS (5)	+3	PREMIER CHOCOLATE CHIP (2)*	+14
QUAKER		VIENNA FINGERS (2)*	+7
BUTTER POPPED CORN (FAT FREE)	0	CHIPS (ALL PER 1 OZ)	
CHEWY CHOC. CHIP GRANOLA BAR (1)	+4	DORITOS TORTILLA	+4
CHEWY CARAMEL APPLE BAR (1)	+4	FRITO-LAY BARBECUE*	+9
CHEWY PEANUT BUTTER BAR (1)*	+5	GIANT POTATO CHIPS*	+10
CHEWY TRAIL MIX GRANOLA BAR (1)	+5	TOSTITOS CRISPY ROUNDS*	+5
RICE CAKES, FAT FREE	0	UTZ POTATO CHIPS, PLAIN OR BBQ*	+8
RITZ		UTZ CRISP ALL-NATURAL*	+5
BITS SANDWICHES (5)	+3	STELLA D'ORO	
BITS W/PEANUT BUTTER (5)	+2	BREADSTICKS (1)	+3
CRACKERS (5)	+3	FAT-FREE BREADSTICKS	0
CRACKERS, SMALL (10)	+3	SESAME BREADSTICKS (1)	+3

* AVOID

Table 50
TRF Scores of Sweet Snacks

BRACH'S	SERVING SIZE	SCORE
CHOC. COVERED ALMONDS	11 PIECES*	+8
CHOC. COVERED RAISINS	34 PIECES*	+11
CLUSTERS	3 PIECES*	+15
JORDAN ALMONDS	10 PIECES	0
HERSHEY'S		
ASSORTED MINIATURES	5" BAR*	+16
BABY RUTH	1 BAR*	+8
KISSES	8 PIECES*	+17
MILK CHOCOLATE	10 BLOCKS*	+18
MILK CHOCOLATE ALMONDS	10 BLOCKS*	+12
MR. GOODBAR	3 BLOCKS*	+14
MR. GOODBAR PEANUTS	3 BLOCKS*	+12
NUGGETS	4 PIECES*	+14
SYMPHONY ALMONDS	4 BLOCKS*	+14
SYMPHONY MILK. CHOC.	4 BLOCKS*	+18
HOSTESS		
FRUIT PIE, APPLE	1*	+22
FRUIT PIE, BLUEBERRY	1*	+23
FRUIT PIE, CHERRY	1*	+24
FRUIT PIE, LEMON	1*	+26
HOHO'S	3 PIECES	+26
MINI-MUFFINS, BANANA	3 PIECES	+3
MINI-MUFFINS, BLUEBERRY	3 PIECES	+4
MINI-MUFFINS, BROWNIE	3 PIECES*	+6
MINI-MUFFINS, CINN. APPLE	3 PIECES*	+5
MINI-MUFFINS, CHOCOLATE CHIP	3 PIECES*	+7
TWINKIES	1 CUP	+4
TWINKIES, CHOCOLATE CAKE	1 CUP*	+5
TWINKIES, DING DONGS	2 CAKES*	+22
TWINKIES, LOW FAT	1 CAKE	+1
TWINKIES, SPONGE CAKE	1 CAKE	+1

* AVOID

Table 50 continued on next page

TRF Rating System

Table 50 continued

KELLOGG'S	SERVING SIZE	SCORE
POP TART, FROSTED	1	+3
POP TART, LOW FAT	1	+1
POP TART, REGULAR	1	+3
M & M's		
ALMOND	1/4 CUP*	+8
PEANUT	1/4 CUP*	+11
PEANUT BUTTER	1/4 CUP*	+18
PLAIN	1/4 CUP*	+12
MILKY WAY, FUN SIZE	2 BARS*	+9

* AVOID

TRF Rating System

TRF Rating System

Table 51
TRF Scores of Sweet Snacks

MINTS	SERVING SIZE	SCORE
AFTER EIGHT	5 PIECES*	+8
ANDES	8 PIECES*	+24
JUNIOR MINTS	16 PIECES	+4
YORK	3 PIECES	+4
NESTLÉ		
ASSORTED MINIATURES	5 PIECES*	+16
BUTTERFINGER	4 PIECES*	+9
CHOCOLATE RAISINS	1 BAG*	+6
CRUNCH	1/4 BAR*	+14
REESE'S		
KIT KAT MINIATURES	1 BAR*	+16
NUTRAGEOUS	1 BAR*	+14
PEANUT BUTTER CUPS	2 CUPS*	+10
SNICKERS	2 BARS*	+10
RUSSELL STOVER		
DARK CHOCOLATE ASSORTMENT	2 PIECES*	+12
JELLIES	5 PIECES	0
ROCKY MELLOW	1/8 PIECE	+5
TASTY KAKES		
BUTTERSCOTCH KRIMPETS	3 CAKES	+5
CHERRY PIE	1 PIE*	+7
CHOCOLATE CUP KAKES	3 CAKES*	+6
CHOCOLATE ICED TASTY KLAIR	1 PIE*	+15
CHOCOLATE KANDY KAKES	2 PIECES*	+10
FRENCH APPLE	1 PIECE	+5
FROSTED MINI-DONUTS	4 PIECES*	+16
GHOSTLY GOODIES	2 PIECES*	+16
JELLY KRIMPETS	2 PIECES	+1

* AVOID

Table 51 continued on next page

Table 51 continued

TASTY KAKES (Continued)	SERVING SIZE	SCORE
KREEPY KAKES	2 CAKES	+4
KOFFEE KAKES	2 CAKES*	+6
KOFFEE KAKES, LOWFAT	2 CAKES	0
LEMON PIE	1 PIE*	+6
SNACK BARS, CHOCOLATE CHIP	1 BAR*	+9
ICED FUDGE BAR	1 BAR*	+6
OATMEAL & RAISIN	1 BAR*	+17
WITCHY GOODIES	2 PIECES*	+16
3 MUSKETEERS, FUN SIZE	2 BARS*	+9
TWIX	1 COOKIE	+5
WHITMAN'S SAMPLER	3 PIECES*	+12

* AVOID

Table 52
TRF Scores of Burger King

BREAKFAST		BURGERS	
BISCUIT*	+7	BACON CHEESEBURGER*	+20
BISCUIT W/EGG*	+11	BACON DOUBLE CHEESEBURGER*	+35
BISCUIT W/SAUSAGE*	+19	BIG KING*	+36
BISCUIT W/SAUSAGE, EGG & CHEESE*	+30	CHEESEBURGER*	+18
CINI-MINI'S (W/O ICING)*	+12	DOUBLE CHEESEBURGER*	+33
CROSSANWICH W/SAUSAGE EGG & CHEESE*	+26	DOUBLE WHOPPER*	+45
CROSSANWICH W/SAUSAGE & CHEESE*	+23	ABOVE, W/O MAYO*	+42
FRENCH TOAST STICKS (5)*	+10	DOUBLE WHOPPER W/CHEESE*	+57
HASH BROWNS, SMALL*	+11	ABOVE, W/O MAYO*	+54
HASH BROWNS, LARGE*	+19	HAMBURGER*	+12
SANDWICHES/SIDE ORDERS		WHOPPER*	+28
BK BROILER CHICKEN*	+13	ABOVE, W/O MAYO*	+25
ABOVE, W/O MAYO	+10	WHOPPER W/CHEESE*	+37
BK BIG FISH*	+21	ABOVE, W/O MAYO*	+34
CHICK N' CRISP*	+14	WHOPPER JR*	+19
ABOVE, W/O MAYO*	+11	ABOVE, W/O MAYO*	+17
CHICKEN TENDERS (4)	+7	WHOPPER JR, W/CHEESE*	+23
ABOVE (5 PIECES)	+9	ABOVE, W/O MAYO*	+21
ABOVE (8 PIECES)*	+15	DESSERTS	
DUTCH APPLE PIE*	+7	VANILLA SHAKE, SMALL*	+8
FRENCH FRIES, SMALL*	+12	ABOVE, MEDIUM*	+10
ABOVE, MEDIUM*	+18	CHOCOLATE SHAKE, SMALL*	+8
ABOVE, KING*	+26	ABOVE, MEDIUM*	+12
ONION RINGS, MEDIUM*	+12	STRAWBERRY SHAKE, SMALL	+8
ABOVE, KING*	+16	ABOVE, MEDIUM*	+10
TARTAR SAUCE*	+6		

* AVOID

Table 53
TRF Scores of Kentucky Fried Chicken

CRISPY STRIPS			
COLONEL'S STRIPS	+7	THIGH W/SKIN	+9
SPICY STRIPS	+8	BREAST W/O SKIN	+4
EXTRA TASTY CRISPY		BREAST W/SKIN	+8
BREAST*	+15	WING W/SKIN	+6
DRUMSTICK	+6	SANDWICHES & OTHERS	
THIGH*	+12	CHICKEN TWISTER*	+14
WHOLE WING	+7	CHUNKY POT PIE*	+26
HOT & SPICY CHICKEN		HOT WINGS*	+17
BREAST*	+15	MACARONI & CHEESE	+5
DRUMSTICK	+5	ORIGINAL RECIPE SANDWICH	+10
THIGH	+4	VALUE BB CHICKEN SANDWICH	+4
WHOLE WING	+8	POTATOES & OTHERS	
ORIGINAL RECIPE CHICKEN		BISCUIT	+6
BREAST*	+13	COLE SLAW	+3
DRUMSTICK	+4	CORNBREAD	+5
THIGH*	+11	MASHED W/GRAVY	+3
WHOLE WING	+7	POTATO SALAD	+4
TENDER ROAST CHICKEN		POTATO WEDGES	+8
BREAST W/O SKIN	+4	VEGETABLES	
BREAST W/SKIN	+8	BB BAKED BEANS	+1
DRUMSTICK W/O SKIN	+2	CORN ON THE COB	0
DRUMSTICK W/SKIN	+3	GREEN BEANS	+1
THIGH W/O SKIN	+4	MEAN GREENS	+1

* AVOID

TRF-Rating System

Table 54
TRF Scores of McDonald's

BREAKFAST		SANDWICHES	
BACON, EGG, & CHEESE BISCUIT*	+17	ARCH DELUXE*	+23
BISCUIT	+6	ARCH DELUXE W/BACON*	+25
BREAKFAST BURRITO*	+17	BIG MAC*	+19
EGG MCMUFFIN*	+11	CHEESEBURGER*	+11
ENGLISH MUFFIN	0	CRISPY CHICKEN DELUXE*	+10
HASH BROWNS	+3	FISH FILET DELUXE*	+12
HOTCAKES	+3	GRILLED CHICKEN DELUXE	+9
HOTCAKES W/MARGARINE*	+8	HAMBURGER	+6
SAUSAGE*	+9	QUARTER POUNDER*	+16
SAUSAGE BISCUIT*	+17	QUARTER POUNDER W/CHEESE*	+25
SAUSAGE BISCUIT W/EGG*	+22	SALADS & DRESSINGS	
SAUSAGE MCMUFFIN*	+15	CAESAR	+5
SAUSAGE MCMUFFIN W/EGG*	+22	FAT-FREE VINAIGRETTE	0
SCRAMBLED EGGS*	+10	GARDEN SALAD	0
CHICKEN MCNUGGETS		GRILLED CHICKEN SALAD	0
CHICKEN MCNUGGETS (4)	+5	RANCH	+4
CHICKEN MCNUGGETS (6)	+7	FRENCH	+4
CHICKEN MCNUGGETS (9)*	+9	DESSERTS	
BARBEQUE SAUCE	0	APPLE DANISH*	+11
HONEY MUSTARD SAUCE	+2	BAKED APPLE PIE*	+6
LIGHT MAYONNAISE	+2	CHEESE DANISH*	+17
FRENCH FRIES		CINNAMON ROLL*	+11
SMALL	+3	CHOC. CHIP COOKIE*	+11
LARGE*	+7	CHOC. SHAKE*	+12
SUPER SIZE*	+8	HOT FUDGE SUNDAE*	+18

* AVOID
Although a TRF Score of +8 to +10 may be acceptable for the main entrees, the TRF Scores of side dishes or desserts should be less than +5.

Table 55
TRF Scores of Pizza Hut
(Pizzas per 2 Slices)

BEEF TOPPING		PORK	
HAND TOSSED*	+20	HAND TOSSED*	+21
PAN*	+20	PAN*	+21
STUFFED CRUST*	+25	STUFFED CRUST*	+29
THIN N' CRISPY*	+20	THIN N' CRISPY*	+25
CHEESE		SUPREME	
HAND TOSSED*	+21	HAND TOSSED*	+21
PAN*	+25	PAN*	+20
STUFFED CRUST*	+21	STUFFED CRUST*	+30
THIN N' CRISPY*	+17	THIN N' CRISPY*	+20
CHICKEN SUPREME		SUPER SUPREME	
HAND TOSSED*	+11	HAND TOSSED*	+19
PAN*	+14	PAN*	+21
STUFFED CRUST*	+25	STUFFED CRUST*	+34
THIN N' CRISPY*	+11	THIN N' CRISPY*	+21
HAM		VEGGIE LOVERS	
HAND TOSSED*	+14	HAND TOSSED*	+12
PAN*	+15	PAN*	+15
STUFFED CRUST*	+25	STUFFED CRUST*	+25
THIN N' CRISPY*	+13	THIN N' CRISPY	+9
ITALIAN SAUSAGE		OTHERS	
HAND TOSSED*	+22	APPLE DESSERT	+2
PAN*	+24	BREAD STICK (1)	+2
STUFFED CRUST*	+31	BREAD STICK SAUCE	0
THIN N' CRISPY*	+25	CAVATINI PASTA*	+12
MEAT LOVERS		CAVATINI SUPREME*	+15
HAND TOSSED*	+19	CHERRY DESSERT	+2
PAN*	+23	GARLIC BREAD	+2
STUFFED CRUST*	+41	HAM & CHEESE SANDWICH*	+15
THIN N' CRISPY*	+29	HOT BUFFALO WINGS (4)	+6

* AVOID

Table 55 continued on next page

Table 55 continued

PEPPERONI		OTHERS CON'T	
HAND TOSSED*	+17	MILD BUFFALO WINGS (5)	+8
PAN*	+17	PERSONAL PAN	
STUFFED CRUST*	+29	CHEESE*	+21
THIN N' CRISPY*	+16	PEPPERONI LOVERS*	+24
PEPPERONI LOVERS		SUPREME*	+26
HAND TOSSED*	+25	SPAGHETTI	
PAN*	+30	SPAGHETTI W/MARINARA	+2
STUFFED CRUST*	+37	SPAGHETTI W/MEATBALLS*	+20
THIN N' CRISPY*	+25	SPAGHETTI W/MEAT SAUCE	+10

* AVOID

TRF Rating System

Table 56
TRF Scores of Subway Sandwiches

COLD SUBS (6")		PIZZA SUB*	+16
BLT	+8	ROASTED CHICKEN BREAST	+3
CLASSIC ITALIAN (BMT)*	+17	STEAK & CHEESE	+9
COLD CUT TRIO*	+14	SUBWAY MELT	+9
HAM	+4	SALADS	
ROAST BEEF	+4	BLT	+8
SUBWAY CLUB	+4	BREAD BOWL	+3
SUBWAY SEAFOOD-LITE MAYO	+8	CHICKEN TACO*	+11
SUBWAY SEAFOOD-REG. MAYO*	+19	CLASSIC ITALIAN BMT*	+13
TUNA W/ LIGHT MAYO*	+14	COLD CUT TRIO	+9
TUNA W/ REG MAYO*	+20	HAM	+3
TURKEY BREAST	+3	MEATBALL*	+10
TURKEY BREAST AND HAM	+4	PIZZA	+9
VEGGIE DELIGHT	+3	ROAST BEEF	+3
DELI STYLE SANDWICHES		ROASTED CHICKEN BREAST	+3
BOLOGNA	+8	STEAK & CHEESE	+8
HAM	+3	SUBWAY CLUB	+3
ROAST BEEF	+3	SUBWAY MELT	+9
TUNA*	+11	SUBWAY SEAFOOD-LITE MAYO	+8
TURKEY BREAST	+3	SUBWAY SEAFOOD-REG. MAYO*	+16
HOT SUBS (6")		TUNA*	+20
CHICKEN TACO SUB*	+12	TURKEY BREAST	+1
MEATBALL*	+12	VEGGIE DELITE	0

* AVOID

Table 57
TRF Scores of Taco Bell

BORDER WRAPS		SAUCES & DESSERTS	
CHICKEN FAJITA*	+12	BORDER SAUCES	0
CHICKEN FAJITA SUPREME*	+16	BURGER SAUCE	+3
STEAK FAJITA*	+12	CHEDDAR CHEESE SAUCE	+3
STEAK FAJITA SUPREME*	+16	CHOCOLATE TACO ICE CREAM*	+17
VEGGIE FAJITA	+9	CINNAMON TWISTS	+1
VEGGIE FAJITA SUPREME*	+12	CLUB SAUCE	+3
BREAKFAST		FAJITA SAUCE	+3
CHEESE QUESADILLA*	+20	GUACAMOLE	-1
QUESADILLA W/BACON*	+24	NACHO CHEESE SAUCE	+4
QUESADILLA W/SAUSAGE*	+22	PICANTE SAUCE	0
COUNTRY BURRITO*	+12	PICO DE GALLO	0
DOUBLE BACON & EGG BURRITO*	+20	RED SAUCE	0
FIESTA BURRITO*	+12	SOUR CREAM	+5
GRANDE BURRITO*	+16	THREE CHEESE SAUCE	+4
HASH BROWN NUGGETS*	+11	**SPECIALTIES**	
BURRITOS		BIG BEEF MEXI MELT*	+14
BACON CHEESEBURGER*	+23	CHEESE QUESADILLA*	+19
BEAN	+8	CHICKEN QUESADILLA*	+21
BIG BEEF SUPREME*	+20	MEXICAN PIZZA*	+19
BURRITO SUPREME*	+15	TACO SALAD W/SALSA*	+29
CHICKEN CLUB *	+21	TACO SALAD W/O SHELL*	+24
CHILI CHEESE*	+12	TOSTADA	+10
GRILLED CHICKEN	+8	**TACOS**	
7 LAYER *	+12	BLT SOFT TACO*	+14
		DOUBLE DECKER TACO	+10
NACHOS & SIDES		DOUBLE DECKER SUPREME*	+17
BIG BEEF NACHO SUPREME*	+16	GRILLED CHICKEN TACO	+7
MEXICAN RICE	+7	GRILLED STEAK TACO	+5
NACHOS	+8	SOFT TACO	+10
NACHOS BELL GRANDE*	+20	SOFT TACO SUPREME*	+15
PINTOS N' CHEESE	+8	TACO	+8

* AVOID

Table 58
TRF Scores of Wendy's

FRESH STUFFED PITAS		SALADS	
CHICKEN CAESAR	+10	CAESAR	+4
CLASSIC GREEK*	+15	DELUXE GARDEN	+3
GARDEN RANCH CHICKEN	+8	GRILLED CHICKEN	+5
GARDEN VEGGIE	+6	GRILLED CHICKEN CAESAR*	+8
PITA DRESSINGS		SIDE SALAD	0
CAESAR VINAIGRETTE	+3	TACO SALAD*	+21
GARDEN RANCH SAUCE	+3	SALAD DRESSINGS	
BAKED POTATO		BLUE CHEESE*	+5
BACON & CHEESE	+7	FRENCH	+2
BROCCOLI & CHEESE	+5	FRENCH (FAT-FREE)	0
CHEESE*	+14	RANCH	+2
CHILI & CHEESE*	+16	RANCH (REDUCED FAT)	+1
PLAIN	0	ITALIAN CAESAR	+3
SOUR CREAM	+8	THOUSAND ISLAND	+3
SOUR CREAM & CHIVES	+8	SANDWICHES	
WHIPPED MARGARINE	+4	BREADED CHICKEN	+10
CHICKEN NUGGETS		BIG BACON CLASSIC*	+25
CHICKEN NUGGETS (4)	+5	CHEESEBURGER (KIDS)*	+11
CHICKEN NUGGETS (5)	+7	CHICKEN CLUB*	+11
CHILI		HAMBURGER (KIDS)	+8
CHEDDAR CHEESE	+7	GRILLED CHICKEN	+6
LARGE	+8	JR. BACON CHEESEBURGER*	+14
SMALL	+6	JR CHEESEBURGER*	+12
DESSERTS		JR. CHEESEBURGER DELUXE*	+13
CHOCOLATE CHIP COOKIE*	+11	JR. HAMBURGER	+8
FROSTY, SMALL*	+10	PLAIN HAMBURGER*	+13
MEDIUM*	+14	HAMBURGER (EVERYTHING)*	+14
LARGE*	+18	SPICY CHICKEN	+9

*AVOID

Tips, Tricks, and Practical Guidelines for Using TRF Scores

TRF scores provide a liberating tool with which to choose from among an endless number of healthful foods. As long as the twenty-four-hour TRF scores are kept under +30, the choice of foods is limited only by one's culinary creativity and personal preferences.

Although the TRF scoring system allows plenty of room for flexibility and choice, it is qualitative, and should not be treated as a mathematical number—adding or subtracting as if so much butter or shortening can be offset with so much fish, etc. Preparing a seafood meal with margarine or shortening defeats the purpose of eating the fish because omega-6 poly-unsaturated fat in margarine or shortening prevents seafood's omega-3 fatty acids from entering various cells such as platelets, white blood cells, or the heart muscle. Saturated and trans fatty acids in a rich dessert can suppress the liver cells' ability to produce LDL-receptors no matter how much olive oil was used in the main dish or in the salad dressing. This is no different from the harmful impact of smoking two packs of cigarettes per day, which cannot be erased, even partially, by living in an air-conditioned house or office or in an area with no air pollution.

The purpose of the TRF scoring system is to provide a valid and worry-free tool to choose healthful meals, not to provide loopholes for "cheating" or "outsmarting" the system. Although a single meal, or a single day, of dietary indiscretion will not bring the world to an end, such deviations should be as infrequent as possible.

The following provides a summary of answers to frequently asked questions about the TRF diet.

Should You Eat Red Meat?

More than 70 percent of people in the United States think that red meat is a contributing factor to heart attack. This is unwarranted. Several recent studies have shown that moderate amounts of lean red meats do not raise LDL cholesterol any more than chicken or turkey. For example, extra-lean ground beef has 7 percent total fat, about one-half of which is saturated. However, about 50 percent of this saturated fat is stearic acid which acts like monounsaturates and does not raise the LDL cholesterol. Thus a quarter pound of uncooked, extra-lean ground beef has a mere 2 grams undesirable saturated fat, which should not affect anyone's blood cholesterol level.

You should, however, avoid greasy red meats, including regular hamburger, ribs, meatloaf, steak, hot dogs, sausages, bacon, or processed cold cuts such as bologna. The problem is not the red meat, but the white fat. Extra lean ground beef (7 percent fat) for hamburgers, meat loaf, and kabobs, or lean London broil, sirloin, and tenderloin, or lean pork products, veal, venison, or buffalo meat, can all provide delicious and healthful meals, provided they are used in small servings of less than 6 oz. Since grilling can make hamburgers made with lean ground beef dry, you can always mix one-fourth to one-half tablespoon of olive oil with it to make it as juicy as regular hamburger, but without the undesirable saturated fats. Chops, whether lamb, veal or pork, are too greasy and have very high TRF scores, unless they are trimmed thoroughly after cooking.

Should You Eat Poultry Meats?

Although chicken and turkey can provide a vast number of delicious and healthy meals, they should not become the "alternative" to lean red meats. Chicken and turkey neither prevent nor promote coronary artery disease. But for people with a high risk of developing coronary artery disease, and for those who already have coronary artery disease, neutrality is counterproductive. This is because these individuals do not have time on their side. By doing "no harm" (remaining neutral and relying on chicken and turkey), they miss the opportunity to move towards the goal of reducing their risk of having a coronary event. When you grill, bake, or broil chicken, you can leave the skin on in order to prevent the meat drying and making it tough and inedible. In these instances, the fat of the skin does not transfer to the meat, but you should remove the skin before eating it. When you cook chicken with other ingredients in a pot or pan, however, these ingredients can absorb some of the melted fat, especially potatoes, carrots, and other vegetables. In these situations you should remove the skin before cooking it.

Should You Eat Seafood?

Seafood provides a vast number of cardio-protective benefits, unmatched by any other food. Since seafood's cardio-protective role is directly related to its omega-3 polyunsaturated fat content and not to its protein or other nutrients, contrary to a common misconception, the fattier the fish, the better it is. Forty to 50 percent of the fat in seafood is omega-3 polyunsaturated fat, and another 20 to 30 percent is monounsaturates. Even a big chunk of this saturated fat is stearic acid, which acts very much like monounsaturates, leaving little coronary-unfriendly saturated fat to worry about. As a rule, the fat content of white fish is substantially less than that in fish with pink or dark meats (Tables 10 and 11).

To achieve the full benefits of omega-3 polyunsaturated fat, you should eat, on average, three to four seafood meals per week. For example, two days a week, say Monday and Thursday, you can eat some kind of seafood for lunch (such as tuna fish sandwiches without mayonnaise). Then, one or two nights per week you can eat a seafood of your choice for dinner. You should not prepare seafood with vegetable oils or fats (which contain a very high concentration of omega-6 polyunsaturated fat), because it defeats the purpose of eating seafood in the first place. Sautéing with olive oil, canola oil, or hazelnut oil (which are all predominately monounsaturated) is the better alternative. Shrimp and many other shellfish have very low fat content, about 1 percent total fat, compared to 30 percent for a choice grade T-bone steak. On the other hand, fish with pink or red flesh contain more fat (usually less than 10 percent), about 40 percent of which is the cardio-protective omega-3 polyunsaturated fat. For this reason, you should try to choose fattier fish, such as salmon, and tuna (Tables 10 and 11).

The cholesterol content of all fish is comparable to, or even lower than, chicken or turkey. Among shellfish, only squid has a moderately high cholesterol content (Table 11), but most people do not eat squid three times a day. As for shrimp, although its cholesterol content is a bit more than chicken or turkey, it can still provide a coronary-friendly meal because of its low saturated fat. In other shellfish such as clams, a large portion of their "cholesterol" content is not actually cholesterol as we know it, but cholesterol look-alikes or sterols, that are poorly absorbed from the intestine. These cholesterol look-alikes, moreover, actually prevent the absorption of cholesterol from the intestine, making them desirable. It is for this reason that the cholesterol content of some shellfish, such as clams or scallops (Table 11), is practically negligible.

Should You Eat Dairy Products and Eggs?

All low-fat dairy products (such as milk, yogurt, or cottage cheese) are excellent nutrients for all ages, except for those with lactose intolerance.

Approximately 50 percent of adult Hispanics, 60 percent of African Americans, 70 percent of Asians, and 50 percent of Middle Easterners are lactose intolerant, as is 10 percent of the white population of the United States. For them, products containing lactose can cause gas, bloating, diarrhea, or abdominal cramps. Lactose-free milk, such as Lact-Aid milk, or combining one or two Lact-Aid tablets with milk and cottage cheese is a reasonable option for lactose intolerant people.

In processed cheeses such as American, cheddar, mozzarella, provolone, parmesan, and Swiss, lactose is fermented and broken down. Therefore, processed cheeses do not cause any symptoms in lactose intolerant individuals. Unfortunately, processed cheeses have very high TRF scores (Table 22). Meals containing cheeses as the main ingredient such as pizzas, ravioli, and grilled-cheese sandwiches are not coronary-friendly. Still, occasional pieces of any cheese should not be viewed as poisonous or a trigger for a coronary event.

For too long eggs have been unfairly and arbitrarily eliminated from our diet because of the unwarranted fear that they may raise blood cholesterol level. This self-perpetuating misconception is almost entirely due to the cholesterol content of each yolk (an average of 220 mg per egg). But total fat content of eggs is about 4 percent—the same as the dark meat of chicken or turkey. And the yoke and the egg white provide wonderfully nutritious meals for people of all ages, especially the young and the elderly. Numerous studies have shown that eating seven to ten eggs per week (without butter or shortenings) does not raise cholesterol levels. The TRF scores of an omelet with two medium-sized eggs cooked with olive oil or canola oil is about +7. This or other egg dishes without the added fat are reasonable choices, two to three times per week, and provide a good deal of flexibility.

What's the Right Amount of Fruits and Vegetables?

During the past twenty-five years in the United States, consumption of fruits and vegetables has increased by 22 percent and 19 percent respectively. Unfortunately, more than half of the vegetables Americans eat are potatoes, half of them fried, which contain a big dose of undesirable trans fatty acids. Dark leafy vegetables and deeply colored fruits (such as all berries, plums, nectarines, and grapes) are rich sources of cardio-protective antioxidants/flavonoids. For this reason, in the TRF diet at least five to seven servings per day of vegetables and fruits are highly encouraged.

What Types of Dietary Fat Should Be Avoided?

You should drop from your diet butter, creams, stick margarine, shortening, cooking fats, lard, and mayonnaise. All of these fats have very high TRF scores. Stick margarines and shortenings not only have a high concentration of saturated fats, but also 15 to 30 percent trans fatty acids, which makes them quite coronary-unfriendly. Given the choice between butter and stick margarine, the best choice is olive oil! Olive oil, canola oil, or hazelnut oil can be used for all cooking needs, but a small amount of soft, trans fatty acid-free margarine (such as Benecol, Brummel & Brown, Smart Balance, or Take Control) or a low-fat variety can be used sparingly. (The TRF score of two tablespoons of Benecol spread is +1, and for Brummel & Brown spread it is +4, compared to an average of more than +16 for many stick margarines.)

Foods prepared with margarines, shortenings, or cooking fats are coronary-unfriendly. For example, a danish for breakfast is no better than eating two fried eggs, plus bacon and buttered bread. Doughnuts, muffins, and croissants also have relatively high concentrations of saturated and trans fatty acids, which also raise their TRF scores. The same is equally true for cakes, cookies, pastries, pies, and doughnuts.

Deep-fried anything—such as deep-fried chicken, seafood, onion rings, french-fried potatoes, or doughnuts—has a high concentration of trans fatty acids and omega-6 polyunsaturated fat, and unacceptably high TRF scores. On the other hand, you can sauté various foods in a nonstick pan using a small amount of olive oil, canola oil or hazelnut oil.

High intake of omega-6 polyunsaturates present in all vegetable oils such as corn, sunflower, safflower, sesame, and soybean oils—contrary to decades of misleading advertising—are also unhealthy. The three major concerns with these vegetable fats are that they: (1) lower HDL cholesterol; (2) increase oxidization of LDL cholesterol—a major disadvantage, since oxidized LDL particles are quite coronary unfriendly; and (3) spark a lingering concern that omega-6 polyunsaturated fat might increase the risk of certain cancers such as breast, colon, and prostate.

Current recommendations to increase consumption of polyunsaturated fat to 10 percent of dietary energy intake were based on the knowledge available thirty years ago. At present, such recommendations are obsolete and have no relevance to cardiovascular health, especially since monounsaturated fats such as olive oil or canola oil are healthful alternatives, and are readily available everywhere at prices comparable to other vegetable oils. Substituting olive oil or canola oil for all other oils and fats in the diet raises the HDL cholesterol and lowers the LDL cholesterol. But more importantly, this simple change in the type (but not necessarily the amount) of dietary fat inhibits the oxidization of LDL cholesterol. Table 59 summarizes the differences between the TRF diet and the current diet recommended by the American Heart Association and the National Cholesterol Education Program.

Fats such as palm oil, palm kernel, or cotton seed oil often used in various baked products have very high concentrations of saturated fats and, proportionately, very high TRF scores (Table 19). Although the amount of these oils in a daily diet is relatively small, when added to other saturated and trans fatty acids in a typical Western diet, you can no longer ignore them. On the other hand, an occasional slice of pie or cake, or a piece of chocolate, would not clog anyone's coronary artery overnight.

Should Eating Out Be Avoided?

Dining out need not necessarily be a "coronary trap." Dishes prepared with creams, butter, margarine, or cooking fat may be appetizing, but they have quite high TRF scores. This is particularly true with cream, butter, and nearly all French sauces, such as béarnaise and hollandaise. The sensible approach is to ask your server if a particular dish can be prepared with olive oil instead of butter, cream, or margarine. At good restaurants, this request is almost always honored. In fact, choosing a seafood entree, especially if it is grilled, lightly sautéed, baked, poached, or broiled (preferably using olive oil), minimizes any concern about hidden and unwanted fats.

In fast food restaurants, grilled chicken or roast beef sandwiches without the added butter or margarine or greasy sauces are reasonable options (see "Fast Foods" at the end of this chapter). As seen in Tables 52 and 54, the TRF scores of various sizes of french fries are high, so choose the smaller size instead of the extra large. Similarly, salads with various cheeses and sauces are no better than hamburgers at these restaurants.

Table 59
The Composition of the Twenty Risk Factor Diet

	% OF ENERGY TRF DIET	% OF ENERGY AHA/NCEP**
SATURATED FAT	<7	<7
OMEGA-6 PUFA	<7*	10
OMEGA-3 PUFA	>2	?
MONOUNSATURATES	15-20	? 3
TOTAL FAT	30-35	<20
COMPLEX CARBOHYDRATES	<55	>65
PROTEINS	15	15
DIETARY CHOLESTEROL	<400 MG	<200 MG
FRUITS & VEGS PER DAY	>5 SERVINGS	>5 SERVINGS

Based on an average of 2,000 calories per day
* Non-hydrogenated vegetable oils only (no margarines, shortening, or cooking fats)
** AHA = American Heart Association; NCEP = National Cholesterol Education Program

Breakfast at fast food restaurants is even worse in terms of its fat content. Still, occasional eggs, bacon, or even sausages, either at home or in restaurants, are not a disaster.

You should also avoid big portions of any meal—anywhere, anytime—because invariably they have too many calories and too high TRF scores. "All you can eat" smorgasbords, buffet dinners, two-for-one, and extra large sizes are notoriously coronary-unfriendly, provide too many calories, very high TRF scores, and are often conducive to overeating everything but the "right stuff."

French, Italian, and even Chinese restaurants in the United States often prepare meals with an inordinate amount of hidden fats. Many Chinese restaurants use peanut oil so excessively that it literally covers every piece of vegetable and meat in the dish, turning it into a most unhealthy meal. Table 60 shows how much fat is absorbed by various foods during Chinese stir-frying. When eating out, it is best to choose a simple entree that is not disguised with, or swimming in, various ingredients. (Tables 19 through 58 provide an easy reference for all of the foods that have high TRF scores which you should avoid.)

Table 60
Amount of Oil Absorbed Per 100 gm
Portion During Chinese Stir-frying

	GRAMS
SHREDDED LOW-FAT PORK	4
FRESH SOYBEAN	5
CUBED CHICKEN	7
GREEN PEPPERS	8
KIDNEY BEANS	9
ONIONS	11
PEA PODS	12
CAULIFLOWER	13
CABBAGE	13
SPINACH	13
MUSHROOM	14
CARROT	14
EGGPLANT	14
BAMBOO SHOOT	15
BROCCOLI	15

Are Fast Foods Out of the Question?

The fast food industry is an American invention that is mushrooming all over the world. In the United States, almost everyone, especially those with young children, visits a fast food establishment at least once a week. Although over two-thirds of people consider fast foods "junk food," this does not seem to deter them from eating them.

Whether we like it or not, the fast food industry is here to stay. Tables 52 through 58 provide TRF scores of menus served at some of the largest fast food chains in the United States. With a few exceptions, similar foods at other fast food eateries have the same TRF scores with only minor variations.

Among the reasons so many people eat at fast food establishments are that they are convenient and informal, the service is fast, and the food is pre-dictable and reasonably tasty (especially for youngsters). But, of equal impor-tance, these foods are affordable, and some actually have nutritional value!

After pressure by citizen groups in the early 1990s, a few fast food chains in the United States began a public relations game, lowering the fat content of a few of their entrees. Some even introduced a few low-fat items to pro-vide consumers with so-called "heart healthy" choices. But by the late 1990s, regrettably, most of the lean items had disappeared from the menus of nearly all fast food eateries. At present, there seems to be an unofficial race among the fast food chains to make their sandwiches bigger or meatier, and by adding various sauces or garnishes, even more calorie- and fat-laden. Many recent items added to menus at fast food eateries are worse than the previous items. Equally puzzling is the silence of public health officials, citizen advo-cacy groups, and the public in general, all of whom seem to have given up.

The TRF scores of some entrees at fast food chains are so unhealthful that, like alcohol or tobacco products, they should be forced to carry a health warning. For example, one Double Whopper with Cheese at Burger King has 67 grams of fat (100 percent of total daily requirement), 26 grams of saturated fat (more than 100 percent), and nearly 3000 mg of salt (60 percent). Overall, the TRF score of this atrocious concoction, not counting any french fries or deserts, is +57. A king-size french fries por-tion adds another 26 points, and a medium milk shake, another 12 points, giving that meal a total TRF score of +95! This is more than the allowed TRF score of all meals for three whole days.

McDonald's and Taco Bell's offerings have also become fattier, and pack much higher TRF scores than they did a few years ago. Among the big fast food chains, only Wendy's resisted the trend for a while, but they too have recently succumbed to the notion that "bigger is better." For example, they have introduced "Cheddar Lovers Bacon Cheeseburger," a dreadful combination with about 50 gm of fat, of which nearly half is sat-urated, and more than 3000 mg of salt. Just as disheartening are the TRF scores of Wendy's Taco Salad and Greek Salad which are +21 and +15, respectively. In contrast, the scores of their Deluxe Garden Salad and Grilled Chicken Salad are quite reasonable at +3 and +5, respectively.

At Taco Bell, very few entrees have TRF scores below +10. A Taco Salad with Salsa scores +29, and a Chicken Club Burrito scores +21. It is not as if they could not lower the fat content, especially saturated and trans fatty acids, but like the rest of the fast food industry, they choose not to.

Kentucky Fried Chicken has managed to turn the harmless chicken into a coronary-unfriendly meal by deep-frying it in cooking fat loaded with saturated fat and trans fatty acids. For example, their Tender Roast Breast without skin has a healthful TRF score of +4. In sharp contrast, Extra Crispy Breast has a coronary-unfriendly score of +15, and Chunky Chicken Pot Pie's score is nearly twice as bad at +26.

SUBWAY sandwiches are another example of good and bad all mixed up. For example, the average consumer may not suspect that a SUBWAY Tuna Sub has a TRF score of +20 and a Seafood and Crab Sub a score of +19—five times higher than a TRF score of Roast Beef or Ham (with TRF scores of +4), and more than six times higher than a Turkey Breast or Chicken Breast Sub (with TRF scores of +3).

Pizza Hut and nearly all other pizzerias, both national and regional, are no better. For example, most people associate the term "vegetarian" with nutritious and healthy foods. At pizzerias, vegetarian no longer means what it implies. Instead, it means a greasy, cheese- or margarine-laden concoction with a few slivers of onions, green peppers, mushrooms, or occasionally black olives. TRF scores of all of these pizzas are very high, especially since most people tend to eat more than one or two pieces. For example, the TRF score of four pieces of Pizza Hut's Veggie Lovers Stuffed Crust Pizza is a disheartening +50, equal to the allowed TRF scores of all foods and snacks for two days.

Recent studies have shown that consumption of fat that has been used for deep-frying in fast food restaurants impairs artery wall function, and the ability of the arteries to dilate properly (Chapter 1). This is because previously used cooking fats have a concentration of oxidized fatty products 400 percent higher than that of unused fat. Thus, fried items at fast food restaurants put consumers in a double jeopardy: too much fat with very high TRF scores, and far too many oxidized fat by-products.

It is also helpful to know in advance which items among fast food menus have low TRF scores using Tables 52 through 58. To reduce TRF scores and caloric content of any item, choose those without (or ask the server to leave out) sauces, mayonnaise, margarine, fried onions, mushrooms, bacon, melted cheese, or "double" anything. Grilled chicken, roast beef or turkey sandwiches without the above items are usually reasonable choices. Baked potato instead of french fries is also another way of cutting down on the unnecessary trans fatty acids. Still, an occasional serving of french fried potatoes (small-size) will not cause irreparable harm to anyone's coronary artery. But when in doubt, use the TRF scores.

Is It All Right to Have Desserts and Snacks?

Desserts are often very calorie-rich and contain hidden margarine, shortening, or butter, which makes them far more unhealthful than most main dishes. Cakes (especially cheesecakes), cookies, pies, tarts, and other pastries all have high TRF scores and should be avoided whenever possible. Even "light" ice creams often are not what "light" implies; they are still loaded with undesirable saturated fat and unneeded calories. But small servings of sorbet, sherbet, or frozen yogurt, garnished with or added to a bowl of various berries or a fruit cocktail, are reasonable choices. Even a few pieces of chocolate-covered almonds or raisins are better than other chocolate-rich snacks or desserts containing high levels of margarine, shortening, or coconut.

Should I Skip Meals?

A recent joint study by the U.S. Food and Drug Administration and the National Heart, Lungs and Blood Institute showed that in the United States, 20 percent of men and women, 51 percent of female high school students, and 18 percent of male students skip breakfast on a regular basis.

People skip breakfast for reasons such as getting up too late for work or school, or to take care of children or the elderly. A large number of people skip breakfast intentionally, and think they are helping themselves by cutting down on their calories. But numerous studies in both laboratory animals and humans have consistently shown that fewer meals lead to weight gain; to lose weight and keep the lost weight off, have three to four separate, but small meals. Often, people who skip breakfast or lunch eat a huge dinner, followed by frequent snacks until bedtime. For many, total calories consumed with dinner and snacks equal or exceed that which they would have eaten in three or four small meals. The large calorie load at dinner, the usual sedentary state after evening meals, and the frequent nibbling or snacking until bedtime, all contribute to more calories.

Skipping meals means we burn fewer calories than we would have during the day, and store more calories as fat at night. Meal skipping also increases the level of certain enzymes within fat cells which will enhance the storage of fat. In addition, skipping meals will reduce the ability of the liver to produce LDL-receptors, and can contribute to higher blood cholesterol levels. Also, when the stomach and the small intestine have not received foods for several hours, the abundant amount of unused digestive enzymes will increase the efficacy with which the next meal is digested and absorbed, thus increasing the total calories that enter our bloodstream. Eating breakfast also contributes to a better attitude towards work, school, and self, more stamina and less tiredness during the day, better maintenance of blood sugar level, less hunger, and less subsequent snacking later in the day.

What If I Can't Remember Whether a Certain Food Is Coronary-friendly or Not?

When in doubt or bewildered about how much of which ingredients are present in your food, or when you are simply wondering "What can I eat?" always use the TRF scores as your guide. Remember that the lower the TRF score of a food or meal, the better it is. Try to keep the TRF scores of breakfast and lunch to less than +5 each. This way, there are far more choices available for dinner (or the main meal). One of my primary goals for developing the TRF system is to provide you with a flexible and practical guide for cardiovascular health. Do *not* turn this flexibility into a rigid or fanatical game of scorekeeping. Try to keep your daily TRF score to less than +30. But if an occasional meal adds another +10 to +15 points to your daily TRF scores, so be it. The goal is long-term consistency, not dietary celibacy.

Part II:
The Twenty Risk Factors:
One by One

(1) Abdominal Obesity

An important feature of obesity is the location and distribution of fat, rather than the actual weight. An obesity pattern with body fat distribution around the waist and inside the abdomen (potbelly or beer belly) is distinctly different from that which involves the chest, arms, or hips. This is because fat cells in and around the abdomen act quite differently from fat cells everywhere else, even though they may look like regular fat cells.

Obesity can be measured in several ways:

(1) *Weight on the basis of height:* Although this tool has been used for over fifty years, it is a most inaccurate way of judging the presence or extent of abdominal obesity. It is a rough estimate based on no specific formula.

(2) *Waist to hip ratio:* This ratio is obtained by measuring the circumference of the natural waistline and the widest part of the hips. The waistline measurement is divided by that of the hips to obtain the waist/hip ratio. Desirable waist/hip ratios are less than 0.90 for men and less than 0.75 for women. Because abdominal obesity is a major risk factor for coronary artery disease, waist/hip ratio (or even waist measurement alone) is preferable to weight/height.

(3) *Body Mass Index (BMI):* Although BMI is less vague a measurement than the older means of determining ideal weight on the basis of height, it is still inaccurate. BMI is presently the most popular means of expressing body weight with a wide international acceptance. You can determine your BMI by dividing your body weight in kilograms by the square of your height in meters. Table 61 provides a wide range of BMIs based on body weight in pounds and height in inches (which is still the popular measurement system in the United States). Normal BMI for men should be less than twenty-five, and for women, less than twenty-four. Although BMI is a more accurate way of determining obesity, waist/hip ratio is still the best tool for assessing abdominal obesity.

Recently the American Cancer Society researchers reported its findings of a fourteen-year study of more than one million adults in the United States (457,785 men and 588,369 women). Among nonsmokers, the body mass indexes associated with the lowest death rates (from all causes) were 23.5 to

25 for men, and from 22 to 23.5 for women. High BMI among white men and women increased their all-cause mortality by 2.5 and twofold, respectively. Although the impact of obesity among African Americans was less pronounced, this difference is partly due to the coexistence of other risk factors among blacks, resulting in deaths before the impact of obesity becomes fully apparent. For a similar reason, obesity seems to affect older persons (more than seventy years of age) less than it does their younger counterparts. Still, because these groups have a higher overall risk of mortality from cardiovascular events and cancers, their obesity should be taken even more seriously.

In humans and most animals, insulin is essential for the metabolism of dietary carbohydrates, fat, and, to a lesser extent, proteins. Humans cannot survive without insulin. Even inadequate or ineffective insulin can cause serious damage in many organs. Abdominal obesity is almost always associated with a decreased ability of various tissues to respond to usual amounts of insulin, a condition called "insulin resistance." Insulin resistance is a major risk factor for coronary artery disease and the development of diabetes. In addition, obese individuals with insulin resistance often have lower levels of HDL cholesterol and higher levels of LDL cholesterol and triglycerides. Even more important, people with abdominal obesity tend to have a higher proportion of small LDL particles which are significantly worse than large particles (Part II, (15)). Children and adolescents with abdominal obesity, like adults, have higher triglyceride and lower HDL levels.

In adults with severe abdominal obesity, the risk of developing coronary artery disease is increased almost ninefold. The risk of stroke is also significantly higher among both men and women with abdominal obesity. A recent study of 28,000 U.S. male health professionals between the ages of forty and seventy-five showed that the risk of stroke was 2.3 times greater in those with the highest waist/hip ratio (W/H ratio greater than 0.97) than in those in the lowest category (W/H ratio less than 0.89). The long-term follow-up of more than 116,000 female nurses in the United States showed almost identical results: the risk of stroke among women with marked abdominal obesity was 2.4 times greater than among those with a W/H ratio less than 0.8.

What You Should Do

Because abdominal obesity significantly increases your risk of hypertension, coronary artery disease, and diabetes, you must try to deal with this serious risk factor. Being slightly to moderately overweight (without abdominal obesity) does not affect the cardiovascular system, but being even slightly overweight increases the risk of a number of cancers, including breast, ovary, cervix, prostate, and colon.

Although a detailed discussion of various aspects of obesity is not within the scope of this book, the following recommendations provide a rational guideline for successful and lasting weight reduction:

(1) *You must reduce your dietary fat and, even more importantly, carbohydrates.* This is essential! The use of TRF scores for foods and snacks provides a convenient way to avoid unnecessary fat in your diet. For those who are more than 50 percent over their ideal body weight, the total daily TRF scores should be less than +20.

The common argument that "calories are calories no matter where they come from" is sensible, but not entirely true. For example, out of every 100 calories in the form of proteins, the body burns 20 calories to facilitate the absorption process, leaving only 80 calories for use. In contrast, out of each 100 calories as fat, the body spends only 2 calories absorbing the fat, leaving 98 calories for use. With carbohydrates the body spends 8 grams out of 100 for the work of the intestine during absorption, leaving 92 calories for use. In other words, fat calories are worth about 18 percent more than protein calories and 6 percent more than carbohydrate calories. Gram for gram, fat has 250 percent more calories than carbohydrates or proteins. Thus all fat-containing foods are more energy dense (pack in more calories) than those without fat or with very low fat.

Although it is easy to avoid visible fat, reducing hidden fat requires more vigilance because it is often disguised and very hard to identify. For example, in many fast food restaurants where salad dressings are added to a garden salad, they can supply as many calories as one roast beef sandwich plus french fries, but with 50 percent more fat. Table 62 provides examples of hidden fats in some common foods.

Table 61
Body Mass Index (BMI) Based on Weight and Height

WEIGHT (LBS)	5'0"	5'1"	5'2"	5'3"	5'4"	5'5"	5'6"	5'7"	5'8"	5'9"	5'10"	5'11"	6'0"	6'1"	6'2"
130	25	25	24	23	22	22	21	20	20	19	19	18	18	17	17
135	26	26	25	24	23	22	22	21	21	20	19	19	18	18	17
140	27	26	26	25	24	23	23	22	21	21	20	20	19	18	18
145	28	27	27	26	25	24	23	23	22	21	21	20	20	19	19
150	29	28	28	27	26	25	24	23	23	22	22	21	20	20	19
155	30	29	28	27	27	26	25	24	24	23	22	22	21	20	20
160	31	30	29	28	27	27	26	25	24	24	23	22	22	21	21
165	32	31	30	29	28	27	27	26	25	24	24	23	22	22	21
170	33	32	31	30	29	28	27	27	26	25	24	24	23	22	22
175	34	33	32	31	30	29	28	27	27	26	25	24	24	23	22
180	35	34	33	32	31	30	29	28	27	27	26	25	24	24	23
185	36	35	34	33	32	31	30	29	28	27	27	26	25	24	24
190	37	36	35	34	33	32	31	30	29	28	27	26	26	25	24
195	38	37	36	35	33	32	31	31	30	29	28	27	26	26	25
200	39	38	37	36	34	33	32	31	30	30	29	28	27	26	26
205	40	39	37	36	35	34	33	32	31	30	29	29	28	27	26
210	41	40	38	37	36	35	34	33	32	31	30	29	29	28	27
215	42	41	39	38	37	36	35	34	33	32	31	30	29	28	28
220	43	42	40	39	38	37	36	34	33	33	32	31	30	29	28
225	44	43	41	40	39	37	36	35	34	33	32	31	31	30	29
230	45	43	42	41	39	38	37	36	35	34	33	32	31	30	30
235	46	44	43	42	40	39	38	37	36	35	34	33	32	31	30
240	47	45	44	43	41	40	39	38	36	36	34	33	33	32	31
245	48	46	45	43	42	41	40	38	37	36	35	34	33	32	31
250	49	47	46	44	43	42	40	39	38	37	36	35	34	33	32

Height

To calculate any Body Mass Index not listed above:
1. Multiply weight (in pounds) by 700
2. Square height in inches (H x H)
3. Divide #1 by #2

All carbohydrates, simple or complex, can contribute to obesity through their fat-sparing action. Since carbohydrates provide about 60 percent of daily calories, cutting their intake by half (even without a significant fat reduction) can still promote weight loss. But ideally, a balanced approach to cut down both carbohydrates and fat intake, while increasing the exercise-related energy expenditure, is not only more effective but can be followed indefinitely without any undesirable side effects. This combination can also prevent the yo-yo syndrome or "weight cycling" that occurs in more than 90 percent of "dieters." The five carbohydrate culprits are: bread, pasta, rice, potato, and sweets (including cakes, cookies, pies, pastries, chocolate, donuts, and ice cream).

All foods with high fat content (except those prepared with olive oil, canola oil, or hazelnut oil) have TRF scores exceeding +10, and many exceed +15 to +20. So when in doubt, always use the TRF scores. For the purpose of obesity management, calories from olive oil or other monounsaturates are not different from butter or margarine. For this reason, you should reduce the amount of all fats and oils, as well as all carbohydrates, simple or complex.

(2) *You must increase your energy expenditure.* Although you can lose weight by dieting without exercise, more than 90 percent of people who lose weight this way will regain it within the first year. It is for this reason that vigorous exercise and physical activity is almost always necessary for successful weight loss and weight maintenance.

In fact, for most people obesity is primarily an *exercise deficiency syndrome.* Although many people claim that they do not have time for exercise, they are often referring to a convenient time. Since there are approximately 1,400 minutes in each twenty-four hours, almost everyone should be able to allocate or set aside about forty of these minutes or roughly 3 percent of their time to care for themselves.

Anti-obesity Drugs

At present there are no obesity drugs with a long-term track record of safety and efficacy. This simple fact should be borne in mind when considering long-term use of any anti-obesity drug, notwithstanding the advertising claims. Although there are a number of promising anti-obesity drugs in the research pipeline, these are at least several years away from being approved as both safe and effective.

Prescription Drugs

One recent drug, sibutramine, marketed in the United States under the trade name Meridia, has been shown to be relatively safe on a short-term basis. Unlike fenfluramine and dexfenfluramine, which could potentially cause heart valve lesions after long-term use (over six months) or result in vascular damage in the lungs, sibutramine does not seem to have these potentials.

One concern with sibutramine is that it may raise blood pressure. Other relatively mild side effects include headaches, insomnia, and constipation. However, as with any new drug it is never safe to assume that side effects of sibutramine are limited to those listed above. Only long-term studies in a large number of individuals can provide adequate information regarding both safety and efficacy.

Sibutramine (like any other anti-obesity drug) does not work by itself and without dietary and lifestyle modifications. You can't take one or two pills and wake up in the morning twenty pounds slimmer. Moreover, sibutramine is a prescription drug and should be taken under close medical supervision. It is also expensive and not reimbursed by many health insurers.

Orlistat, marketed as Xenical, is another prescription drug promoted for weight loss and weight management. Orlistat blocks the function of an intestinal enzyme—lipase—which is necessary for the breakdown and absorption of dietary fats. When the action of lipase is blocked, a good part of dietary fat passes through the intestine unabsorbed (which may cause loose bowel movements or even diarrhea). In a recent European study of 688 obese adults, participants were placed on low-calorie diets and Orlistat, 120 milligrams three times per day. After one year, the Orlistat group lost 10 percent of their body weight, compared with 6 percent for those who were not given Orlistat. However, as soon as they stopped taking Orlistat they experienced a rebound effect, which resulted in their regaining nearly all of the lost weight in a short time. Is it worth taking a drug three times a day for one year to lose only 4 percent of body weight (10 percent for the drug, minus 6 percent for the placebo)? For a 200-pound person, 4 percent is approximately 8 pounds after one year of daily Orlistat. This is hardly a breakthrough or even a modest improvement in obesity treatment.

Table 62
Percent of Calories from Fat

FOOD	CALORIES FROM FAT
BEANS	4
MOST SHELLFISH	5
BREAST OF TURKEY (W/O SKIN)	7
MOST WHITE MEAT FISH*	10
SALMON, TUNA, OR MACKEREL*	14-18
1 PERCENT MILK	17
BREAST OF CHICKEN (W/O SKIN)	17
DARK TURKEY (W/O SKIN)	23
TOP ROUND, BEEF, LEAN	29
2 PERCENT MILK	36
TENDERLOIN, BEEF, LEAN	41
DARK CHICKEN (W/O SKIN)	42
BREAST OF CHICKEN (W/SKIN)	44
GROUND TURKEY	45
WHOLE MILK	50
EXTRA LEAN HAMBURGER	53
DARK CHICKEN (W/SKIN)	56
TURKEY OR CHICKEN HOT DOGS	70
MOST PROCESSED CHEESES	75
BEEF HOT DOGS	80
POTATO OR CORN CHIPS	80

* Depending on the type of fish and its fat content, the percentage of calories from fat may vary slightly.

Over-the-counter Drugs, Herbs, and Supplements

Taking 200 mcg of chromium twice per day seems to have a significant impact on improving the body's response to insulin, especially among people with abdominal obesity, whether diabetes is present or not. As such, chromium, along with the dietary and lifestyle modifications discussed above, might be a helpful aid in a reasonable weight loss program.

Several over-the-counter appetite suppressants use phenylpropano-lamine as the active ingredient. At manufacturers' recommended doses, these products are relatively safe but not effective unless combined with both diet and exercises. Rare major side effects include stroke, heart attack, and severe irregularities of heart rhythm, which can be fatal. Minor side effects include nervousness, sleep disturbance, elevated blood pressure, dizziness, headache, and nausea. Overall, these products do little towards coping with the problem of obesity or its underlying causes.

Various herbs, ginseng, DHEA, melatonin, and a host of other supplements do not have any appreciable weight loss effect unless accompanied by the two essential principles of weight loss and weight maintenance: decreased energy intake and increased exercise level.

Abdominal, as well as generalized, obesity is a chronic disease that takes years to set in, and therefore requires sustained long-term treatment. As with any other chronic disease, as soon as the treatment is stopped it will recur. We must also acknowledge that if it were easy to treat, everyone would have done it. So, to repeat: no matter what approach you choose, it must include the two pillars—reduce energy intake (calories in the diet) and increase energy output (exercise).

(2) Low Birth Weight

Low birth weight, and in many instances low weight during early infancy, is associated with increased risk of coronary artery disease, hypertension, diabetes, kidney failure, and thyroid disorders in adult life.

A recent study from India showed that the prevalence of coronary artery disease among men and women over forty-five years of age whose birth weight was less than 5.5 pounds was 11 percent. In sharp contrast, the prevalence among persons with birth weight greater than 7 pounds was only 3 percent. In other words, the risk was more than 3.5 times greater among those with the lowest birth weight. The highest rate of coronary artery disease (20 percent) was seen among people whose birth weight was less than 5.5 pounds and whose mothers also weighed less than 100 pounds. In another study from the United Kingdom, the prevalence and severity of coronary artery disease was greatest in those with the lowest recorded birth weight; the risk for people who had weighed less than 6.5 pounds at birth was more than five times greater than for those who weighed more than 7.5 pounds at birth.

Low birth weight also doubles the risk of diabetes in adulthood. In the U.S. Nurses' Study, which included more than 69,000 women, birth weight of less than 5 pounds was associated with an 83 percent higher risk of diabetes. Contrary to a common misconception, higher birth weight in this or other studies was associated with a lower risk of diabetes (except among those whose mothers had gestational diabetes).

Low birth weight is often related to health and socioeconomic factors affecting pregnant women. Some of these factors include poverty, poor education, lack of family or social links, smoking, drinking, drug abuse, and lack of (or very erratic) prenatal care. All of these factors can affect the nutritional status and health of the mother and the fetus she carries. In the United States, low birth weight is far more common among African Americans than among their white counterparts, which is not due to genetic or racial differences. It is because of poor prenatal care (for some of the reasons listed above), compounded by a large number of underage pregnancies.

The association of low birth weight and coronary artery disease is independent of other cardiovascular risk factors. A large number of studies have shown that malnutrition in the fetal stage and infancy can result in the later development of several chronic diseases. Other risk factors in adult life expedite and worsen the impact of low birth weight on coronary artery disease.

Fetal malnutrition, for example, contributes to lower production of a compound called elastin in the arterial wall. Since elastin plays a major role in the pulsation and dilation of the arteries, deficient elastin makes the arteries stiffer and less likely to dilate properly when needed. The stiffness of the arteries in adult life is a major contributor to hypertension, kidney failure, stroke, and heart attacks.

Fetal malnutrition, with or without other contributing factors, can also cause alterations (mutations) in a vast number of genes. Many of these mutations remain dormant but slowly over the years contribute to the insidious development of various chronic diseases in adult life. Mutated genes have a significant impact on cardiovascular diseases. For example, there are over 350 different mutations affecting LDL receptors in the liver. Such mutant receptors are unable, or have a lower capacity, to clear LDL cholesterol from the bloodstream, which results in high blood cholesterol levels.

An enzyme called "lipoprotein lipase" is responsible for clearing triglycerides from the bloodstream. A minor mutation in this enzyme has been shown to increase the risk of heart attack nearly fivefold. Other genetic mutations occurring during the fetal stage can contribute to a vast number of abnormalities which collectively increase the risk of chronic heart disease in adults who were underweight as newborns.

What You Should Do

The growth and development of the fetus inside the uterus, long before the cradle, may have a significant impact on the future development of cardiovascular and other diseases during adult life. Obviously we cannot ask for a recall or turn the clock back and change our nutritional status while we were in our mother's womb. From the public health standpoint, however, we must make every effort to prevent fetal malnutrition if we are to substantially reduce the risk of many chronic disorders, including various cardiovascular diseases, in future generations. Sadly, the tragedy of famine and malnutrition in Africa, Bangladesh, Iraq, and elsewhere will have a devastating impact on the future health of all these populations.

If you were underweight at birth, it is not inevitable that you will have various chronic diseases. Genetic mutations or susceptibilities to chronic diseases acquired as a result of fetal malnutrition and low birth weight are neither familial nor hereditary. In other words, they are not the sort of problems that are passed on from generation to generation. They are random events occurring during fetal life and therefore are limited to those affected individuals and not their siblings or offspring. Adults with low birth weight should be tested for coronary risk factors periodically, and treated vigorously to preempt or modify the impact of each risk factor. Even in the absence of any major risk factors, you should still adopt a healthy lifestyle (including a diet based on the TRF system, exercise, weight control, no smoking, and stress management) to minimize the health impact of your low birth weight.

Most health care providers are unaware that low birth weight is a major risk factor for coronary artery disease, heart attack, stroke, hypertension, diabetes, and kidney or thyroid diseases. All of these are serious diseases with serious complications. Aside from educating the health care providers, readers who had low birth weight should bring this to the attention of their physicians and request screening for these diseases from time to time.

(3) High Blood Pressure

High blood pressure, or hypertension, affects people all over the world. At least sixty-five million Americans have hypertension. In 80 percent of hypertensives, high blood pressure has no readily identifiable cause. This is called "essential hypertension" or "idiopathic hypertension" (meaning the cause is unknown). The other 20 percent of hypertensives have a wide range of causes, including kidney diseases, sedentary lifestyles, abdominal obesity, hardening of the arteries, narrowing of the artery of one or both kidneys, certain tumors of adrenal glands, and, very rarely, excessive dietary sodium combined with low potassium intake.

Even essential hypertension is not exactly without a cause. Recent studies have found several genetic abnormalities in people with essential hypertension. Some of these involve various enzymes or biochemical compounds that regulate blood pressure. Such defects or mutations result in dysfunctional or nonfunctional enzymes, thereby derailing the regulatory processes that keep blood pressure normal.

As noted in (2), malnutrition during fetal life can also affect the formation of elastin, a substance that plays a major role in the pliability and dilating ability of the arteries. Developments in molecular biology and DNA technology give hope that, step by step, we are getting closer to discovering every cause of hypertension. These developments have also provided incentives for the pharmaceutical industry to come up with targeted drugs that can be matched to individual needs.

Because of the sheer size of the population with high blood pressure all over the world, the number of people who suffer from its complications is enormous. Effective methods of controlling blood pressure can protect millions of people each year from needless strokes, heart attacks, kidney failures, blindness (because of damage to retinal arteries), and heart failure.

A recent long-term study of 19,000 men and women with hypertension showed that a diastolic blood pressure (the bottom number) of over 85 increased the risk of heart attacks by about 35 percent and the risk of stroke by about 45 percent. In a collaborative study, researchers tracked 124,774 participants from both the People's Republic of China and Japan for an average of seven years. Among these individuals, nearly 1,800 suffered strokes, 55 percent of which were fatal. Overall, the risk of a stroke among those with the highest blood pressure was thirteen times higher than in those with the lowest blood pressure. In fact, each five-point drop in diastolic blood pressure reduced the risk of a stroke by 40 percent.

In the largest international collaborative study of hypertension to date, researchers followed 450,000 individuals for an average of sixteen years. Among those with a diastolic blood pressure of 102 or greater, the risk of stroke was five times more than in those with a diastolic blood pressure number of less than 75. For hypertension sufferers aged forty-four to sixty-five, the risk of stroke was five times higher, while for older persons it was two times higher. This study confirmed that the devastating complications of high blood pressure are not limited to "old folks." Younger people in their prime are affected even more severely. Current studies strongly suggest that the optimal blood pressure should be below 130/80 and that the risk of various cardiovascular complications dramatically increases at blood pressures greater than 150/100.

Long-term hypertension can cause small "mini-strokes" which lead progressively to dementia. In a long-term French study, doctors treated 1,238 hypertensives vigorously with two or three anti-hypertensive drugs. Another 1,180 were treated less vigorously (with one anti-hypertensive drug). The hypertensive individuals who were treated vigorously had 50 percent less risk of dementia than the "control" group (those treated less vigorously, which, regrettably, is how most hypertensives are treated in the United States). Overall, if a thousand hypertensives were adequately treated for a period of five years, about twenty cases of dementia could be prevented. In a twenty-year population-based study of 999 older men, Swedish investigators also found a significant link between hypertension and dementia. Since there is no effective treatment for dementia, controlling high blood pressure as early as possible becomes even more imperative.

For some hypertensive individuals, identifying and treating the underlying cause may cure their hypertension. For a vast number of others, however, hypertension may remain a chronic, lifelong disorder that requires dietary and lifestyle changes and, often, daily use of anti-hypertensive drugs.

In some hypertensives, blood pressure goes up and down; periodically, it may even be normal, giving them a false sense of security. Unfortunately, this kind of unstable hypertension is not something you can ignore. Intermittent periods of pulsatile and forceful jetstreams of blood lashing against atherosclerotic plaques in the coronary and cerebral arteries (hardened arteries) can significantly increase your risk of a heart attack or stroke if left untreated. You cannot dismiss, ignore, or undertreat high blood pressure, whether it is stable or unstable.

Diet

Salt

For most people with high blood pressure, dietary salt is not a problem. But the guidelines provided in Chapter 2 ("Supplemental Vitamins and Minerals") provide a rational and scientific basis for salt reduction in salt-sensitive people such as African Americans, the obese, or the elderly.

Fruits and Vegetables

A recent study called the Dietary Approaches to Stop Hypertension showed that a diet low in saturated fat but rich in fruits and vegetables (eight to ten servings per day) and low-fat dairy products can have a modest impact on blood pressure. On this diet, the average drop in systolic blood pressure (the top number) was 5.5, and the average drop in diastolic pressure was three. Although for a small number of borderline cases these average drops may be adequate, for a vast number of individuals with moderate to severe hypertension, these are very small changes with very little practical benefit. However, in spite of its limited blood pressure-lowering effect, such a diet does provide other cardio-protective and anti-carcinogenic benefits.

Since the average number of servings of fruits and vegetables in the U.S. diet, and in most Western diets, is about four to five servings a day, doubling this should not be a difficult undertaking. Eating cereals with berries, raisins, peaches, or other fruits, or toasted whole wheat bread in the morning with 1 percent milk or low-fat yogurt along with an orange, an apple, or a banana—all are easy and quick choices. Raisins or other fruits instead of sweet snacks are reasonable and tasty midday alternatives. For lunch, any low-fat meat sandwich or meal with a salad and some vegetables is practical, even when eating at a fast food restaurant. For dinner, sensible and healthy choices include seafood, poultry, or lean meat with two or three servings of vegetables, with or without salad and whole wheat bread, rice, or pasta. For dessert, either fruit or frozen yogurt is a good option, and for snacks later at night, another serving of fruit can round out a day's dietary requirement for eight to ten servings of fruits and vegetables.

Seafood

You can also reduce your blood pressure by increasing omega-3 fatty acids from seafood. Here, three to four seafood meals per week provide a practical way to reduce not only blood pressure but also the risk of cardiovascular events. For lunch, a tuna fish sandwich two days a week, without mayonnaise (or with the fat-free variety), or just tuna with mustard or salsa to make it zesty, is reasonable. This would then allow for two dinners per week of seafood, preferably those with high levels of omega-3 fatty acids (Tables 10 and 11).

Potassium

Numerous studies have provided compelling evidence that increasing dietary potassium is more effective than decreasing salt intake in lowering blood pressure. Although most people can get an adequate amount of potassium from their diet, in those who are taking diuretics (which eliminate both sodium and potassium in the urine), supplemental potassium is wise. Unlike sodium, the margin of safety for blood potassium levels is somewhat narrow and thus your doctor should supervise your supplementation. Some "light" salts and salt substitutes contain potassium as a replacement for sodium. Their regular use in cooking and in the salt shaker helps lower dietary sodium while at the same time increasing the potassium intake.

Calcium

The blood pressure-lowering effect of supplemental calcium is relatively small and unpredictable. However, calcium supplementation, especially for older persons, has other important benefits.

Exercise

Regular exercise four to five days per week has a significant blood pressure-lowering effect, exceeding that of salt restriction. Regular exercise is perhaps the most important lifestyle change that can dramatically reduce the risk of various cardiovascular events.

Herbal Remedies

In spite of various hollow claims of herbal promoters and retailers, none of the available herbs has shown any significant anti-hypertensive effects. Herbs with minor anti-hypertensive effects are ginkgo, hawthorn, and garlic. Licorice, on the other hand, may cause severe sodium retention, potassium depletion, and exacerbation of hypertension. For this reason, you should avoid licorice products.

Vitamins

A Boston University study showed that long-term use of daily vitamin C supplements (500 milligrams per day) reduced systolic blood pressure by an average of ten points. However, it did not change the diastolic blood pressure. By preventing oxidization of nitric oxide (a potent dilator of blood vessels) in the bloodstream, vitamin C may prevent the constriction of the arteries and lower blood pressure.

Anti-hypertensive Drugs

At present, there are a vast number of effective and safe anti-hypertensive drugs that have been extensively evaluated which your doctor can prescribe. Treatment of hypertension is not a do-it-yourself sort of health care. Hypertension is a serious disease that demands serious attention and vigorous intervention. Anti-hypertensive drugs are quite effective in dramatically reducing or preventing the risk of strokes, heart attacks, and cardiovascular disabilities in both men and women of all ages. The higher the blood pressure and the greater the number of other associated risk factors, the larger the benefit of anti-hypertensive therapy. This is because individuals with several risk factors have an extremely high risk of developing catastrophic cardiovascular events, and effective treatment of their hypertension may make an enormous difference.

What You Should Do

Hypertension, perhaps unfortunately, causes no symptoms in most individuals. Unlike a sore throat, flu, arthritis, or other painful disorders, many cardiovascular diseases in their early stages are painless. Because there is no immediate reward such as that which comes with alleviating a symptom, many people are reluctant to adhere to a lifelong treatment of their hypertension. Poor compliance with recommended treatment is perhaps the worst risk factor for developing complications of hypertension. If your blood pressure is higher than 130/85, you should be treated. Blood pressure does not have to be 240/150 before action is taken. More than 70 percent of people who suffer strokes or heart attacks have a "borderline" hypertension (blood pressure less than 150/95).

Although a vast number of effective and safe anti-hypertensive drugs are available today, we have, regrettably, done a poor job of adequately managing hypertension, especially among the older population. In a recent two-year study of eight hundred hypertensive men, 40 percent still had blood pressure of higher than 160/90 despite an average of more than six hypertension-related visits to their doctors per year. In fact, blood pressure was normalized in less than one-third of these men.

Although over 65 million Americans have high blood pressure, not everyone will suffer a cardiovascular event. Clearly, coexistence of other major coronary risk factors contributes to the deleterious impact of hypertension. Furthermore, there are wide differences among various populations, as is seen by comparing blood cholesterol levels. For example, at a similar level of blood pressure (such as 150/90), the risk of a cardiovascular event for Americans or northern Europeans is at least three times greater than for southern Mediterraneans or Japanese. This highlights the fact that the intensity of treatments for hypertension (like a host of other disorders) may vary greatly from person to person, and therefore should always be "tailor-made" under medical supervision.

(4) Chronic Infections

For several decades it was believed that ulcers of the stomach or duodenum (the first portion of the small intestine) were primarily due to excessive acid. Today we know that is not necessarily so. A germ called helicobacter pylori causes 50 to 60 percent of gastric or duodenal ulcers, and about 50 percent of stomach cancers. Eradication of these germs from the stomach not only helps cure the ulcers, but also prevents their recurrence; more importantly, it reduces the risk of stomach cancer.

For several decades it was assumed that elevated blood cholesterol was the principal cause of coronary artery disease. Today, we know that is untrue. Coronary artery disease is a chronic inflammatory process in the arterial wall, in some ways similar to arthritis which is a chronic inflammatory process of the joint surfaces. Some infections can cause arthritis, and others may contribute to the inflammation of the arterial wall.

A common respiratory tract germ called "chlamydia pneumoniae" is an important risk factor for coronary artery disease. In fifteen different studies dealing with atherosclerosis (hardening of the arteries) involving coronary and carotid arteries or aorta, researchers found c. pneumoniae infection in more than half the cases. In contrast, only 5 percent of normal arteries showed any evidence of c. pneumoniae infection. This strikingly higher risk in infected individuals—a tenfold increase—strongly suggests that c. pneumoniae has a role in atherosclerosis and coronary artery disease.

Scientists have found c. pneumoniae inside coronary and carotid artery plaques in several ways. In one study from the University of Utah, 79 percent of coronary artery plaques obtained during surgery showed evidence of infection with c. pneumoniae, whereas normally only 4 percent of arteries were infected. In another study from the University of Washington, Seattle, 60 percent of samples from carotid artery plaques tested positive for c. pneumoniae.

A thirteen-year follow-up of over 19,000 Finnish men and women, with an average age of forty-three at the onset of the study, showed that among those with a history of chronic bronchitis (many of which are secondarily infected with c. pneumoniae), the risk of developing coronary artery disease was nearly 50 percent greater than in those without chronic bronchitis. This finding also explains, in part, why individuals with various chronic lung diseases tend to have a much greater risk of coronary artery disease and stroke.

In a study from the United Kingdom, 213 patients who had suffered heart attacks participated in a double-blind study. After eighteen months of observation, those who had the highest levels of antibodies to c. pneumoniae (a marker for the infection) were four times more likely to suffer coronary events (including additional heart attacks, angioplasties, and coronary bypass surgery) than similar patients without antibodies to c. pneumoniae. Perhaps the most compelling evidence that c. pneumoniae is not just a bystander was that c. pneumoniae-positive patients who received azithromycin (an antibiotic with potent anti-c. pneumoniae effect) had a risk of recurrent coronary events equal to that of patients who did not have the germ.

In a recent Argentinean study, researchers using a different antibiotic reduced the occurrence of coronary artery disease from 10 percent in the placebo group (given no antibiotics) to only 1 percent in the treated group.

Another study from Germany showed that among individuals with coronary bypass grafts, 25 percent of the vein grafts (taken from patient's legs) that had reclogged were infected with c. pneumoniae. In contrast, only 5 percent of their other veins showed any evidence of infection with this germ. The findings of this study suggest that the vein grafts become infected with c. pneumoniae after surgery, which contributes to an accelerated atherosclerosis in the vein graft.[22]

The following case history illustrates the impact of c. pneumoniae infection. Mr. Robert S was forty-six when he had his first heart attack and required balloon angioplasty to open up his clogged coronary artery branches. Four months later, his arteries were reclogged, and he experienced frequent chest pain when he walked from his car to his office less than fifty yards away. He underwent coronary bypass surgery with two grafts from his leg veins. Three months later, one of the grafts clogged again and he suffered frequent chest pain and shortness of breath. He had been on a cholesterol-lowering drug and three other medications to keep his blood pressure under control. At this point, his blood antibody level for c. pneumoniae was very high at 526 (any value higher than 64 indicates infection with c. pneumoniae). Instead of further surgery, he continued his previous drugs but also went on a diet with TRF scores of less than +20 per day and took a three-week course of Zithromax, an antibiotic with a strong anti-c. pneumoniae effect. Within the first ten days of treatment his symptoms improved, and in the subsequent three-and-a-half years he has had no further angina or reclogging of his coronary artery. His most recent angiogram (pictures of his coronary artery) showed that the previously clogged graft is more than 30 percent open, and his other graft is fully functional. His anti-c. pneumoniae antibody is now at thirty-two.

Another indicator of smoldering inflammations or infections is a protein in the bloodstream called "C-reactive protein," which is produced by the liver. Normally, the blood level of C-reactive protein is less than 0.40 mg/dl. In the absence of an acute illness, an elevated blood level of C-reactive protein is indicative of a smoldering or chronic infection somewhere in the body.

Several recent studies have shown that raised levels of C-reactive protein signal higher rates of coronary events, similar in magnitude to the risk associated with elevated blood cholesterol levels. A raised C-reactive protein level, in the absence of acute infections or inflammatory processes (such as rheumatoid arthritis, lupus, and ulcerative colitis), may point to the existence of an ongoing inflammatory process inside atherosclerotic plaques of coronary and carotid arteries. Since an ongoing inflammation often makes the plaques unstable and vulnerable to rupture (causing heart attack), health care providers should take a rise in C-reactive protein levels seriously.

What You Should Do

The role of infections (or any other risk factor) in coronary artery disease cannot be viewed in isolation. Because coronary artery disease is almost always multifaceted, infection with c. pneumoniae or other germs usually works in tandem with coexisting coronary risk factors. Therefore, you should not focus on these infections and dismiss the other major coronary risk factors listed in Table 4. Even if you eradicate c. pneumoniae infection, other risk factors continue to wreak havoc and damage your coronary artery unless they are corrected as well.

At present, blood testing for c. pneumoniae is relatively expensive but available through most laboratories. One major drawback of the test is that it may give a false negative result in up to 20 percent of patients who have been infected and have evidence of the germ in their coronary plaques. Nevertheless, because we can treat c. pneumoniae, you should be tested for this infection if you already have coronary artery disease.

You should also be tested if you have multiple coronary risk factors or a history of chronic respiratory tract disorders, even in the absence of any apparent coronary artery disease.

Should we give antibiotics to all individuals with positive blood antibodies against c. pneumoniae? Although one hundred million Americans have abnormal blood cholesterol levels, not all require cholesterol-lowering drugs. Similarly, treating a vast number of people with antibiotics for three weeks (and in some cases up to three months) is neither appropriate nor cost effective. However, the test for C-reactive protein may provide some guidance. In c. pneumoniae-positive individuals, a positive C-reactive protein test strongly argues in favor of an active, rather than a dormant, c. pneumoniae infection. Such individuals should be offered at least a two-week course of an appropriate antibiotic. This is essential if the infected individual is being scheduled for any coronary artery procedure, especially angioplasty or bypass surgery. For those who require these procedures on an emergency basis, the blood tests should be done the same day. If they (c. pneumoniae and C-reactive protein) are both positive, treatment should be started as soon as possible. At present, studies are underway to determine the most suitable antibiotics, dose, and duration of treatment.

Even at low doses, aspirin can reduce the C-reactive protein level significantly, but has no impact on c. pneumoniae. It is not clear whether this anti-inflammatory effect of low-dose aspirin alters the course of c. pneumoniae and its impact on coronary artery disease. Still, it does constitute another reason why most men and women over forty-five years of age should take a daily, low-dose aspirin. Pravachol, a cholesterol-lowering drug, also decreases C-reactive protein level. Recent data show that, in people with elevated blood cholesterol and a raised C-reactive protein level, Pravachol seems to reduce the risk of a future coronary event by more than 45 percent, much better than the 30 percent risk reduction seen among those with elevated blood cholesterol who do not have a raised C-reactive protein. This additional benefit is due to Pravachol's anti-inflammatory action.

(5) Elevated Blood Fibrinogen

Fibrinogen is a protein in the bloodstream that is necessary to form blood clots. Fibrinogen can stick to the inner lining of an artery like a piece of chewing gum, and form the basic skeleton of a clot. Once deposited and adhered to the arterial wall, it signals blood platelets to clump and stick to this framework. In turn, this combination traps red and white blood cells from the bloodstream and creates a clot or thrombosis. As the thrombosis matures, other constituents or compounds in the bloodstream such as calcium or iron may be trapped or deposited in the clot, making it firmer and more established.

Eighteen recent studies have shown that an elevated blood fibrinogen (more than 250 mg/dl) increases the risk of coronary artery disease approximately two to three times. Very high fibrinogen levels are associated with even greater risks (as much as six times higher) of cardiovascular events. In a long-term follow-up of fifteen hundred persons in the Framingham Heart Study, for every 56 mg/dl increments in baseline blood fibrinogen, the eighteen-year risk of a cardiovascular event in men rose by 34 percent. The risk for women was only slightly less than that for men.

People with elevated blood fibrinogen levels often have a number of other coronary risk factors that further increase their risk of heart attacks or strokes. For example, a high percentage of their LDL particles are the small, dense variety that are particularly coronary unfriendly. In addition, they have lower HDL cholesterol and higher triglyceride levels. Raised fibrinogen levels also increase blood viscosity. It is this combination— abnormal blood cholesterol levels, increased clotting potential, and higher blood viscosity—that makes elevated fibrinogen an important risk factor for coronary artery disease and heart attack.

In a recent Scottish Population Study, researchers tracked 11,629 men and women aged forty to fifty-nine for an average of 7.6 years. Elevated blood fibrinogen, especially among men, was one of the strongest predictors of all coronary artery disease. The impact of a raised fibrinogen level was even more important than high blood pressure, diabetes, smoking, sedentary lifestyles, elevated blood cholesterol, and body mass index. In women, too, the risk was nearly as important.

What You Should Do

Although genes partly determine blood fibrinogen level, an individual's lifestyle can affect it too. Eating saturated fats or trans-fatty acids (butter, cream, margarine, shortening, and cooking fats), having abdominal obesity, sedentary lifestyles, chronic infections (bronchitis, colitis, sinusitis), and too many red blood cells, all increase fibrinogen levels.

Perhaps the most effective way you can reduce your blood fibrinogen level is to eat more seafood, fruits, and vegetables, get regular vigorous exercise, lose weight, and treat chronic infections appropriately.

Among cholesterol-lowering drugs, niacin lowers blood fibrinogen levels significantly. The fibrinogen-lowering effect of niacin is parallel to its cholesterol-lowering effect, and therefore you may need higher doses (more than 1.5 to 2 grams per day) to achieve a good response. Of the statins (Part II, (15)), pravastatin (Pravachol) at doses of 40-80 mg per day lowers fibrinogen by about 10 percent. Other statins, however, do not lower fibrinogen levels significantly. So if you require cholesterol-lowering drugs and have a high fibrinogen level, pravastatin should be the preferred drug, whether you take niacin or not.

(6) Abnormal Blood Platelets

As noted, an acute heart attack is due to the development and expansion of a clot within the lumen of one or more branches of the coronary artery. This coronary thrombosis is made up largely of fibrinogen (a clot-promoting protein in the bloodstream), as well as clumps of blood platelets that adhere to the site of a tear or injury in the inner wall of the artery. Without vascular injury or clumping of the platelets, a coronary thrombosis or heart attack will not occur.

Vein clots, referred to as phlebitis, have relatively few platelets but plenty of fibrinogen and trapped red blood cells. The tendency to develop phlebitis is often increased significantly when the blood flow through the veins, especially in the legs, is slowed down. This can occur in varicose veins or during long periods of inactivity such as long flights, recovery from a broken leg or hip, hospitalizations, major surgeries, and certain illnesses.

To initiate and sustain clumping, platelets produce a protein called "adhesion protein." Adhesion protein helps platelets stick together and to the inner lining of the artery. Ordinarily, all platelets have the inactive form of this adhesion protein on their surface. But when they come in contact with certain compounds in the bloodstream such as oxidized LDL cholesterol, the adhesion protein is activated, making platelets "sticky." Activated platelets, especially too many of them (more than 250,000 per ml), also produce a number of toxic products that stir up turmoil inside coronary plaques (Chapter 1).

Recently two inherited variations of platelet adhesion protein have been identified which, with the slightest provocation, make platelets much more likely to clump and stick to the arterial wall. Persons with these abnormalities—called "platelet polymorphism"—have a high risk of developing premature heart disease. In platelet polymorphism, the DNA sequence of the adhesion protein is different by only a single amino acid. Yet this seemingly minor difference or mutation causes a sixfold increase in the risk of coronary events among people under sixty years of age.

What You Should Do

If you have any risk factor for coronary artery disease, you should get a platelet count. Those with premature coronary artery disease (or a family history of it) should also have special tests to check for platelet polymorphism. What can be done for abnormal platelets?

Aspirin

Aspirin, even in low doses of 80 to 100 mg per day, destroys an enzyme inside platelets called "COX-1." Because COX-1 helps to activate the platelets' adhesion protein, most platelets exposed to aspirin lose their ability to produce activated adhesion protein. But people with platelet polymorphism are resistant and unresponsive to low doses of aspirin. Red blood cells can also activate platelets even in people who take low-dose aspirin. Boosting the dose of aspirin to 325 mg once every two weeks can effectively abolish this red cell-related activation and clumping of platelets.

In adults with or without a history of coronary artery disease, low-dose aspirin can reduce the risk of a heart attack by about 30 percent. This is as good as that of most currently available cholesterol-lowering drugs, at a fraction of the cost. In the United States, hospital death rates from heart attacks vary by as much as 30 percent, depending on whether patients are cared for in one of the "top fifty hospitals" or elsewhere. This difference, however, is largely due to early use of aspirin (and the use of beta blocker drugs) in the "top fifty hospitals."

Regrettably, despite compelling evidence that aspirin saves countless lives, more than a third of physicians and healthcare providers do not take aspirin themselves, and even fewer advise their patients to take it. In a recent study, the death rate at six months following a heart attack among those not taking aspirin was twice that of individuals taking aspirin. Yet in the United States 50 percent of individuals with coronary artery disease do not take aspirin. Aspirin use among African Americans, who have a high risk of catastrophic cardiovascular events, is even more dismal: only 35 percent of black men and 13 percent of black women take aspirin. This is a tragic case of collective neglect by everyone involved.

There is a consistent seasonal variation in the rate of heart attacks; they are nearly 50 percent more common in winter than in summer. These variations are seen despite geographic and climatic differences, so escaping to Florida or Arizona for the winter does not help, unfortunately. Studies from Australia have also shown that fatal or nonfatal heart attacks are 20 percent to 40 percent more common in their winter (June through

August) and spring (September through November) than during other times of the year. To some extent these seasonal variations are due to the shorter duration of light per day, lower levels of physical activity, negative affect (Part II, (9)), and higher incidence of flu, but also in the changes in platelets that enhance clumping and stickiness. Here, too, both aspirin and omega-3 polyunsaturates from seafood provide considerable protection.

Not only does aspirin reduce the risk of clot formation, but by improving the function of the artery's inner lining it increases the blood circulation and oxygen supply to the heart muscle. The case for aspirin's cardio-protective benefits is so compelling that all men over the age of thirty-five and women over forty-five should be strongly urged to take a low dose of aspirin (81 mg) every day, provided they are not allergic to it. And you should boost this low-dose once every two weeks. The risk of any stomach irritation, even in those with preexistent dyspepsia, with such a low-dose is negligible.

In addition to COX-1, a number of biochemical compounds (some of which are present in variable quantities in everyone's bloodstream) can also activate platelets. Low-dose or even high-dose aspirin cannot prevent platelet activation as a result of these compounds. A number of new anti-platelet drugs have been developed that counteract the action of some of these compounds and reduce the risk of platelet activation. At best, the efficacy and the safety of these agents are equal to those of aspirin, yet the drugs are far more expensive (approximately $3 a day for Plavix, one of the newer anti-platelet drugs, versus only a few cents for aspirin). Still, for those who cannot take aspirin (due to allergy, gastric irritation, or other reasons), these new anti-platelet agents provide safe and effective substitutes to lower the risk of heart attack or stroke.

Seafood

Another effective way to improve the function of your platelets and make them coronary-friendly is to increase your intake of omega-3 fatty acids from seafood (Chapter 2, "Omega-3 Polyunsaturated Fat"). This requires an average of three to four seafood meals per week over a long period. Since margarine, shortening, and vegetable fats interfere with the entry of omega-3 fatty acids into the platelets, seafood should not be cooked with vegetable-source fats. Olive oil, canola oil, and hazelnut oil are reasonable alternatives.

(7) Too Many Red Blood Cells

Very often people assume that rosy cheeks mean good health. Regrettably, this is not always so. Chronic sun exposure, excessive alcohol intake, obesity, chronic lung diseases, and too many red blood cells in the bloodstream can make your face reddish, rusty, or plethoric. Normally, there are approximately 4.5 to 5.5 million red blood cells per milliliter of blood. For most people, the volume of red blood cells that settles at the bottom of a test tube (called "hematocrit") is between 42 and 45 percent of the whole blood volume (the remainder is the serum or plasma). In people with too many red cells, or "too much" blood, the hematocrit can comprise 48 percent to 55 percent of the blood.

In people with too much blood (hematocrit greater than 45 percent), the blood flow in the arteries, like congested highways, is slowed down, so that vital organs may not receive adequate amounts of the oxygen carried by red blood cells. The problem of poor oxygen delivery is even more relevant during periods of high oxygen demand such as vigorous exercises, or with various stresses such as anger and hostility (Part II, (9)).

Healthy coronary or cerebral arteries are resilient enough to adapt partially and accommodate overcrowding by red cells. But arteries affected by atherosclerosis (hardening of the arteries) become stiff and lose their ability to dilate and accommodate this overcrowding. Thus, the task of delivering oxygen to vital organs during physical or emotional stresses becomes even more problematic in people with atherosclerosis.

Figure 7
Relation of Hematocrit Levels (HTC) to Cardiovascular Mortality

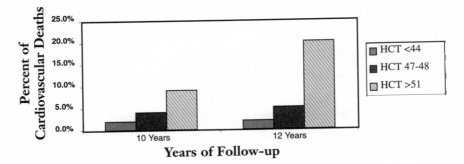

The volume of red blood cells accounts for approximately 70 percent of the blood viscosity. Thus any increase in hematocrit can significantly increase blood viscosity, making blood flow through smaller arteries more difficult. It is for this reason that people with too many red blood cells may experience bouts of dizziness, confusion, forgetfulness, visual disturbances, impotence, shortness of breath, and high blood pressure. They might also develop episodes of mini-strokes, which can eventually result in dementia. Several studies have shown that the risk of coronary events increases progressively as the hematocrit is raised from 42 percent to 48 percent and beyond. As seen in Figure 7, when the hematocrit exceeds 51 percent, the risk of cardiovascular mortality increases nearly nine times as compared to those with a hematocrit below 44 percent.

What You Should Do

Many disorders can increase the number of red blood cells. They include chronic lung diseases or bronchitis, a sedentary lifestyle, obesity, excessive alcohol or tobacco use, aging, hemochromatosis (an excess of iron), and benign or premalignant bone marrow disorders. If you have an elevated hematocrit, your doctor should investigate all of the above. Once the doctor has ruled out those disorders, the most effective and the easiest approach to lower your hematocrit is to donate a unit of blood every several weeks until the hematocrit drops to the 42 to 44 percent level. Afterward, periodic blood donation (perhaps every three to four months) would prevent your hematocrit from creeping up again.

Regrettably, some blood banks may be reluctant to use donated blood from people with high hematocrit for transfusion because of concerns about the cause. In these cases, the procedure is no longer called blood donation, which is free to the donor; instead, it is called "therapeutic phlebotomy," or blood letting, which carries a service fee covered by most health insurance policies. The blood taken from these people is discarded.

But the message here is: those with rosy cheeks should share their fortunes (of too many red blood cells) with those who desperately need them by giving blood to blood banks that accept high-hematocrit blood. Regular blood donation is a noble goal that may save two lives—the donor's and the recipient's.

(8) Elevated Blood Homocysteine

Over the past several years more than a hundred studies have shown that elevated blood homocysteine level is a major risk factor for a host of cardiovascular diseases. Like fibrinogen, homocysteine is a protein, not a fat. Everyone has homocysteine in his or her blood, but the kidneys maintain it at a normal level in two ways. First, the body breaks down 50 percent of homocysteine with the aid of vitamin B-6 and eliminates the harmless by-products in the urine. The body converts the other 50 percent to an essential amino acid called "methionine," with help from folic acid (vitamin B-9) and vitamin B-12. Methionine, however, can be recycled and converted back to homocysteine.

Although deficiencies of vitamin B-6, folic acid, and vitamin B-12 can interfere with the smooth operation of these natural pathways of release and result in accumulation of homocysteine in the bloodstream, such deficiencies are uncommon disorders in developed countries. Aging, especially when associated with poor nutrition and low blood levels of folic acid or vitamin B-12 and chronic kidney diseases, can also raise blood homocysteine levels. Eating too much red meat can increase homocysteine while seafood will decrease levels in the blood. Sulfanomide anti-bacterial agents also raise the homocysteine blood level by 30 to 50 percent.

Inherited genes are by far the most common reasons for elevated blood homocysteine level, accounting for over 90 percent of cases. One generation passes abnormalities of the enzymes responsible for the breakdown of homocysteine to the next. For example, approximately 10 percent of the population in Great Britain and the United States have a genetic defect in the enzyme that is responsible for breaking down homocysteine through the folic acid pathway. This recent discovery suggests that at least one out of ten people in the United States and Great Britain (as well as many other populations) are genetically programmed to have an elevated blood homocysteine level.

Homocysteine is a potent oxidant of LDL cholesterol. It can also directly injure the inner lining of blood vessels. Importantly, homocysteine is a major cause of clot formation within coronary and brain arteries and is a frequent culprit in phlebitis of various veins.

Unfortunately, doctors rarely test for blood homocysteine level, in large part because they are unaware of its tremendous impact on the cardiovascular system. In addition, many laboratories cannot measure homocysteine levels accurately. For this reason, blood homocysteine measurements should always be performed by special laboratories that perform this procedure routinely and accurately.

Another confusing factor is that many laboratories use obsolete and erroneous values for "normal" blood homocysteine level, and consider 5 to 15 or even 5 to 17 micromoles per liter as normal. In truth, the upper limit for blood homocysteine level should not exceed 9 micromoles per liter. Recent studies have shown that a homocysteine blood level above 14, which still falls within the "normal" range of some laboratories, increases the risk of coronary artery disease 500 percent.

As the homocysteine levels go up from 5 or 6, cardiovascular mortality progressively increases almost linearly (Figure 8). For example, the annual cardiovascular mortality at a blood homocysteine level of 6 is approximately 150 per 100,000 population, whereas at 11 it is nearly 500 per 100,000—a threefold increase.

In a Scandinavian study, researchers followed up for nearly five years with 587 men and women with established coronary artery disease. During this period, 25 percent of those with homocysteine levels of more than 15 died, compared to only 4 percent of those with levels of less than 9, a 600 percent difference. A recent national survey of 3,766 healthy males and 4,819 healthy females in the United States showed that the average blood homocysteine level was 9.6 in males and 8 in females. The findings of this survey were consistent with cross-country data, confirming that current upper limits of "normal" levels of blood homocysteine must be revised downward to less than nine.

At all blood levels of homocysteine, women are nearly twice as likely as men to develop vascular complications, including phlebitis, heart attack, stroke, and hardening of the arteries of the legs. In a recent study of young women between the ages of fifteen and forty-four who had developed strokes, homocysteine levels above 11 were associated with a 300 percent higher risk of stroke. Adjustment for other risk factors such as blood cholesterol level, blood pressure, and smoking did not change this strong association. In another study, the risk of stroke among middle-aged men increased progressively with rising blood homocysteine levels. In a three-year follow-up of 28,263 post-menopausal women in the Women's Health Study, an elevated homocysteine level more than doubled the risk of cardiovascular events. Undoubtedly, longer periods between follow-ups, such as seven to ten years, will increase the rates of cardiovascular events much further.

Figure 8
Cardiovascular Mortality

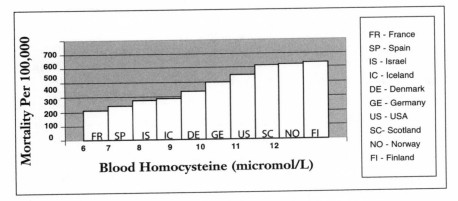

Ms. Joan E was thirty-seven when she experienced chest pain and short-ness of breath, which were attributed to "anxiety and stress." Her father had died at the age of fifty-one after his second heart attack, and her forty-three-year-old brother had experienced a "massive coronary" after two failed angioplasties, requiring coronary bypass surgery. Although her HDL cho-lesterol was 38 (for women, normal values should be greater than 55) and her LDL cholesterol was 125 (normal values should be less than 100), both were dismissed as "within the acceptable range." Because of persistent angina, two years later she quit her teaching job at a local community college. Cardiac catheterization showed that two branches of her coronary artery were more than 80 percent clogged, and she was advised to have coronary bypass surgery. At that time her blood homocysteine level was 21 (and her brother's was 24). Her LDL, HDL, and triglycerides were all still abnormal. She was started on a variety of interventions including a diet with TRF score of about +20 per day, low doses of aspirin along with 800 IU vitamin E per day, progressively greater levels of exercise, niacin (to raise her HDL and lower her LDL and triglycerides), and triple therapy with vitamin B6, folic acid, and vitamin B-12 to lower her homocysteine level. Within three months her LDL, HDL, triglycerides, and homocysteine levels were normal, and she was able to walk on the treadmill three miles a day without angina. She also went back to her teaching position. (Her brother also started triple therapy and lowered his homocysteine to 10 within four months.)

This case illustrates that everyone with premature coronary artery disease (before the age of fifty-five), and especially those with a strong family history of cardiovascular events, must take active measures and, if necessary, insist on being tested for major coronary risk factors including homocysteine.

Three recent studies have shown that elevated blood homocysteine levels significantly increase the risk of Alzheimer's disease. In the most recent study, investigators at the University of Oxford looked at 164 patients aged fifty-five or older with a diagnosis of Alzheimer's disease. They were found to have significantly higher blood homocysteine along with lower folic acid and vitamin B-12 levels than the control population (without Alzheimer's disease). The importance of these studies is that with simple, practical, and very inexpensive measures (such as daily supplementation with folic acid, B-12, and B-6), we may potentially prevent this catastrophic disease in a large number of people, or perhaps slow down the rapid deterioration in those already affected.

Cardiovascular events and strokes are uncommon among children. But among children with elevated homocysteine levels, the risk of stroke is more than four times higher than in children with normal blood levels.

What You Should Do

An elevated homocysteine level is a major risk factor for various cardiovascular diseases as well as Alzheimer's disease. Since approximately 10 percent of the population may have high blood homocysteine levels, you should have your homocysteine level checked if you fall into any of the following categories:

(1) Anyone with a history of coronary artery disease, stroke, hardening of the arteries, peripheral vascular disease ("poor circulation"), or phlebitis

(2) Adults with a family history of cardiovascular disease

(3) Men and women over the age of forty with any major coronary risk factor

(4) All adult diabetics and persons with chronic kidney disease

(5) All individuals over the age of forty with a family history of Alzheimer's disease

(6) Children of parents with high homocysteine levels

If you have an elevated homocysteine level (over 9), you should follow a diet with a total daily TRF score below +30. Such a dietary regimen is automatically low in red meats, a rich source of methionine, that is converted to homocysteine. Because dietary proteins, from either animal or plant sources, contribute relatively little to blood homocysteine level—no more than 10 to 20 percent—you cannot rely on diet alone to lower your homocysteine level. Still, eating deeply colored fruits and vegetables that contain vitamin B-6 and folic acid is helpful in bringing it under control. Fortification of cereals with folic acid can also lower homocysteine by 1 to 2 points. Unfortunately, vegetables and fruits have no vitamin B-12.

Nearly 70 percent of people with elevated homocysteine will respond to supplemental folic acid at doses of 1-2 mg, along with 1 mg of vitamin B-12 twice a day. Those who fail to respond may require the addition of vitamin B-6 at doses of 50-100 mg twice daily.

There are several reasons for taking significantly higher doses of folic acid and vitamin B-12. First, not all vitamin B-12 and folic acid preparations are readily absorbed from the intestine, and some people take them haphazardly. Second, 20 percent of older people in the United States have mild vitamin B-12 deficiency, which may be due to their inability to absorb the vitamin adequately. Lastly, since genetic defects in the enzymes responsible for breaking down homocysteine make results variable, individuals may not respond to low doses of vitamin B-12 and folic acid. Higher doses can overcome these problems. But with a good response within three to six months the dose can be reduced slowly.

(9) Negative Affect

During the past decade numerous studies in laboratory animals and humans have shown a direct relationship between certain psychosocial factors and development of cardiovascular diseases. These psychosocial factors range from depression, hostility, and anger to overcrowding, poor social environment, and difficult interpersonal relationships.

For example, a certain breed of mice that is susceptible to hardening of the arteries responds quite differently to a high-fat, high-cholesterol diet when the mice are subjected to various stresses. Coronary plaques similar to those that occur in humans were found far more often in mice housed five to a cage than in mice housed individually in their own cages. Negative affect has two components:

(1) Acute, short-term symptoms such as frequent episodes of sadness, depression, or anger, sometimes over trivial matters.

(2) Chronic, long-term symptoms which may range from a pessimistic outlook, cynicism, and defensiveness to outright hostility and a "bad attitude." Hostility, anger, and depression have the most potent impact on coronary artery disease. Contrary to a common misconception, type-A personality (the "go-getter" type) has no significant association with coronary artery disease.

Negative affect is quite common among the U.S. adult population and that of many other countries. In a large, nine-year follow-up study from Finland, people with high hostility scores were three times more likely to die from cardiovascular diseases than those with low scores. Another recent study showed a direct relation between hostility scores of populations in various American cities and the incidence of cardiovascular diseases. The "city of brotherly love," Philadelphia, had the highest hostility score and, not surprisingly, one of the highest cardiovascular disease rates among major cities studied.

The recent Baltimore Epidemiological Catchment Area Study showed that persons with at least one episode of major depression were approximately two to eight times more likely to have a heart attack. Among those aged eighteen to forty-four who had no history of depression at entry into the study, only 1 percent developed heart attacks during the thirteen-year follow-up. In contrast, 8 percent of those with a major depressive episode did so. In the forty-five to sixty-four age group, the heart attack rates were 8 percent and 17 percent among those without a history of depression and those with such a history, respectively.

In a forty-year follow-up of male medical students who graduated from Johns Hopkins University, the risk of a heart attack among those who had experienced an episode of clinical depression was more than twice those without a history of depression. Adjusting for other traditional risk factors such as age, smoking, hypertension, blood cholesterol levels, obesity, level of physical activities, and family history of heart attacks did not change these findings.

Two recent long-term studies have also shown that negative affect increases the risk of stroke by more than 60 percent. Similarly, the overall risk of death from various causes—including accidents, cancers, or infectious diseases—is significantly greater among depressed persons.

Unfortunately, negative affect is quite prevalent among individuals who have already developed coronary artery disease, affecting nearly 50 percent of this group. For eight years, researchers in Belgium tracked more than three hundred men and women between the ages of thirty-one and seventy-nine who had coronary artery disease. Those with depression had a death rate that was more than four times greater than the death rate for those without. Negative affect in these individuals is often unrelated to the severity of, or disability from, their disease. It reflects an unmasked psychological state that predated their heart attack or stroke. Understandably, the preexistent negative affect is further aggravated by their heart disease and a "why me?" attitude of bewilderment or anger.

In spite of its well-documented impact, negative affect is one of the least recognized and least treated coronary risk factors. This is not limited to one country. It is sadly an international failure of mental health care.

Negative affect is associated with the excessive release of adrenaline-type "stress factors" into the bloodstream from the adrenal glands and the nervous system. Stress factors lower HDL cholesterol, increase blood triglycerides and homocysteine levels, cause spasm of coronary and cerebral arteries, and raise blood pressure. They can also greatly increase blood levels of a number of clotting agents. Adrenaline-type compounds activate blood platelets so that they are more likely to stick together and initiate clot formation inside the arteries. The spasm of coronary arteries reduces blood flow, and hence oxygen supply, to the heart muscle. A combination of several of these biological events in response to bursts of unremitted anger or sadness can cause dangerous and sometimes fatal irregularity of the heart rate, or can cause a tear in coronary plaques, resulting in a heart attack.

Of course, negative affect can make people apathetic and therefore they ignore or delay seeking medical attention. Such individuals also tend to have less healthy, more sedentary lifestyles, and just don't care for themselves in general. Some may also abuse drugs, including alcohol and tobacco products, which further compounds the problem.

Most of these unhealthy lifestyles go toward explaining the findings of a large number of studies that negative affect is associated with a significant increase in the rates of certain cancers including colon, pancreas, lung, and breast. Unfortunately, cancers in these individuals, much like other organic diseases, are usually discovered at later stages when a cure is more problematic.

What You Should Do

Negative affect is a common psychiatric disease all over the world. In the United States nearly 20 percent of the adult population has this disease, few of whom are recognized or treated. Fortunately, most individuals with depression or negative affect can be treated successfully. A major hurdle is that a large number of such people refuse to acknowledge that they have "a problem" and are unwilling to seek help, especially from psychiatrists. For these people, a sympathetic and tolerant health care provider can make a large, life-saving difference. If you feel prolonged sadness, frustration, impatience, defensiveness, aggressiveness, anger, explosiveness, or depression, or simply feel as if you have hit bottom, please talk to your doctor. People with negative affect almost always have various biochemical abnormalities in the brain. Today, there are a vast number of safe and effective drugs that can dramatically improve these chemical imbalances and bring equilibrium to the brain's neurotransmitters. Negative affect is essentially a neurotransmitter-deficiency disease, much like diabetes is an insulin-deficiency disease.

Over-the-counter herbs such as Saint John's Wort and Kava Kava, in spite of bloated claims of efficacy, have no significant impact on negative affect, especially among people who have already suffered a cardiovascular event. These people need genuine, effective care, and their problem should not be trivialized by questionable herbal therapy. Still, for those who can't afford to see a psychiatrist or buy modern-day anti-depressants, Saint John's Wort may offer some benefits. The problem is that you can't be sure if the contents listed on the outside of the bottle are indeed inside the bottle. More often than not, the potency, purity, and efficacy of Saint John's Wort vary greatly from brand to brand, or even from bottle to bottle of the same brand. The same is equally true for Kava Kava.

Meditation, stress management, and psychotherapy may also be valuable tools in dealing with negative affect. In addition, active participation in religion may contribute to a healthier lifestyle, more serenity and peace of mind, and a sense of purpose that often may prove as valuable as psychotherapy. Although religion and medicine should be kept separate, health care providers and patients need not separate themselves from religion. It is essential to look at negative affect as you would look at high blood pressure, diabetes, elevated homocysteine, or any other coronary risk factor. All are major risks that will not go away by themselves.

(10) Smoking

Each year about 420,000 people die in the United States as a result of tobacco-related illnesses. This is comparable to wiping out the entire population of a midsize city. In Europe, smoking accounts for 1.2 million deaths each year. And the problem is just as dire elsewhere; sadly, it is only getting worse.

In the United States, passive smoking, or breathing secondhand tobacco smoke, is responsible for nearly 57,000 deaths each year. Among these, 37,000 deaths are due to cardiovascular events.

The evidence now is overwhelming that smoking contributes to coronary artery disease, as well as a host of other health problems. Regular, passive smoking that results from such environments as living with a smoker doubles women's risk of coronary artery disease. Among children who live with at least one smoker, HDL cholesterol level is 10 percent lower than it is in children not exposed to passive smoking. Recently, researchers exposed healthy subjects fifteen to thirty years of age to environmental tobacco smoke for more than one hour each day to see how their arteries functioned. In passive smokers, the ability of their arteries to dilate was half as much as in non-smokers, and identical to that of regular, active smokers. The findings of this study strongly suggest that human arteries (including coronary and cerebral) have a threshold for tobacco smoke by-products. Once this threshold is reached, even with smoking "just a few" cigarettes or with exposure to passive smoking, they lose a substantial part of their ability to dilate when needed.

Sadly, about 90 percent of smokers pick up the habit before they turn eighteen, and smoking rates among young people all over the world are on the rise. The trend is particularly disturbing in former Soviet bloc countries, Asia, and Latin America. This trend toward tobacco use at younger ages and for prolonged periods is a forerunner to a vast epidemic of tobacco-related disabilities and deaths in the future.

Tobacco smoke contains over 1,200 chemical compounds, some of which have yet to be identified or studied. The cardio-toxic, carcinogenic, and other harmful effects of tobacco are not limited to carbon monoxide and nicotine. Some of the other components of tobacco smoke are potent oxidants and carcinogens. Tobacco smoke alters many biological markers in the human body that can directly contribute to coronary artery disease. Some of these toxic effects include:

- increased oxidization of LDL

- increased white blood cells

- increased fibrinogen

- increased stickiness and clumping of platelets

- spasm and constriction of the arteries

- decreased HDL cholesterol level

Cigars, Pipes, and Low-tar, Low-nicotine Cigarettes

Although many cigars or pipe smokers assume that cigars or pipes are less harmful alternatives to cigarettes, they are mistaken. There are at least three reasons why:

First, many cigar and pipe smokers claim that they do not inhale. But they do! Their blood nicotine levels (or urine cotinin level, a by-product of nicotine) may be as high as that of cigarette smokers. Cigar and pipe smokers inhale some endstream smoke (through the mouth) and a large amount of sidestream smoke (smoke in the air, through the nose), especially in rooms with poor ventilation.

Second, as saliva moves to and from the pipe stem and cigar butt, it brings into the mouth nicotine and a vast number of other compounds, some of which are clearly carcinogenic. Nicotine is readily absorbed from the mouth and the stomach while other compounds can cause irritation and cancers of the lips, tongue, oral cavity, larynx, throat, esophagus, and stomach.

Third, smoking pipes or cigars instead of cigarettes is not a "better" choice, or even the "lesser of two evils." The only minor difference is that people smoke cigars and pipes less frequently than cigarettes. On the other hand, a cigar contains several times more tobacco than a cigarette, and it is smoked for a very long time as compared with an average of five to seven minutes for a cigarette.

As noted, even shorter daily exposure to tobacco smoke, whether from cigarettes, cigars, or passive smoking, is unsafe. In a recent study, 225 men who had smoked only cigars for an average of sixteen years were compared with 14,200 other men who had never smoked any tobacco products. Stogie smokers who averaged two cigars per day had an 87 percent higher risk of dying of cancer and an 89 percent higher risk of dying of various cardiovascular diseases. Is this a "safer" alternative to cigarettes?

Smoking low-tar, low-nicotine cigarettes also provides no major advantage over regular varieties. Part of the problem here has to do with the smoker. Many smokers who switch to low-tar or low-nicotine brands soon learn to seal off perforations in the filter with their fingertips. This reduces the airflow through the cigarette and sends a less diluted smoke to the lungs. Another problem is that some smokers increase the number of cigarettes they smoke instead of decreasing it, which also defeats the purpose of switching. People who have switched to low-tar or low-nicotine brands tend to develop cancers deep in the lung tissue, whereas smokers of regular brands develop cancers of the bronchial tree. This is mainly due to the fact that, for more satisfaction, light-brand smokers deeply inhale, which deposits carcinogen particles in deeper portions of the lungs.

What You Should Do

Decades of observation have clearly shown that tobacco is harmful when used as directed. The health and human cost of smoking is so staggering that it defies any estimate. Recently the U.S. tobacco industry agreed to pay $205 billion to the individual states over the next twenty-five years to compensate them for their anticipated tobacco-related health expenditures to Medicare and Medicaid recipients. But the cost of providing healthcare for all tobacco-related diseases (not counting the 420,000 lives lost annually) is many times greater.

No matter how long you have smoked, stopping now is the right thing to do. Unfortunately, quitting smoking, as smokers know, is a difficult undertaking; otherwise more would have done it. Clearly, no single method is suitable for everyone. What has worked for a friend, coworker, or family member may not work for you.

Nicotine Gum and Patches

The Food and Drug Administration (FDA) has approved over-the-counter nicotine gums such as Nicorette and nicotine patches such as Nicoderm CQ and Nicotrol, largely because the majority of smokers attempting to quit are unlikely to see a counselor or physician. Unfortunately, in spite of the vast amount of misleading advertising, the six-month quit rates for users of these products is only about 10 percent—hardly a success story. Although for "healthy" smokers these products may be safe in the short-term, in people with cardiovascular disease it may be problematic to receive large amounts of nicotine throughout the day with nicotine gum or through the slow-release nicotine patches.

Since the six-month quit rates for nicotine gums and patches are so low, some smoking counseling centers advocate a combination of both. Unfortunately, the quit rates of this dual approach have improved only an additional 6 to 7 percent. In spite of their relatively poor quit rates, the use of nicotine gums, patches, or a combination of the two may be one of the few options for those who have been unable to quit without a "nicotine fix."

Nicotine nasal spray is available today in the United States by prescription only. The rationale is that using one or two puffs per hour (a somewhat impractical approach) allows for a rapid absorption and high blood levels of nicotine.

The nicotine inhaler is another prescription device. It is not exactly an inhaler in the same way that asthma products are. With the nicotine inhaler, most of the nicotine in the vapor is absorbed through the lining of the mouth and does not reach the lungs. Both the nasal spray and nicotine inhaler are reported to double the six-month quit rate, but the nose and throat irritation caused by these products is a major drawback.

Other Smoking Cessation Aids

Some studies have suggested that hypnosis, acupuncture, or psychotherapy might be helpful in quitting smoking. Most of these studies were poorly designed; the methods have low short-term and long-term quit rates and are impractical for many smokers.

Smoking cessation aids such as over-the-counter herbs and products obtainable only through toll-free numbers or the Internet are generally useless; occasionally they are even dangerous. They are designed to take advantage of gullible, and sometimes desperate, consumers. Although an occasional smoker may be able to quit (a placebo effect), the failure rate is too high to justify the waste of one's money on these questionable products.

Anti-depressant Drugs as Smoking Cessation Aids

Recently some studies have suggested that certain anti-depressant drugs such as nortriptyline (Pamelor) and bupropion (Zyban and Wellbutrin) are helpful in smoking cessation. But because of side effects associated with larger doses, nortriptyline has not been used extensively for this purpose. Two recent double-blind studies examined the efficacy and safety of bupropion at doses of 150-300 mg per day for six to eight weeks. In one multicenter study of 615 subjects, short-term quit rates were 40 percent. A year later, 22 percent of smokers who had taken bupropion for six to eight weeks still had not resumed smoking. As modest as these results seem, they are considerably better than those for other interventions. (Remember, the long-term quit rate for smokers using nicotine patches or nicotine gums is about 10 percent.)

In a second study involving 893 cases, a nine-week course of sustained-release bupropion was compared with a nicotine patch, bupropion plus a nicotine patch, and a placebo pill. The quit rates at twelve months were 15.6 percent for the placebo group, 30 percent for the bupropion group, and 35 percent for the group that received both bupropion and a nicotine patch. This study essentially validated the findings of the first one and confirmed that at least a third of smokers can be helped to kick their habit.

Bupropion (Zyban or Wellbutrin) may work by increasing the availability of certain neurotransmitters in the brain. Among other actions, nicotine increases the number of functioning neurotransmitters in the brain. By mimicking nicotine's action on the brain cells, bupropion can reduce or stop smokers' frequent cravings for nicotine. Bupropion also minimizes the irritability, depression, and other emotional disturbances associated with quitting, and makes life a bit easier for smokers and people around them.

Although a single 150 mg dose of bupropion is adequate for most smokers, a heavy, long-term smoker may do better with 150 mg twice per day. The drug is started seven to ten days before the actual quit date to ensure that enough of the drug has begun to act on brain cells; you continue it for six to eight weeks to allow for a smooth nicotine withdrawal. Interestingly, smokers who take bupropion are less likely to gain weight than using other approaches.

(11) Sedentary Lifestyle

Over the past decade, a wealth of information has reaffirmed what everyone intuitively knows: vigorous physical exercise has a vast number of health benefits. Unfortunately, less than 25 percent of the U.S. population gets any exercise on a regular basis. This dismal figure also pertains to the populations of most other developed countries.

Being a couch potato is not a benign lifestyle. It is a self-inflicted and deadly disease. The U.S. Centers for Disease Control and Prevention attributes 250,000 deaths each year to lack of exercise. This is more than all deaths due to accidents, suicides, and HIV infection *combined.*

Regular exercise reduces the risk of cardiovascular events in both men and women by at least 50 percent. Regular exercise also reduces the risk of several cancers, including breast, ovarian, prostate, and colon. People who exercise on a regular basis reduce their risk of maturity-onset diabetes (type 2) by nearly 300 percent.

Regular physical exercise has a vast number of beneficial effects on cardiovascular health, as listed in Table 63. Men and women of all ages benefit from regular exercise. For example, an eight-year study of 3,120 healthy women showed that physical fitness (as assessed by treadmill testing) dramatically affected cardiovascular health. The age-adjusted death rate from cardiovascular disease among the most fit women in the study was 8 in 10,000 persons each year, as compared to 74 among the least fit women—a more than 900 percent difference.

In the U.S. Nurses' Study, scientists monitored more than 84,000 women for eight years. Women who exercised regularly (even brisk walking) had a 54 percent lower combined risk of heart attack and stroke than their sedentary counterparts.

A recent, long-term (twenty-five-year follow-up) study from Sweden showed that men who exercised on a regular basis were 70 percent less likely to die from cardiovascular disease than were sedentary persons. In another twenty-two-year follow-up study of 2,014 middle-aged Norwegian men, the risk of dying from cardiovascular disease among those who exercised regularly was 53 percent lower than that of nonexercising men.

Finnish researchers studied the relationship of leisure-time physical activities and death from all causes in 16,000 male and female Finnish twins. After an average follow-up of seventeen years, among the twin pairs who were healthy at the beginning of the study the relative risk of death from causes other than accidents, violence, or suicide was 34 percent less for occasional exercisers and 56 percent less for regular exercisers. This study confirms that longevity is not necessarily genetically predetermined, and that lifestyle is a paramount factor.

A study of 4,311 older British men (average age, sixty-three) who were free of any cardiovascular problems at the beginning of the study showed that regular physical exercise reduced cardiovascular mortality by 34 percent and noncardiovascular mortality by 52 percent. According to another ten-year study from the Netherlands featuring men between the ages of sixty-four and eighty-four at the start of the study, the risk of dying from cardiovascular disease or cancer was 30 percent lower for those who participated in moderate activities such as walking or cycling for more than twenty minutes every day than it was for nonexercisers.

Among men and women with preexisting coronary artery disease, regular exercise is just as important as any heart medication. In addition to the other benefits listed in Table 63, exercise helps to open up side channels (collaterals) in the coronary artery, which improves blood circulation to the heart muscle. Studies have consistently shown that regular exercise decreases death rates from coronary artery disease among these individuals by 30 to 50 percent.

A common misunderstanding is to confuse thinness or leanness with health. They are *not* the same. In a recent eight-year follow-up of 21,925 men between the ages of thirty and eighty, physically unfit, lean men had twice the risk of all-cause mortality as fit, lean men. In fact, unfit, lean men had a much higher risk of cardiovascular-related death than did men who were fit but obese. In other words, what counts is fitness, not leanness.

The Vulnerable Weekend Athlete and the Occasional Exerciser

Almost everyone—young or old, fit or unfit—can and should exercise. As Arthur Fiedler, the late conductor of the Boston Pops, once said, "He who rests, rots!" Unfortunately, occasional bursts of exercise are not only useless, but may actually be harmful. Weekend athletes have more aches and pains, pulled muscles, shinsplints, and heel problems than people who exercise regularly.

Researchers recently compared the impact of exercise on the oxidization of LDL cholesterol in two groups of college students. In students who were not long-term exercisers, the oxidization of LDL cholesterol actually increased after occasional exercise sessions. In contrast, among track team members who had been regular exercisers for more than two years, LDL oxidization was reduced considerably. Why this 180-degree difference in response? The reason is that during all physical activities the body produces many oxidants (free radicals). The body's ability to procure antioxidants and cope with the oxidants increases in regular exercisers but not in occasional or weekend exercisers.

It is unfortunate that the benefits of exercise, or any other healthy lifestyle, cannot be saved in a bank so that you could withdraw dividends on a long-term basis. In reality, the benefits of exercise are limited to days or weeks. Exercise—like eating, sleeping, and good hygienic practices—is necessary for good health and requires frequent repetition. "What have you done for me lately?" is the body's response to the assertion, "I used to be very athletic."

Although the risk of an exercise-induced heart attack is very low, each year one out of 2,500 men over the age of forty suffers a heart attack while exercising. Overall, it is estimated that anywhere between 4 percent and 20 percent of all heart attacks occur after a bout of moderate to heavy exertion, especially among the least fit individuals. This explains why the most important aspect of any exercise program is to avoid sudden, strenuous exertions, especially for unfit or nonexercising individuals. For example, the risk of a heart attack after a bout of strenuous physical activity such as shoveling snow for a fifty-year-old, sedentary, "out of shape" man is more than *10,000 percent greater* than it is for a regularly exercising and well-conditioned man of the same age. For the unfit, it is a lot smarter and safer to pay the neighbor's high schooler to clear the driveway than to risk a massive heart attack.

The annual incidence of exercise-related deaths in the United States is approximately one death per 100,000 young male athletes and one per 700,000 young female athletes. For middle-aged men, the risk is one per 18,000. Looked at from another perspective, the risk per total hours of exercising, it seems even more miniscule: For men between the ages of twenty and thirty-nine, the risk is one per 4 million hours of exercise; between forty

Table 63
Health Benefits of Regular Exercises

CARDIOVASCULAR BENEFITS	**DECREASES:**
	RISK OF HEART ATTACK BY 50 PERCENT
	RISK OF STROKE BY >35 PERCENT
	LDL CHOLESTEROL BY 10 TO 15 PERCENT
	TRIGLYCERIDES BY 20 TO 30 PERCENT
	ABDOMINAL OBESITY
	POST-EXERCISE HEART RATE
	BLOOD PRESSURE
	FIBRINOGEN
	INSULIN RESISTANCE
	THE NUMBER OF SMALL, DENSE LDL PARTICLES
	INCREASES:
	HDL CHOLESTEROL BY 10 TO 20 PERCENT
	TPA (A POTENT CLOT-BUSTER) BY >20 PERCENT
ANTI-CANCER BENEFITS	**DECREASES:**
	RISK OF BREAST CANCER BY 50 PERCENT
	RISK OF COLON CANCER BY 50 PERCENT
	RISK OF PROSTATE CANCER BY >30 PERCENT
OTHER BENEFITS	**DECREASES:**
	RISK OF PREMATURE AGING
	RISK OF DIABETES
	RISK OF PROSTATE ENLARGEMENT
	RISK OF VARIOUS INFECTIONS
	MUSCLE WASTING
	OSTEOARTHRITIS
	OSTEOPOROSIS
	CHRONIC FATIGUE SYNDROME
	RISK OF DEMENTIA
	CONSTIPATION AND IRRITABLE BOWEL

Table 63 continued on next page

Table 63 continued

OTHER BENEFITS	INCREASES:
	STAMINA
	WELL-BEING
	SEXUAL FUNCTIONS
	SELF-WORTH
	APPETITE
	LEAN BODY MASS
	HEALTHFUL LONGEVITY
	IMMUNE SYSTEM

and forty-nine, it is one per 1.3 million hours; and between sixty and sixty-nine, the risk is one per 900,000 hours. For women, the risk at all ages is even lower than for men. Even for people who have previously suffered heart attacks, in a supervised program the risk of exercise-related death is extremely low at one per 784,000 hours. And the risks vary among different types of exercises: for instance, the risk of a sudden cardiac death is nearly seven times higher for jogging (associated with profuse sweating, magnesium loss, and dehydration) than for other forms of exercise.

The intensity and duration of exercise must be individualized, and increased only gradually. Exercise regimens should take into account physical ability, age, gender, presence and severity of any cardiovascular disease or other medical problems, the environment (e.g., hot and humid versus indoors and air-conditioned), time of day (there is more risk of an exercise-induced heart attack in the early morning), tiredness, and physical or medical limitations. What is reasonable for a twenty-five-year-old man is not necessarily applicable to a fifty-five-year-old. In addition, the level of physical activity possible for a fifty-five-year-old healthy person is hardly applicable for a fifty-five-year-old with preexisting coronary artery disease, diabetes, high blood pressure, or a host of other risk factors. Men older than forty and women older than fifty with any major coronary risk factor should have an exercise stress test (or exercise echocardiogram—an ultrasound version of the exercise stress test) before the start of an intensive exercise program.

What You Should Do

You should look at regular exercise the same way that you look at eating or sleeping: as a necessary part of your life. Since there are 1,440 minutes in each twenty-four hours, it is not unreasonable to set aside forty or fifty of those minutes for exercise. For most sedentary people, the greatest reduction in overall mortality occurs when they move to the next level of physical activity (light), or to 40 percent of their maximum capacity. However, the common assertion that people should exercise at 60 percent to 70 percent of their maximum capacity is true for conditioned and fit persons, especially those under sixty.

The amount of calories you burn using different equipment or exercise machines can vary quite significantly. Among the more popular indoor exercise machines, treadmills burn more calories and put more aerobic demands on your heart than do cross-country simulators or stair climbers. Stationary bikes are about one-third less efficient (at comparable levels of intensity) than treadmills and 15 to 20 percent less efficient than other machines. So before purchasing an exercise machine, you must test various machines several different times to be sure that you choose one that is right for your temperament, needs, and, most importantly, long-term adherence.

The single most important aspect of exercising is to do it safely and choose an exercise program that is fun, or at least not detestable. You should always start slowly, three or four times a week, and then over time gradually increase both the intensity and duration of each exercise session. For years, exercise physiologists have used the heart rate as the standard indicator of exercise intensity. For people without heart disease, exercise should be intense enough to increase the heart rate to between 60 and 80 percent of the maximum heart rate. (Maximum heart rate is calculated as 220 minus a person's age. Thus the maximum heart rate for a fifty-five-year-old person is 220 - 55 = 165, and the desirable, exercise-induced rate is 60 to 80 percent of that, which is between 100 and 132 beats per minute.) But people with coronary artery disease have no need for this type of intense exercising.

To be effective, exercise has to be sustained for thirty or more minutes (plus a warm-up and cool-down of five to ten minutes each). Window shopping, swimming two laps and then stretching out to sunbathe, regular office or house chores, gardening, painting, mowing, golf, taking the house pet for a leisurely walk—such activities are not rigorous enough or sustained enough to be of much value (except perhaps for the elderly, those with severe cardiovascular diseases, or people with physical disabilities). On the other hand, brisk, long walks; jogging; rowing; biking; lap swimming; aerobic or aquatic exercises; "Jazzercising"; handball; racquetball; and bodybuilding are all reasonable alternatives. Older persons should incorporate gentle resistance training exercises into their routine. Two recent studies suggest that breaking the exercise time into two fifteen- to twenty-minute periods is as cardio-protective as sustained exercise. The main drawback of this approach is the difficulty of finding enough time in the day and the necessary discipline, commodities that are hard to come by.

(12) Diabetes

Diabetes is the consequence of inadequate insulin in the body. Almost every active cell in the body—especially those of the heart, brain, liver, and muscles—needs glucose for its work. Because insulin is essential for the entry of glucose (sugar) into all human tissues, the failure of the pancreas to produce an adequate amount of insulin after eating results in the accumulation of glucose in the bloodstream instead of in various tissues where it is needed. Unfortunately, high blood sugar (hyperglycemia) has many undesirable effects on practically every organ, including the brain, eyes, heart, and kidneys. The internationally accepted standard for diagnosing diabetes is a fasting blood glucose level (after an overnight fast) higher than 126 mg/dl on two separate days, or any random blood glucose higher than 200 mg/dl. Relying on fasting blood sugar, however, will miss a large number of people with diabetes. This is because many people with normal fasting blood sugar may have very high levels after a meal. For this reason, a glucose tolerance test (a blood sugar level obtained two hours after ingesting 75 grams of glucose) may be very useful. In this test, two hours after ingestion, blood sugar should be less than 140 mg/dl.

When the blood sugar remains high for days or weeks, some glucose seeps into the interior of the red blood cells in the bloodstream. Inside the red blood cells glucose binds with hemoglobin—the oxygen-carrying protein of the red blood cells. This process (the binding of glucose with hemoglobin, or any other protein in the body) is called "glycosylation." An elevated glycosylated hemoglobin (more than 6 mg/dl) positively identifies about 99 percent of poorly controlled diabetes.

In type 1 diabetes, insulin-producing glands of the pancreas are almost completely destroyed or inactive. The destruction of insulin-producing glands could be a consequence of viral diseases—which are sometimes dismissed as regular colds or flus—or can be the result of auto-immune disorders. The process usually begins in childhood or adolescence. Nearly all of these cases require insulin therapy.

Type 2 diabetes, or maturity-onset diabetes, occurs later in life, usually after the age of forty. It constitutes nearly 90 percent of diabetes cases. The problem in this type of diabetes is not so much a true insulin deficiency as it is a lack of resistance on the part of various tissues—especially the muscles and the liver—to insulin. In other words, these individuals are "insulin resistant." Since they usually do not require treatment with insulin, type 2 is also referred to as "noninsulin dependent diabetes."

Among adults in the United States, nearly 15 percent of whites and 25 percent of African Americans have type 2 diabetes or insulin-resistance syndrome. The San Antonio Heart Study recently reported a dramatic rise in the incidence of type 2 diabetes among both Mexican Americans and the white population in the San Antonio area. Within a ten-year period, the incidence of diabetes more than doubled among Mexican Americans and tripled among non-Hispanic whites. The trend remained significant even after adjustment for various risk factors, including ethnicity, socioeconomic status, gender, and age. It is almost surely due to the growing epidemic of obesity and sedentary lifestyle. In a recent report from the U.S. Centers for Disease Control and Prevention, researchers found a worrisome 76 percent rise in diabetes among men and women in their thirties over the past decade. In addition to the possible culprits listed above, long-term consumption of trans fatty acids (common in deep-fried foods from the mushrooming fast food industry) starting in childhood may be a contributing factor.

Today 15 million Americans have type 1 and 2 diabetes, a number that may exceed 25 million by the year 2010. More than 60 percent of Pima Indians in the United States, compared to less than 2 percent of Apache Indians in Chile, develop type 2 diabetes or insulin resistance by the time they reach the age of forty. We know that type 2 diabetes is a consequence of genetic and environmental factors combined with permissive dietary and lifestyle practices. Recent data from the United States, Europe, Asia, and South America have shown that low birth weight (less than five pounds) doubles the risk of type 2 diabetes. Similarly, the risk of type 2 diabetes is significantly increased among individuals whose mothers had gestational diabetes.

More than a third of children of a diabetic parent (especially if the parent is the father) will develop type 2 diabetes. The percentage of affected persons may exceed 50 percent among obese and sedentary offspring. But even among these individuals, the onset of diabetes is not inevitable. Indeed, dietary and lifestyle changes can reduce the risk to less than 10 percent among genetically susceptible individuals. For example, in a six-year follow-up of 8,633 nondiabetic men between the ages of thirty and seventy-nine when the study began, those who were the least physically fit had more than a 300 percent higher risk of developing type 2 diabetes. A sedentary lifestyle, abdominal obesity, and excess carbohydrate or energy intake all contribute to insulin resistance and type 2 diabetes.

Elevated blood glucose directly damages the endothelial lining. But it also binds with LDL proteins in the same way that glucose binds with hemoglobin. Unfortunately, glycosylated LDL cholesterol is quickly oxidized in the bloodstream. Although in nondiabetic adults less than 2 percent of LDL is oxidized in the bloodstream, in diabetics up to 10 percent of LDL particles can be oxidized. The problem is that oxidized LDL particles are no longer recognized and taken up by the liver's LDL receptors, and hence they pile up in the bloodstream. High concentration of oxidized LDL is a potent toxin for endothelial cells in the entire arterial system (including the arteries of the brain, eyes, kidneys, and lower extremities) and contributes to various complications of diabetes. Cardiovascular complications account for 80 percent of all diabetic deaths.

Diabetics also have higher triglycerides and lower HDL levels, both of which make a bad situation even worse. An additional concern with HDL cholesterol in diabetics is that it too can become glycosylated and lose its potency as an antioxidant and a transporter of cholesterol from the arteries to the liver (Part II, (14)). Under these circumstances, even "normal" levels of HDL may be inadequate and unable to provide any protection for the cardiovascular system, especially when other major coronary risk factors are also present.

What You Should Do

Diabetes, especially when it is inadequately controlled, is at least twice as bad as an elevated blood cholesterol level in causing various cardiovascular complications. Because diabetes can affect practically every organ and cause devastating complications, it must be treated vigorously whether it is type 1 or type 2. Unfortunately, the care of diabetes requires daily—and, for some type 1 diabetics, hourly—recourse to a variety of interventions. Most complications resulting from diabetes are preventable. The problem is that they are not prevented when and how it counts most: as early as possible and on a sustained basis.

Type 2 diabetes often goes together with abdominal obesity and a sedentary lifestyle. No dietary measures or anti-diabetes drug can effectively control the problem unless these two hugely important factors are corrected.

The main focus of diabetes management is to reduce blood sugar and prevent glycosylation of LDL cholesterol and vascular damage. A dietary program with a TRF score of less than +30 per day (Chapter 3) is ideal for nearly all diabetics. Since the omega-6 polyunsaturates (vegetable oils, margarine, and shortenings) increase oxidization of LDL particles, you should make every effort to decrease your intake or eliminate them from your diet altogether. Because saturated fats contribute to a further reduction in LDL receptors (and rise in LDL cholesterol), you should also avoid them. You can achieve both of these goals when you keep daily TRF scores of all foods below +30 and preferably closer to +20. The use of olive oil will not only reduce the oxidization of LDL cholesterol but also help to reduce insulin resistance. Because seafoods are not energy dense and contain cardio-protective omega-3 polyunsaturated fat, they are the most desirable sources of protein for diabetics. Unlike complex carbohydrates, simple carbohydrates contribute to the aggravation of diabetes and are, therefore, undesirable for diabetics of all ages. You should also avoid certain complex carbohydrates (starches) such as white bread, bagels, pasta, rice, and potato that the body quickly breaks down and converts to simple sugars in the intestine. Small amounts of table sugar or honey, however, have no deleterious impact when you use them infrequently.

All diabetics, whether type 1 or 2, must take vitamin E in doses of 400 to 800 IU daily and 200 to 500 mg of vitamin C per day. The use of antioxidants is even more important in younger diabetics who endure the ravages of high blood sugar for many years. Certain prescription drugs such as ACE inhibitors (ramipril or lisinopril, etc.) can significantly reduce the cardiovascular, retinal, and kidney damage so often seen in diabetics. Unfortunately, less than 20 percent of diabetics in the United States are taking these life-saving drugs.

Diabetics with elevated triglycerides or cholesterol disorders require a far more intensive intervention than nondiabetics with these conditions. Even in diabetics with minimal cholesterol elevation, cholesterol-lowering measures can reduce the very high risk of coronary events by 30 percent. Since nearly one in five people with cardiovascular disease also has diabetes or insulin resistance, aggressive cholesterol lowering in this group may require a multipronged attack. Because of the increased rate of oxidization of almost any tissue in diabetics, you should not rely solely on vitamin E or vitamin C to deal with the large oxidant load. Moreover, not all oxidants are necessarily neutralized by vitamin C or vitamin E (it would have made everyone's life a lot easier if they were!). For this reason, all diabetics should enrich their diet with many servings of dark green, leafy vegetables and deeply colored fruits such as berries, plums, nectarines, peaches, and figs. Drinking one or two glasses of a mixed vegetable juice such as V-8 is also a reasonable alternative to colas or other drinks with meals.

Two recent long-term studies, the U.S. Nurses' Health Study (women) and the U.S. Physicians' Study (men), showed that diabetic men and women who had one to two alcoholic drinks daily had a 58 percent and 55 percent lower risk of coronary deaths, respectively, when compared with nondrinkers, even after adjustment for a number of major coronary risk factors. These data suggest that if you are a diabetic, you should consider having one or two drinks (wine, cocktails, or light beer) with dinner. But since alcohol decreases insulin resistance, you may have to lower the nighttime dose of your insulin or other anti-diabetic medication to prevent hypoglycemia (low blood glucose).

Diabetes is a serious disease with a high risk of serious or fatal cardiovascular complications. Thus the treatment of diabetes should never be a do-it-yourself approach. Since the requirements of each diabetic may vary even from one day to the next, treatment strategies should always be individualized under the supervision of a physician. Whether the choice is insulin or oral anti-diabetes drugs, diabetics always need a variety of interventions to prevent cardiovascular, neurological, kidney, eye, and other serious complications.

(13) Elevated Blood Triglycerides

While triglycerides have no cholesterol, they are still a major risk factor for coronary artery disease. Triglycerides in the bloodstream have two sources: about 80 percent come from absorbed dietary fat, and the remainder are made in the liver (primarily from dietary carbohydrates) and released into the bloodstream.

Although triglyceride levels of less than 200 mg/dl are considered "desirable," this cut-off point should be lowered to less than 100 mg/dl. For example, in a fifteen-year follow-up of 492 individuals with coronary artery disease between the ages of thirty and eighty at the beginning of the study, those with triglyceride levels of more than 100 mg/dl had twice the incidence of coronary events when compared with those whose initial triglyceride levels were less than 100 mg/dl. In another study, researchers measured fasting triglyceride levels of 340 men and women who left six Boston area hospitals after their first heart attack. After adjusting for other coronary risk factors, people with elevated triglyceride levels had a 300 percent higher risk of heart attack. The Framingham Heart Study, the Paris Prospective Study, the Copenhagen Male Study, and seventeen other population-based studies all clearly show that an elevated blood triglyceride level is a significant independent risk factor for coronary artery disease.

People with elevated triglyceride levels often have low levels of HDL cholesterol (Part II, (14)), and a greater number of small, dense LDL particles (Part II, (15)). Both of these associated abnormalities increase the harmful effect of elevated triglycerides. Persistent elevation of triglycerides can also contribute to "fatty liver," a disorder in which a large number of triglycerides accumulate in the liver. If left untreated, fatty liver can progress to cirrhosis of the liver.

What You Should Do

At present, the guidelines set by the National Cholesterol Education Program provide three tiers of triglyceride levels: desirable is less than 200 mg/dl, borderline is 200-400 mg/dl, and high is greater than 400 mg/dl. Today this whole classification is obsolete. The desirable values I have introduced (Table 3) for various cholesterol and triglycerides are based on a large number of new studies published since National

Cholesterol Education Program guidelines were released several years ago. Accordingly, your normal fasting blood triglyceride level, very much like your level of LDL cholesterol, should be below 100 mg/dl. Any value above this cutoff point is abnormal.

The backbone of an effort to lower triglycerides is diet and exercise-induced weight loss, especially in those with abdominal obesity. The most important aspect of a diet to lower blood triglycerides is to reduce dietary fat and simple carbohydrates such as all sweets, including candies, cookies, cakes, pies, pastries, doughnuts, chocolates, jams, jellies, table sugar, carbonated beverages, honey, or even sweet fruits such as raisins, dates, and grapes. You should also avoid certain complex carbohydrates that the body readily breaks down in the intestine and converts to sugar. Some of these include white bread, white rice, white pasta, and potato. Whole wheat, sourdough, or dark breads, wild rice mixed with vegetables, or whole wheat pasta (in small portions) are good alternatives.

When dietary carbohydrates are 60 percent or more of your daily calories as recommended by some proponents of low-fat, low-cholesterol diets, it can often increase your blood triglycerides by as much as 20 to 30 percent, making a bad situation even worse. Since dietary fat ordinarily contributes 80 percent of blood triglycerides, people with high triglyceride levels should cut down all dietary fats. The only exception to this rule is omega-3 polyunsaturated fats from seafood, which lower triglyceride levels by 20 to 30 percent (see below).

Perhaps the most compelling aspect of a diet with a low TRF score is the ability to eat plenty of seafood. Seafood's omega-3 fatty acids are nearly as effective in lowering triglycerides as any of the currently available drugs, but without the side effects. In the first several weeks of treatment of high triglycerides by dietary modification, you should eat at least four to five seafood meals per week with no added fat of any kind. Because it is the omega-3 fat in seafood that lowers triglycerides, not its protein, fatty fish (Chapter 2, "Omega-3 Polyunsaturated Fat") are preferable to low-fat, white fish. This dietary change alone should lower your triglycerides by at least 20 to 30 percent.

Fortunately, most people with elevated triglycerides do not have very high levels. For them, abdominal obesity, sedentary lifestyle, insulin resistance or diabetes, excessive alcohol intake, and poor dietary practices readily account for their problem. Although estrogens can raise the liver's output of triglycerides in women, the change is relatively small (in the order of 5 to 10 percent). In women with very high triglyceride levels, however, the use of estrogens (oral contraceptives or estrogen replacement therapy) can exacerbate the problem to a much greater extent. Estrogen replacement therapy by means of skin patches (transdermal estrogens) has no significant impact on triglycerides or cholesterol levels. This is because estrogen enters the bloodstream slowly and in quantities not sufficient to stimulate the liver to overproduce VLDL particles enriched with triglycerides.

Other approaches to lower your triglycerides include:

Fish Oil

For those who do not like seafood (how could anyone dislike seafood?), initially two to three fish oil capsules three times per day may provide an effective alternative. Many fish oil products, however, contain various impurities, including a high level of trans fatty acids that may be counterproductive. But certain fish oil capsules made by reputable pharmaceutical companies under the name of Max-EPA and Promega have much lower concentrations of trans fatty acids or other impurities.

Another advantage of eating seafood over taking fish oil capsules is that by substituting fish, which is less energy dense, for foods that are energy dense (such as red meat, pizza, and fried chicken), individuals with high triglyceride levels can also lose some of their abdominal obesity. Since seafoods replace other meals, unlike fish oils which are taken as supplements, they are better in dealing with high triglyceride levels.

Exercise and Weight Loss

Because abdominal obesity contributes to insulin resistance and raised levels of triglycerides, even a 5 to 10 percent weight loss can be an essential part of lowering your triglycerides. Regular exercise complements and improves the efficacy of dietary intervention to lower triglycerides. It also helps with weight loss, abdominal obesity, and insulin resistance. Clearly, sedentary or obese individuals, with or without a preexistent cardiovascular disease, should not start a vigorous exercise program the day their high triglyceride levels are diagnosed. For many this is impractical, and for some it may even be dangerous. Still, everyone with a high triglyceride level must engage in some form of exercise and slowly increase both the duration and intensity of the workouts.

Triglyceride-lowering Drugs

At present there are several drugs with proven efficacy in lowering triglycerides, but they have certain side effects that may dictate the choice of one over the other.

Appropriate doses of niacin decrease LDL cholesterol and triglycerides by about 30 percent, while they can increase HDL by the same percentage. Unfortunately, niacin has some side effects which limit its use, especially at high doses. To avoid niacin's side effects, initially it should be taken in very small doses (not exceeding 250 mg), two or three times per day. Over the next several weeks the dose can be gradually increased to reach 1500-2000 mg per day. A recent niacin formula allows for a single night-time dose of up to 2000 mg. But here too the drug should be started at a small dose and increased gradually over a six-to-eight week period (Chapter 2, "Supplemental Vitamins and Minerals").

Gemfibrozil and "Fibrates"

Gemfibrozil and other fibrates are very effective in lowering triglycerides. They are reasonably safe when used for one to two years. At low doses, they can lower triglycerides by as much as 30 to 40 percent. As triglycerides are lowered, the HDL levels can rise by approximately 10 percent. Two recent studies have shown that a new type of fibrate (Tricor) can increase blood levels of homocysteine by 46 to 56 percent, whereas gemfibrozil (which is also far less expensive) does not have a similar detrimental side effect. Clearly, in people with elevated blood homocysteine or any kidney disorder (which raises blood homocysteine level), Tricor should be avoided.

Statins

High doses of available statins (Part II, (15)) can lower triglycerides by 20 to 60 percent and at the same time lower LDL cholesterol levels. At higher doses, however, they are usually far more expensive than niacin or gemfibrozil. In urgent cases, the use of high doses of statins such as

Lipitor or Zocor (60-80 mg per day) combined with gemfibrozil is appropriate. At high doses, statins reduce the liver's production of VLDL particles enriched with triglycerides, thereby helping to lower blood triglyceride levels.

If you have high triglycerides, in addition to the above measures, you should stop drinking all alcoholic beverages. You should also take vitamin E at doses of 800-1000 IU per day, and a low dose of aspirin (81 mg per day), to counteract the increased clottability of the blood often associated with high triglycerides.

Over-the-counter Drugs and Supplements

There are currently no effective over-the-counter drugs other than niacin that can lower triglycerides. As noted earlier, niacin is effective only at high doses (more than 1500 mg per day). This high dosage should never be taken without a physician's or health-care provider's supervision. Lower doses of niacin simply have no appreciable impact, and are essentially useless for this purpose.

Fish oil supplements are readily available without a prescription and are quite effective. Beyond niacin and fish oil, there are no other effective nonprescription drugs or supplements to treat high triglyceride levels.

A large number of people with elevated triglycerides require a variety of interventions, with diet and lifestyle changes on one side, and therapy with two or more lipid-lowering drugs on the other. Although the risk of side effects associated with high doses of triglyceride-lowering drugs cannot be ignored, co-therapy with two or three drugs at low doses is not only more effective, but has far fewer side effects. For example, low doses of gemfibrozil (600 mg twice a day) combined with one of the statins, or niacin (less than 2000 mg per day) and fish oil provide an excellent response with very few side effects.

(14) Low HDL Cholesterol

For decades we have promoted the notion that the "bad" LDL cholesterol is the major culprit in heart attacks and strokes. But a low level of the "good" HDL cholesterol is an even greater culprit, especially among women.

The National Cholesterol Education Program determined the current "desirable" or "normal" HDL cholesterol levels nearly a decade ago. On the basis of these guidelines, an HDL level greater than 35 mg/dl for men and greater than 45 mg/dl for women is "normal." Recent studies have shown that these values are no longer valid and need upward revision. In fact, the risk of having a heart attack is more than 50 percent higher for both men and women with HDL levels currently accepted as "normal." In Table 3, I have introduced up-to-date normal values for different types of cholesterol and triglycerides. Thus for men the normal HDL level should be greater than 45 mg/dl, and for women greater than 55 mg/dl.

Using the new cut-off points for HDL cholesterol, at least 50 percent of men and 70 percent of women with coronary artery disease have low levels of HDL cholesterol. In a recent study of 8,200 men and women with documented coronary artery disease, 30 percent had total cholesterol levels below the current "normal" level of 200 mg/dl. Among this group, 52 percent had HDL cholesterol levels below 35 mg/dl even though their total cholesterol was "normal." In fact, for women low HDL levels are far more important than elevated LDL levels; nearly twice as many women with coronary artery disease have low HDL as those who have elevated LDL levels.

The risk of heart attacks in both men and women progressively increases with lower levels of HDL cholesterol. For each 5 mg decrease in HDL level beyond the new normal values (greater than 45 mg/dl for men and greater than 55 mg/dl for women), the risk of coronary artery disease increases by 30 to 50 percent. Thus, an HDL cholesterol of 30 mg/dl in men or 40 mg/dl in women more than doubles the risk of cardiovascular events. Another major concern is that people with low HDL levels who develop coronary artery disease often have multivessel disease involving several branches of coronary artery, which dramatically increases their risk of a future heart attack. A low HDL level also increases the risk of reclogging following coronary angioplasty fourfold.

Figure 9
Rate of Coronary Artery Disease by HDL Level

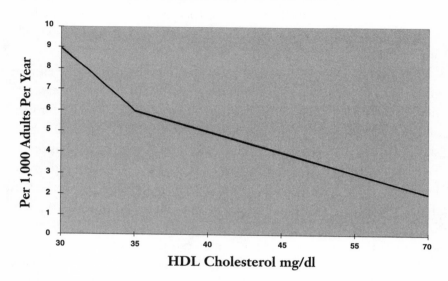

HDL Cholesterol mg/dl

Why Do Some People Have Low HDL Cholesterol Levels?

For most people, a low HDL cholesterol level has multiple genetic, lifestyle, or dietary causes:

- In many, a low HDL level is in part due to a genetic defect in the production of HDL cholesterol. For example, Japanese children consistently have higher HDL levels than their Western counterparts, an advantage that is continued into their adult life. The more severe forms of HDL deficiency almost always have a familial and genetic component, and a family history of coronary artery disease in several members, usually under the age of forty-five. Mr. Howard L, thirty-two years of age, was first seen for evaluation of what he thought was "indigestion" (which was in fact angina) after walking or playing with his two children in the backyard. His father had died at the age of forty-nine with a heart attack, and his older brother suffered his first heart attack at the age of thirty-five (and died at the age of forty). Aside from his strong family history of premature coronary artery disease, Mr. L also had abdominal obesity, a sedentary lifestyle, an LDL cholesterol level of 110 (which he proudly thought was "very good" and held up as his ticket to salvation!). But his HDL cholesterol was 28 (his brother's HDL after his second heart attack was 25 and remained untreated). Mr. L had a heart scan (an ultrafast CT scan) that showed a moderate amount of calcium deposits in his coronary artery, clear evidence of relatively advanced coronary artery disease. Six months after Mr. L was placed on a diet with a TRF score of about +20 and a variety of interventions to change his multiple risk factors, his HDL had risen to 47, his LDL was down to 85, and his homocysteine, which was 17, dropped to 8. He had also become a regular exerciser without experiencing chest pain on exertion, and lost 14 pounds in weight. At this point, his risk of a premature heart attack had decreased from more than 70 percent to less than 10 percent (Part III will tell you how to determine your own risk).

- Regular, vigorous exercises can raise HDL cholesterol by an average of 10 to 15 percent. The flip side of this is that sedentary people lower their HDL levels by 10 to 15 percent.

- Abdominal obesity almost always lowers HDL by 10 to 20 percent. General obesity, however, is not necessarily associated with lower HDL levels. People with abdominal obesity and low HDL levels also have a high percentage of small dense LDL particles which are particularly atherogenic (Part II, (15)), making a bad situation even worse.

- Bad dietary habits can lower HDL cholesterol by 10 to 20 percent. For example, eating lots of carbohydrates, in particular simple carbohydrates, lowers the HDL production. A recent study among children and adolescents with elevated blood cholesterol levels showed that children who ate too many carbohydrates had HDL cholesterol levels that were about 20 percent lower than children whose carbohydrate intake was relatively low. In adults, limiting dietary carbohydrate intake to no more than 45 percent of total calories while increasing monounsaturates will frequently raise HDL cholesterol by about 10 to 20 percent.

- Elevated blood triglycerides are almost always associated with low HDL cholesterol levels. By lowering triglyceride levels, you can increase HDL by 20 percent (Part II, (13)).

- Dietary intake of omega-6 fatty acids (vegetables oils and fats), particularly those that contain trans fatty acids (margarines, shortenings, and cooking fats), can lower HDL by 5 to 10 percent.

- Smoking can lower HDL cholesterol by more than 10 percent. Conversely, smoking cessation can raise HDL levels by 10 to 15 percent within a few weeks.

- Estrogen deficiency in post-menopausal women can lower HDL by 10 to 15 percent. On the other hand, oral estrogen replacement therapy can raise HDL by 10 to 15 percent. Estrogen skin patches, however, barely raise HDL cholesterol levels (by 2 to 5 percent) (Appendix B).

- Gender difference in blood levels of an enzyme produced by the liver called "hepatic lipase" is a significant contributor to lower HDL and higher LDL levels in men but not women (even after allowance is made for all other variables such as age, hormonal status, and weight). The higher levels of this enzyme in men account for almost 97 percent of the gender difference in HDL levels. Intensive cholesterol-altering interventions can reduce blood levels of this lipase and raise the HDL levels.

- Long-term intake of steroid hormones, including cortisone-like compounds, anabolic steroids, testosterone, DHEA, and androsterone can lower HDL levels by 5 to 10 percent.

What Does HDL Cholesterol Do? [23]

HDL cholesterol has a vast number of cardio-protective benefits:

- It barters with LDL and exchanges some of its own triglycerides for LDL's cholesterol load, and carries that cholesterol to the liver for disposal. This is called "reverse cholesterol transport" from tissues to the liver.

- It also blocks LDL particles and white blood cells from trespassing into the walls of the coronary artery, an important measure in preventing coronary artery disease. In a way, it acts like a doorman that prevents undesirables from entering the arterial wall.

- It facilitates the repair of any injury to the inner lining of the arteries. HDL also reduces the clumping and oxidization of LDL particles by approximately 50 percent. This potent antioxidant role is perhaps HDL's most cardio-protective virtue.

What You Should Do

The best way to raise your HDL cholesterol is to correct all the ten factors I listed earlier that lower its levels in the blood. Among these, a sedentary lifestyle, abdominal obesity, elevated triglycerides, smoking, and dietary habits are the primary culprits.

Regular, vigorous exercise is practically mandatory as a component of any intervention to raise your HDL. Exercise can increase HDL cholesterol by 10 to 20 percent. However, there may be even greater improvements when abdominal obesity and raised triglycerides are also brought under control with exercises and dietary changes. In people who have high HDL levels, regular, vigorous exercises can increase the HDL levels to a greater extent than in those who have low HDL levels. Thus, someone with an HDL of 25 should not expect exercise alone to raise the HDL to normal levels.

Since smoking lowers HDL cholesterol by 5 to 10 percent, this is another major reason for quitting. Quitting smoking promptly (within two to three weeks) raises HDL levels by greater than 10 percent.

Diet plays a significant role in improving HDL levels. In this regard, raising dietary monounsaturates (olive oil, canola oil, or hazelnut oil) is a far better option than a high carbohydrate, low-fat, or vegetarian diet. Recent data from investigators at Columbia University in New York showed that among children and adolescents, a high dietary intake of simple carbohydrates lowered their HDL levels by about 20 percent. The same is true in adults or older persons.

Low fat diets consistently lower HDL percent cholesterol levels in adults. Unfortunately, many healthcare providers have the bad habit of unleashing a stale sermon on the virtues of a low-fat, low-cholesterol diet to everyone with cholesterol disorder. No matter how well intended, this is still a counterproductive recommendation that often makes a bad situation even worse.

A dietary plan based on the TRF scoring system (with TRF scores of +20 to +30 per day for all foods and snacks) fulfills all the dietary requirements for raising your HDL cholesterol by 10 to 15 percent. The addition of one or two glasses of wine (or one or two cocktails) with dinner may contribute to a further 10 to 15 percent increase in HDL level. For people who are not overweight or diabetic, three glasses of orange juice each day may also raise their HDL by 10 to 20 percent (Chapter 2, "Beverages").

Drugs to Raise HDL Cholesterol

Niacin (at doses of 1500-2000 mg/dl) is the most effective HDL-raising drug we have (Chapter 2, "Supplemental Vitamins and Minerals"). Since many individuals with low HDL cholesterol levels also have elevated LDL cholesterol, the use of statins (Part II, (15)) is an effective, double-edged approach to lower LDL levels and at the same time raise HDL by 7 to 10 percent. Fibrates also can raise HDL levels by 5 to 10 percent, especially as triglyceride levels are lowered (Part II, (13)).

Since one of the major functions of HDL cholesterol is to protect LDL cholesterol from oxidization, anyone with low HDL levels should take a daily dose of 400-800 IU of vitamin E. At these doses, vitamin E can reduce oxidization of LDL by 40 percent, picking up some of the responsibilities of HDL. In a way, vitamin E becomes an HDL-helper, or a "poor man's" HDL. Fish oils or seafoods in general can raise the HDL level slightly as they lower triglycerides. Chromium supplements (Chapter 2, "Supplemental Vitamins and Minerals") may also increase HDL levels by improving insulin resistance, but the increase is limited to 5 to 7 percent.

(15) Elevated LDL Cholesterol

After four decades of research, the evidence is quite compelling that elevated blood cholesterol is a major risk factor for coronary artery disease and stroke. This association has been shown across all populations worldwide—in countries with very low, as well as those with very high, prevalence of coronary artery disease.

In the Multiple Risk Factor Intervention Trial, researchers followed up 362,000 middle-aged men for an average of six years. As seen in Figure 10, there was a progressive increase in the risk of death from coronary artery disease as cholesterol levels rose from low to high levels. During the six-year follow-up, the death rate among those with a cholesterol level of 260 mg/dl was 14 per 1,000 men as compared to 4 per 1,000 men among those with a cholesterol level under 180 mg/dl: a 350 percent difference. This and a large number of other studies have shown that desirable total cholesterol levels for both men and women should be less than 180 mg/dl, and preferably closer to 150. For LDL cholesterol, the corresponding values should be less than 100 mg/dl, and closer to 80 mg/dl.

Figure 10
Relation of Blood Cholesterol Levels to Age-adjusted Risk of Death for Coronary Artery Disease

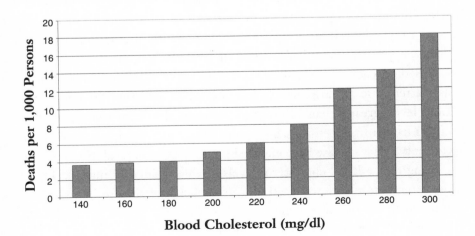

Not Everyone with Elevated Blood Cholesterol Develops Coronary Artery Disease

Recently scientists reported the findings of a twenty-five-year follow-up of 12,500 men between the ages of forty and fifty-nine years from seven countries (five European, the United States, and Japan). As seen in Figure 11, mortality from coronary artery disease correlated well with blood cholesterol levels across the board, even in countries with traditionally low rates of coronary artery disease. At any given level of LDL cholesterol, however, the risk of coronary artery disease and its complications varied among different populations. For example, a cholesterol level of 210 mg/dl in middle-aged Japanese males was associated with a 4 percent risk of death from coronary artery disease within twenty-five years. The risk associated with the same cholesterol level in Mediterranean men was 5 percent, whereas in Americans it was 12 percent, and for northern Europeans it was 15 percent. In fact, northern Europeans with a blood cholesterol level of 190 mg/dl have twice the risk of Mediterraneans with a blood cholesterol of 250 mg/dl. This is an enormously important finding, illustrating why similarly elevated blood cholesterol levels among various populations do not necessarily impart similar risks or require similar interventions. The relative sensitivity of different populations to cholesterol also explains why cholesterol reductions to a set level would not provide equal protection against coronary artery disease in all populations, or even among all individuals in a given population. The relevance of blood cholesterol levels to coronary artery disease applies to both men and women of all age groups.

Based on current cholesterol values, 60 percent of people with coronary artery disease have total cholesterol levels exceeding 200 mg/dl, and LDL levels greater than 130 mg/dl. But using the more accurate guidelines I have introduced in Table 3, more than 80 percent of people with coronary artery disease have elevated total cholesterol levels (in excess of 180 mg/dl) or LDL cholesterol levels (greater than 100 mg/dl). Thus, any intervention to lower LDL cholesterol should aim for levels below 100 mg/dl, and not accept the current "borderline" (up to 160 mg/dl) or "desirable" (less than 130) levels as normal.

In the United States, more than one hundred million Americans have elevated LDL cholesterol levels exceeding the 100 mg/dl cut-off point.

Figure 11
Relation between Total Blood
Cholesterol and Rate of Death

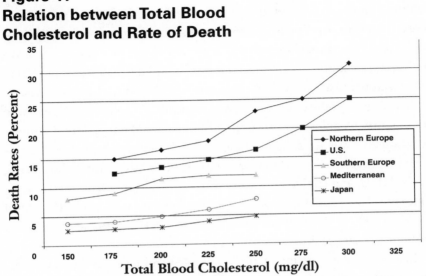

Fortunately, not everyone with an elevated blood cholesterol level develops coronary artery disease; more than two-thirds do not. About twenty million people in the United States have advanced coronary artery disease, and an equal number have early or silent coronary artery disease. Using the new guidelines introduced in Part I, Chapter 1, approximately 80 percent (or about thirty-two million) of Americans with early or advanced coronary artery disease have elevated blood cholesterol levels. People with elevated blood cholesterol and coronary artery disease, however, nearly always have coexisting risk factors as well.

What separates the sixty-eight million Americans with elevated blood cholesterol who do not have coronary artery disease, from the thirty-two million who do? There are at least two explanations:

First, LDL particle size is certainly a big factor. Whether for genetic or a variety of dietary and other lifestyle reasons, those who have a preponderance of small, dense LDL particles are several times more likely to develop coronary artery disease than those with large LDL particles.

Second, since coronary artery disease has many causes, the fewer risk factors an individual has, the smaller chance he or she has to develop coronary artery disease. The coexistence of several risk factors also explains, in part, the differences in how different populations around the world respond to high cholesterol levels.

Fluctuations in Blood Cholesterol

Blood cholesterol levels always fluctuate from day to day or week to week. This is in part due to the constant bartering among various lipoproteins as they exchange cholesterol or triglycerides with one another. In addition to these continuous internal adjustments and fluctuations, a number of other factors can also contribute to variation in blood cholesterol levels.

Recently I conducted a study among healthy hospital employees who were not on a cholesterol-lowering drug or diet. We took blood samples on a weekly basis for four weeks and sent duplicate samples to two different laboratories. More than 90 percent of the time, total cholesterol, LDL, HDL, and triglycerides varied by at least 10 percent during those four consecutive weeks. In other words, a person's total cholesterol level could be 200 mg/dl one week, and 220 mg/dl or 180 mg/dl another week, without any cholesterol-lowering intervention.

Because of the wide fluctuations in cholesterol levels in the same individual from week to week, we should not rely on one reading to classify the cholesterol status of anybody as normal or abnormal. Also, because of these inherent variabilities, we should not pass judgment on the efficacy or failure of any cholesterol-altering diet or medication solely on the basis of one blood test.

Does the LDL Particle Size Matter?

LDL cholesterol particles in the bloodstream, like oranges or eggs, come in various sizes. In general, however, we lump them all into two groups:

(1) *Large LDL particles, or type A:*
   Relatively speaking, these particles contain more triglycerides than cholesterol in their core, but their outer shell is essentially identical with their smaller siblings. However, since their core is enriched with triglycerides, their particle size is enlarged by about 10 percent.

(2) *Small, dense LDL particles, or type B:*
   The core of these LDL particles has more cholesterol and less triglycerides, making them slightly but distinctly denser and smaller than their larger kin.

The LDL particle size is enormously important in the development of coronary artery disease. People with a predominantly large variety (type A) are far less likely to develop coronary artery disease, even if their blood cholesterol levels are elevated. On the other hand, people with predominantly small, dense LDL particles (type B) have a higher risk of developing coronary artery disease, even when their blood cholesterol levels are normal. This is because small LDL particles trespass through the inner lining of coronary (or cerebral) arteries more easily than the larger ones. In addition, they are also more oxidizable, making them quite coronary-unfriendly.

The predominance of small, dense LDL particles (type B), even with "normal" LDL cholesterol levels, increases the risk of coronary artery disease by 300 to 500 percent. More importantly, among men with elevated LDL cholesterol, type B LDL increases their risk of coronary artery disease by more than 600 percent. For example, Mr. Martin S was admitted through the emergency room to the cardiac intensive care unit for monitoring after he experienced a bout of chest pain during his forty-second birthday dinner at a local restaurant. His father had died of a massive heart attack at the age of forty-four. His electrocardiogram and blood tests in the emergency room suggested a possible heart attack. The coronary angiogram taken the next day showed 50 to 60 percent blockage of two major branches of his coronary artery, but no true heart attack. Four weeks after discharge from the hospital his LDL cholesterol was 128, his HDL was 36, and his triglycerides were 324. Regrettably, his cardiologist had told him that his blood cholesterol was fine. In addition, his fasting blood glucose was 129, his homocysteine measured 18, and his hematocrit level was 51. Not only were all of these values abnormal, most of his LDL particles were of the small, dense variety, increasing his risk of heart attack several times further. He began treatment with the TRF diet, in addition to the following multifaceted approach: low doses of aspirin; vitamin E (to decrease oxidization of his LDL particles); niacin (to lower his LDL cholesterol and triglycerides, and to raise the HDL as well as reduce the number of small LDL particles); exercise four to five times a week; triple therapy with folic acid and vitamin B-12, as well as vitamin B6 to lower his homocysteine, and blood donation to lower his hematocrit. Over four years later, he has had no further symptoms, his blood tests are normal, and his angiogram shows a slight decrease in the blockage of his coronary artery to less than 50 percent.

All of these improvements have dramatically lowered his risk of a heart attack. Mr. S is an example of a large number of people with genetic tendencies that cause devastating coronary artery disease at a young age. But most, if not all, of these genetic misfortunes are modifiable with early and aggressive intervention.

Direct measurement of LDL particle size is currently available only through a few laboratories in the United States, and is relatively costly. Within a year or two it should become more widely available and less costly. People with low HDL cholesterol (even if they have an "acceptable" LDL cholesterol level) should ask their physician to test their LDL particle size, especially if they have a family history of premature cardiovascular events.[24]

Naturally Low Blood Cholesterol vs. Cholesterol Lowering

Admittedly, not all individuals with elevated LDL cholesterol develop coronary artery disease (approximately 30 percent do). Yet it is that element of uncertainty—not knowing exactly who, when, and how it develops—that makes cholesterol lowering critical in the prevention of a future heart attack. Here, the high probability of benefit from reducing LDL cholesterol outweighs the very low likelihood of treatment-related side effects, almost all of which are essentially minor or self-limiting. Since individuals with several risk factors have an extremely high risk of developing a major cardiovascular event resulting in disability or death, they must be more proactive and start cholesterol lowering as early as possible.

The cardio-protective benefits of cholesterol lowering measures, even when the LDL can be lowered by 40 to 60 percent, are limited to an approximately 30 percent reduction in the risk of heart attack. In other words, each 1 percent cholesterol reduction up to 30 percent is associated with 1 percent risk reduction. Any additional cholesterol-lowering beyond 30 percent does not appear to confer a significant further benefit, and may even be associated with some drug-induced side effects.

On the other hand, in the Multiple Risk Factor Intervention Trial study of 362,000 men without a previous history of coronary artery disease, the six-year risk of the disease in someone with a blood cholesterol level below 180 mg/dl was 70 percent less than those whose blood cholesterol levels were 30 percent higher (greater than 260 mg/dl). In other words, for each 1 percent lower cholesterol, the risk of coronary artery disease was reduced by 2 percent. Why is there a 200 percent disparity in the risk of coronary artery disease among those who are fortunate enough to have naturally low blood cholesterol levels and those whose high blood cholesterol levels are brought down to normal with treatment? The answer is actually in the question!

Undoubtedly, long-term exposure of coronary and cerebral arteries to high levels of cholesterol may initiate and promote the process of coronary artery disease. Thus, for many, ten, twenty, or thirty years later the impact of cholesterol-lowering efforts may prove to be too little, too late. More alarming is the fact that the first manifestation of coronary artery disease in one-third of all who have it is a heart attack. In other words, once atherosclerosis and coronary artery disease has set in, cholesterol-lowering measures may slow down the progression of coronary artery disease in a third of treated individuals, and perhaps eventually produce some minimal regression in an even fewer people. But these or any other measures cannot make the vessels normal again. Although cholesterol-lowering reduces the risk of a heart attack by 30 percent, correction of other coronary risk factors provides even greater additional protection.

What Does Cholesterol Lowering Do?

Cholesterol-lowering provides three distinct benefits. These benefits do not necessarily coincide; some occur within weeks, whereas other benefits require months or years of sustained treatment to have a tangible impact. In chronological order, the benefits are:

The Immediate Benefit

Approximately 2 to 5 percent of LDL particles in the blood are oxidized. The number of oxidized LDL particles is much higher (up to 10 percent) in diabetics, in people with small, dense LDL particles, and in people with a low antioxidant reserve (often due to low intake). Cholesterol lowering, along with other measures (see below), reduces the number of LDL particles so that there are fewer oxidized particles in the bloodstream to cross into the arterial wall and start new coronary plaques or aggravate the existing ones.

The addition of vitamin E can significantly enhance the efficacy of cholesterol-lowering in restoring the functions of the inner lining (endothelium) of the arteries. Whereas coronary arteries of individuals with high cholesterol tend to constrict in response to various daily stresses, reducing cholesterol and taking vitamin E reverses this process and allows the arteries to dilate instead of constricting.

The improvement in the functions of the endothelium of the arteries usually occurs within a few weeks of the start of a cholesterol-lowering program. Conversely, withdrawal of treatment and subsequent elevation of blood cholesterol levels results in the return of endothelial dysfunction within two weeks. This rapid reversal of fortunes illustrates the importance of long-term adherence to an effective treatment program. A number of coronary risk factors such as smoking, a sedentary lifestyle, high levels of lipoprotein(a), triglycerides, or homocysteine, and low levels of HDL cholesterol, often sabotage the restoration of the endothelial function.

The Mid-range Benefit: Stabilization of Coronary Plaques

An elevated LDL cholesterol level contributes to its progressive accumulation in the wall of coronary and cerebral arteries. As fat-laden plaques bulge, their protective cap becomes thinner and weaker compared to plaques that contain less fat and more smooth muscle cells or scar tissue. Coronary plaques with a thin cap are four times more likely to erode or rupture and cause heart attacks than plaques that are more fibrous and have a thicker cap. When the blood cholesterol level drops for a sustained period, very few or no further LDL deposits occur, and within six to twelve months the plaques become more stable and less prone to erosions or rupture.

The Long-term Benefit: Regression or Shrinking of Coronary Plaques

Long-term cholesterol-lowering facilitates the removal of some fatty deposits from the wall of the arteries. This reverse transport of cholesterol out of the artery's wall is primarily the responsibility of HDL cholesterol. As the cholesterol content of the plaques drops, they shrivel up slightly, contributing to the widening of the artery's lumen. The improvement or reduction of the size and bulging of coronary plaques is called "regression."

Unfortunately, regression is very time-dependent and, even after many years, may be in the order of 1 to 2 percent only. For most people, this regression in the size of coronary plaques amounts to no more than the thickness of two or three sheets of typing paper. In fact, regression of coronary lesions has little relevance to, and is not the main goal of, cholesterol-lowering therapies.

What You Should Do

If you have elevated blood cholesterol, with or without coronary artery disease, lowering your LDL cholesterol helps to:

- Improve the endothelial function
- Prevent the development of new coronary plaques
- Stabilize the existing coronary plaque

However, you cannot achieve all these objectives by cholesterol-lowering drugs alone. You must almost always address and correct all the other coronary risk factors. Since nearly 100 million Americans have elevated blood cholesterol, what is needed is a safer, more effective, and practical approach to cholesterol lowering that nearly everyone can follow without hardship.

Exercise

As noted in Part II, (11), a sedentary lifestyle increases your risk of coronary artery disease by 50 percent, along with significant increases in the risk of various cancers including breast, colon, and prostate.

Vitamin E Supplements

Although vitamin E at a dose of 400-800 IU per day has no impact on blood cholesterol levels, it does reduce the oxidization of LDL, VLDL, and lipoprotein(a), and lowers your risk of coronary artery disease by nearly 40 percent. This is an incredibly inexpensive, safe, and effective way to lower your risk of a heart attack or stroke. Although vitamin E cannot be expected in a short time to have a significant impact on advanced coronary artery disease, even in these cases it can reduce the development of new plaques in other segments of coronary artery, and in the long-term might well decrease the risk of a new catastrophic heart attack.

Aspirin

As noted in Part II, (6), the use of low-dose aspirin (81 mg per day) can reduce your risk of a cardiovascular event by approximately 30 percent. This is an added benefit to cholesterol-lowering measures. However, by improving the endothelial function, aspirin reduces the trespassing of LDL particles into the arterial wall.

Table 64
Other Non-dietary Interventions to Improve Cholesterol Profile

INTERVENTION	% RISK REDUCTION
LOW-DOSE ASPIRIN (81 MG/DL)	30
NORMALIZING LDL CHOLESTEROL	30
NORMALIZING TRIGLYCERIDES	30
NORMALIZING BLOOD PRESSURE	30
NORMALIZING BLOOD HOMOCYSTEINE LEVEL	30
WEIGHT REDUCTION	30
SMOKING CESSATION	30
LOW-DOSE ALCOHOL (1-2 DRINKS PER DAY)	40
LOW-DOSE ESTROGEN REPLACEMENT THERAPY	40
NORMALIZING HDL CHOLESTEROL	50
STRESS MANAGEMENT, TREATMENT OF NEGATIVE AFFECT**	50
REGULAR, SUSTAINED EXERCISE, 4-5 TIMES PER WEEK	50
ADEQUATE CONTROL OF DIABETES	50
MEDITERRANEAN DIET WITH TRF SCORE <+30 PER DAY	70
TOTAL	560

* Some benefits of reducing or eliminating multiple risk factors may overlap, but they are mostly additive. Control or elimination of other major and minor coronary risk factors (Chapter 1) provide even more protection.
** A recent study from Duke University showed that stress management in people with coronary artery disease lowers the risk of a coronary event by 74 percent.

Estrogen Replacement Therapy in Post-menopausal Women
(Appendix B)

Cholesterol-altering Drugs
Niacin: (Chapter 2, "Supplemental Vitamins and Minerals"; Part II (13))

Cholestyramine (Questran, Lo-cholest, and Others)

Cholestyramine is a nonabsorbable compound taken two to three times per day, usually in the form of a powder. But its gastrointestinal side effects and unappealing taste limit its usefulness. At present, there is little justification to use these compounds, especially considering their side effects, relatively high cost, and low effectiveness.

Statins

Perhaps one of the most important developments in the past twenty years in the field of medicine has been the introduction of various statins—medications that can reduce blood cholesterol levels significantly and safely. All statins block the production of new cholesterol by liver cells and increase the number of LDL receptors, both of which lower the LDL cholesterol by 30 to 60 percent. They also lower triglycerides in a dose-dependent manner by 10 to 60 percent, and increase the HDL by 5 to 10 percent (higher doses are not more effective). Statins reduce the inflammation in and around coronary plaques, so that they become less vulnerable to rupture, which causes heart attacks.

At present, six statins have been approved by the FDA and are available by prescription only. There are subtle differences among these drugs with respect to their cholesterol-lowering potencies and other cardiovascular benefits. Table 65 shows the LDL-lowering potency of these six drugs.

Table 65
Cholesterol Lowering with Current Statins by Percentage
(Per 1 oz)

DRUG (MG/DAY)	0.3	10	20	40	80
CERVISTATIN (BAYCOL)	28-30	-	-	-	-
ATORVASTATIN (LIPITOR)	-	37-40	43-46	50-53	55-60
PRAVASTATIN (PRAVACHOL)	-	18	22-24	30-32	-
SIMVASTATIN (ZOCOR)	-	26-28	32-35	39-41	46
FLUVASTATIN (LESCOL)	-	-	16-18	22-24	30
LOVASTATIN (MEVACOR)	-	-	23-25	30-32	40

As shown in Table 65, a substantial cholesterol-lowering occurs with low doses of statins. Subsequent increments, such as doubling or tripling the dose, are not necessarily associated with two to three times greater reductions in your LDL. For this reason, most individuals with elevated LDL cholesterol require relatively low doses, which further improves statins' safety and cost effectiveness. Some individuals with defective LDL-receptors, however, require relatively larger doses to achieve a significant cholesterol-lowering effect.

The cost of statins for each 30 percent cholesterol reduction is quite variable (Baycol being the least expensive and Mevacor the most expensive). Thus, in choosing a statin, various factors should be considered, including cost, blood cholesterol level, overall health of the individual, and the availability of these statins in the formulary of your health maintenance organization or health insurer.[25]

Over-the-counter Cholesterol-lowering Supplements

Since nearly 100 million Americans have abnormal blood cholesterol levels, many entrepreneurs have pounced on the vulnerability of this huge population. After reviewing the available data in mid-1997 and again in the fall of 2000, the United States Food and Drug Administration concluded that the nature of abnormal blood cholesterol levels and its potential complications were such an immensely important public health issue that over-the-counter marketing of cholesterol-lowering agents was an unsafe and ineffective way of treating the problem. As a result, the Food and Drug Administration strongly opposed the development, marketing, and sale of any over-the-counter cholesterol-lowering supplement.

But despite the Food and Drug Administration's rational and wise position, there are still many over-the-counter cholesterol-lowering aids. Some of these contain small amounts of statins or niacin, and some contain various fibers. Garlic, ginseng, and a variety of other herbs are also promoted for lowering blood cholesterol levels. Even if one or more of these agents could lower blood cholesterol by a few percentage points, the effect is too trivial to be truly meaningful. It may also distract people with cholesterol disorders from seeking safe and effective treatment to prevent catastrophic cardiovascular events, especially if they have other coexisting coronary risk factors. For this reason, reliance on these supplements to improve cholesterol disorders and reduce your risk of a cardiovascular event is a dangerous gamble that very few will win.

Heart attacks and strokes are mostly preventable catastrophes. This simple fact should be enough to discourage anyone from using questionable, ineffective, or unproven supplements to prevent or treat these serious diseases. Unfortunately, millions of people both in the United States and elsewhere are oblivious to this truth. The misleading testimonials, sleek advertisements, and profit motives fill the void where there are few knowledgeable and dedicated health care providers.

How Low Should Your Cholesterol Be?

Although an LDL cholesterol of under 100 mg/dl significantly reduces your risk of a heart attack, it is not always necessary to get cholesterol below this level. An undue emphasis on lowering LDL cholesterol far below 100 mg/dl, without dealing with the other nineteen major and twenty minor risk factors (Tables 4 and 5), may be numerically satisfying but may not offer a significant cardiovascular benefit. Table 66 summarizes the indications for statin use among people with elevated cholesterol.

Table 66
Persons Who Should Be on Statins*

- ANY ADULT WITH CAD AND LDL CHOLESTEROL >100 MG/DL

- ANY ADULT WITH A FAMILY HISTORY OF PREMATURE CAD (BEFORE THE AGE OF 55) AND LDL CHOLESTEROL >100 MG/DL

- ANY ADULT WITH TYPE B LDL (SMALL, DENSE PARTICLES) AND LDL >100 MG/DL

- ANY ADULT WITH MULTIPLE RISK FACTORS FOR CAD AND LDL >100 MG/DL

- ANY ADULT WITH DIABETES (TYPE 1 OR 2) AND LDL >100 MG/DL

- ANY ADULT WITH LOW HDL CHOLESTEROL (<45 IN MEN, <55 IN WOMEN) AND LDL CHOLESTEROL >100 MG/DL

- ANY ADULT WITH CHRONIC KIDNEY DISEASE AND LDL >100 MG/DL

- CHILDREN AND ADOLESCENTS WITH FAMILIAL CHOLESTEROL DISORDER AND A HIGH RISK OF DEVELOPING PREMATURE CAD

* Only if they fail to respond to dietary and lifestyle modifications

(16) Elevated Lipoprotein(a)

As noted in Chapter 1, lipoprotein(a) is made up of an LDL-molecule to which a coronary-unfriendly protein called "apoprotein(a)" is attached. This combination makes lipoprotein(a) a double-edged sword: in addition to LDL's misdeeds, it adds insult to injury by increasing the risk of forming microscopic clots (thrombosis) within coronary plaques. These small clots play a major role in the progression of early coronary lesions into advanced clogging of the artery.[26]

In people with chronic kidney dysfunction or failure, blood lipoprotein(a) levels go up significantly and contribute to the high risk of cardiovascular complications. Recent studies have suggested that kidney dysfunction slows down the breakdown of lipoprotein(a). In some individuals with lupus (a systemic auto-immune disease) and rheumatoid arthritis, lipoprotein(a) is also elevated.

In a recent study, researchers examined coronary plaques which were surgically removed from seventy-two patients with coronary artery disease. All specimens contained lipoprotein(a). Of particular interest was the fact that in 90 percent of the specimens, many white blood cells had surrounded the lipoprotein(a) particles, some of which were oxidized and gobbled up by these white blood cells. White blood cells inside the plaques produce certain enzymes that literally digest and weaken the plaques, making them quite unstable and more vulnerable to crack or rupture, a process that is the precursor of a heart attack.

What You Should Do

Unlike all other lipoproteins, lipoprotein(a) is largely unaffected by dietary changes (except for a small 10 to 20 percent reduction with high intake of seafood omega-3 polyunsaturated fat), exercises, weight reduction, and other lifestyle modifications. Caseine (a protein in cheese also available as a dietary supplement) can lower lipoprotein(a) by greater than 20 percent depending on how much is used on a regular daily basis. Large doses are, unfortunately, not practical as daily supplements. Trans fatty acids (found in such products as margarine, shortenings, cooking fats, deep fried items, and pastries) can actually raise lipoprotein(a) by 10 to 20, yet another reason to avoid them.

Among medications, only niacin at doses above 1500 to 2000 mg per day can lower lipoprotein(a) by up to 30 percent. High doses of estrogen-replacement therapy in women can also lower lipoprotein(a) by up to 20 percent. Thyroid hormone (for those with underactive thyroid) and anabolic steroids also can lower the lipoprotein(a) level by 10 to 20 percent (Appendix A).

Because an elevated lipoprotein(a) is far more atherogenic when the LDL cholesterol level is also high, you should strive to lower LDL cholesterol to under 100 mg/dl. A dietary program with TRF scores between +20 to +30 per day with a high intake of seafood, avoidance of trans fatty acids (margarines, shortenings), vitamin E at doses of 400-800 IU per day, and a low-dose aspirin (81 mg per day) are all helpful. Just as important, lipoprotein(a) further aggravates the impact of homocysteine, smoking, high hematocrit, and elevated fibrinogen (all of which increase clotting potential). Thus if you have an elevated lipoprotein(a) you should be tested for all these risk factors.

(17) Age

Because nearly 80 percent of heart attacks occur between the ages of thirty-five and sixty-five, we have always focused our attention on this age group. The two groups on either side of this large majority—the very young and the elderly—have been somewhat ignored.

Since coronary artery disease is a slow developing process, it is most uncommon for children and young adults to develop manifestations of atherosclerosis. Exceptions to this rule are children who have a familial disorder in which their liver has few or no LDL receptors. Since more than 70 percent of LDL particles in blood circulation are removed by these LDL receptors, their absence (or multiple mutations in their protein structure which make them dysfunctional) results in very high blood cholesterol levels often exceeding 500 mg/dl, as well as premature coronary artery disease.

Because a large number of children may have inherited coronary risk factors or genes that produce faulty LDL receptors, coronary artery disease may silently start and progress in this age group. In a landmark study, a total of 2,876 male and female subjects between the ages of fifteen and thirty-four, who had died of external causes, were autopsied (Table 1). Among the youngest age group (fifteen to nineteen years), more than half of the coronary arteries contained signs of atherosclerosis and early plaque formation. The prevalence of these lesions was even higher among those twenty to thirty-four years of age. This study confirmed the view that coronary artery disease begins early, and not when people are in their forties and fifties. In fact, in a previous study of children between the ages of ten and fourteen, more than 50 percent had microscopic evidence of early plaque formation. A recent study from the University of California, San Diego, showed that fatty streaks in the arterial wall may begin in fetuses, and are more common when maternal blood cholesterol levels are high. These observations reaffirm my repeated contention that prevention of a future heart attack must begin early, long before it has progressed to an irreversible stage.

Screening of Children and Adolescents for Cholesterol Disorders

Although screening of all adults for cholesterol and blood pressure is universally accepted, screening children and adolescents still generates a lot of emotional debate. The controversy regarding cholesterol screening in this age group focuses on the following reservations:

(1) *Measurement of cholesterol and lipoproteins is subject to the same drawback and inaccuracies as adults.* Although this is a pertinent concern, it has not stopped us from screening adults and treating them when we find abnormal levels. As is true for adults, no child or adolescent should be diagnosed as having "high cholesterol" on the basis of a single measurement. Among other reasons, this is because blood tests might be done during an acute illness, the week of a birthday, Halloween, or other major occasion when they feast on chocolates and greasy foods which skews the results. Children's blood levels can be distorted by a single testing. Dragging children to a doctor's office after a soccer, basketball, or hockey game should also be avoided to reduce variability in cholesterol measurements.

(2) *Children's "normal" blood cholesterol levels are unknown.* As I showed in Table 3, normal or desirable cholesterol levels in children and adolescents should not be different from someone who is twenty-five, forty-five, or fifty-five years old. This is not an unprecedented revelation: blood levels of sugar, sodium, potassium, calcium, and kidney or liver function tests are all measured similarly across various age groups.

(3) *Children or adolescents with elevated cholesterol will not necessarily become adults with elevated cholesterol or have heart attacks.* Even if we use the currently accepted "normal" cholesterol levels, a third of children and adolescents with elevated blood cholesterol will go on to have high levels as adults. Another third will have "borderline high" values (200-240 mg/dl). Using the more accurate levels I introduced in Table 3, the data suggest that well over two-thirds of children with abnormal cholesterol levels will carry their disorder into adulthood. Conversely, among children and adolescents with normal blood cholesterol, only 20 percent go on to develop abnormal levels as adults; about 80 percent will maintain their normal cholesterol profile. The high probability of an elevated cholesterol carrying over into adult life should be enough to call for vigorous screening and appropriate preventive measures in children and adolescents.

There is no doubt that abnormal blood cholesterol levels beginning in childhood or adolescence are more likely to cause cardiovascular diseases in adult life than normal levels. Recent data from the Bogelusa Heart Study of 204 children and young people who died of noncardiac causes showed that as the number of coexistent coronary risk factors in these youngsters increased, the prevalence and severity of coronary artery disease among them increased several fold. Among youngsters with three or more coronary risk factors, 7.2 percent had already developed advanced coronary lesions when compared with .6 percent for those with no risk factors. A much higher percentage of the former had early signs of fatty deposits in their coronary artery and aorta. As shown in Table 1, coronary artery disease among adolescents and young adults in the United States is frightfully common.

It is difficult to isolate elevated cholesterol as a factor for future risk of cardiovascular diseases in children. Obesity, smoking, sedentary lifestyle, poor dietary habits, and whatever changes in diet or lifestyles they adopt as adults will all impact their future risk. Still, as with any other chronic disorder in children or adolescents, such as asthma, high blood pressure, or diabetes, abnormal cholesterol values cannot be ignored, especially when there are other coexistent risk factors. The coronary risk factors for children and adolescents are largely the same as those that predispose middle-aged and older persons to cardiovascular events.

(4) *Screening all children is expensive.* If we spend money to discourage smoking, alcohol, and drug abuse, or to promote vaccines and seat belts, we ought to spend a fraction of our healthcare resources to arrest the epidemic of coronary artery disease. Unless we do so, a vast number of today's children and adolescents will go on to have massive heart attacks when they are in their thirties, forties, or fifties. This is a moral health care imperative, and a social responsibility regardless of the emotional posturing of politicians or the penny-wise and pound-foolish attitude of managed care companies. Just as preventing youngsters from smoking, drinking, or using drugs will save money and lives in the long run, so too will education about and prevention of coronary artery disease at an early age.

(5) *Even if we find abnormal cholesterol levels, it is difficult to treat youngsters effectively.* Children (as well as adults) are not aware of, and suffer no discomfort from, their abnormal cholesterol levels. Unlike a sore throat or an ear infection, treating an abnormal cholesterol level is not associated with any immediate or tangible relief. Children and adolescents have a short time horizon—next day, or the next Saturday night. Thus it is difficult to make a case for recommendations aimed at preventing a heart attack thirty or forty years down the road. But that is precisely what is needed. Instead of ignoring the problem, we ought to face it squarely, just as we deal with smoking, alcohol or drug abuse, obesity, and depression in this age group. It should be self-evident that ignoring abnormal blood cholesterol levels won't make them go away. We have no choice but to change our laid-back and passive approach if we are to save lives in the future.

The management of abnormal blood cholesterol in children is a family affair; it begins with educating and encouraging parents, and even other siblings, to follow the guidelines suggested in previous chapters. Children emulate their parents and older siblings. There is no doubt about the impact of dietary and lifestyle practices on children and adolescents. The evidence is overwhelming that humans are programmed to like sweets and dislike bitter-tasting foods from birth. Other tastes such as salty, spicy, or fatty foods are acquired. Frequent exposure, familiarity, and social or cultural settings can all influence our tastes for and choice of foods. For example, when given a choice between a spicy snack and a sweet one, nearly half of all Mexican children over the age of seven will pick a spicy one but less than 1 percent of American children do the same. This is because very few American parents feed their toddlers spicy foods. Regrettably, they often reward, bribe, or console their children with sweets laden with invisible fat, most of which is saturated fat and trans fatty acids.

Parents who watch child-oriented commercial television tend to purchase more sugared cereals and candies than those who watch commercial-free children's programs. Part of this, of course, is the influence of commercials on parents, but it also means that impressionable children lured by these commercials talk their parents into buying the advertised products, even though most parents know they are not healthful.

In a recent national survey, 80 percent of parents with children between the ages of six and eleven were familiar with the Food Guide Pyramid developed by the United States Department of Agriculture. Only 37 percent of parents, however, said that they followed the guidelines in preparing their children's meals. In other words, what many parents do is not necessarily based on what they know. If parents set a good example and provide a sensible diet, it may help modify or alter the course of their children's cardiovascular destiny.

An easy way of changing the dietary pattern of youngsters is to change the family diet so that it is as close to a TRF score of +30 per day as possible. No matter how severe the cholesterol disorder is, it serves no purpose for parents to engage in a constant struggle with their children over occasional Big Macs, donuts, chips, or chocolate bars. This can be a frustrating battle that parents usually lose.

A recent report from the Child and Adolescent Trial for Cardiovascular Health showed that overweight and obese children have a much higher risk of serious cardiovascular events as adults than other children. Among the more than 5,100 children and adolescents studied, overweight children had higher blood pressure and LDL cholesterol, had lower HDL cholesterol, and engaged in much less physical activity. Contrary to a common, self-serving assumption that chubby children will "outgrow" their weight problem, only 5 percent of overweight children attained normal weight during the follow-up period. Almost identical findings were reported recently by investigators of the Minneapolis Children's Study, who followed-up 679 children from age seven for a period of sixteen years.

Changing dietary preferences of a child, overweight or not, should be handled with patience, reason, and consistency, not emotionally or with harsh discipline and inflexibility. It may take a few months of fussing and griping before most youngsters gradually accept or adapt to a new diet, provided it is not rigid or punitive. Occasional treats ("junk foods") should not only make children happy, but also help them to better understand and appreciate their parents' reasonableness. Usually, the biggest problem is to convince the parents that they, too, need to change their dietary practices in order to make their youngsters' transition easier; this is often more of an obstacle than changing children's finicky or junk-eating habits.

Regrettably, many meals served at school cafeterias are perfect examples of what children should *not* eat. Packing a nutritious meal at home for one or two youngsters is not very time consuming. If they take time to shave, shower, fix their hair, and dress for work, parents should have an extra few minutes to spend on their children's well-being and future health.

Children with moderate and severe abnormalities of their cholesterol, if they have a family history of premature cardiovascular diseases, should be referred to a cholesterol specialist. Although, in the past, pediatricians shied away from treating children with this kind of problem vigorously, this is no longer acceptable or justified. Recent studies have shown that statins (Part II (14)) are highly effective and safe in lowering blood cholesterol in adolescents and young people with high blood cholesterol levels.

Which Children and Adolescents Should Be Screened?

The following recommendations, based on more than one hundred published studies in the past decade, provide a scientific and rational basis for screening children and adolescents:

- Children with a family history (parents, grandparents, uncles, aunts, siblings, or cousins) of coronary artery disease, stroke, or peripheral vascular disease, especially if they occurred before the age of fifty-five

- Children with a family history of abnormal cholesterol

- Overweight or obese children, and those who have any other coronary risk factor

- All children at age ten and again at age fifteen

What to Screen For?

As noted in Chapter 1, a simple measurement of total cholesterol is at best a waste of time. It may also mislead parents into a false sense of security. If we are to do anything useful, we must obtain a total lipid profile, consisting of total cholesterol, LDL cholesterol, HDL cholesterol, and triglycerides. As with adults, here too the ratio of total cholesterol to HDL cholesterol is a reasonable index to judge the status of an individual. The normal ratio should be less than 4, and preferably closer to 3.5.

As in adults, a single cholesterol profile is not very helpful. Children and adolescents show even more variability in their blood cholesterol levels than adults. A minimum of two cholesterol profiles several weeks apart are required before putting a youngster's cholesterol level in the normal or abnormal category. Fluctuations over or under 180 mg/dl for the total, and over or under 100 mg/dl for LDL cholesterol, are common in children and have no biological significance. Thus, a total or LDL cholesterol level that jumps up and down should not be a source of concern, as long as these values are not consistently abnormal.

What You Should Do

If you have children with abnormal cholesterol levels, the first step is to start them on a diet with TRF scores of less than +30 per day. This flexible dietary approach allows for a vast number of choices, and also meets the goals of recommended dietary allowances for energy, protein, fat, and various micronutrients. Such a diet will not interfere with the psychological or physical maturation of a child. More importantly, a diet based on TRF scores eliminates unwarranted concern over levels of various fats, or cholesterol in a given food or snack, which could make meals an unpleasant experience for children and their parents. A major hurdle is getting children to eat seafood, especially if the parents don't eat or like seafood. Starting with a "mild" fish such as flounder, or lake trout, broiled or sautéed in olive oil, perhaps once or twice a week may be a good strategy. Over the next several weeks you can add tuna or salmon for one or two other meals.

To reinforce and encourage children to follow the diet, periodic input and supervision by a health care provider may prove helpful. The caveat here is that the health care providers should become familiar with the TRF system in order to avoid regressing into obsolete dietary recommendations. It is essential to remember that the purpose of dietary intervention is to reduce the risk of future cardiovascular disease and not merely to show a numerical drop in total or LDL cholesterol levels so as to please the parents or pediatricians.

As with adults, children must be encouraged to exercise on a regular basis, both at school and after school hours. No amount of dietary change can be a substitute for vigorous and regular exercises. Participating in sports also helps reduce the likelihood that youngsters will take up smoking, drinking, or drugs, or that they will develop obesity. Remember that the majority of exercising children and adolescents grow up to be exercising adults.

Children and adolescents with elevated LDL cholesterol also require supplemental vitamin E (200-400 IU per day). For children who have a family history of premature coronary artery disease, other familial risk factors should also be looked for and treated accordingly. For youngsters under the age of eighteen who have slight to moderate elevation of LDL cholesterol (less than 160 mg/dl), cholesterol-lowering drugs may not be necessary. But for those with familial cholesterol disorders (such as high levels of LDL and triglycerides or low levels of HDL), they should always be referred to a lipid clinic with experience in dealing with pediatric disorders, at least for an initial consultation. Most of these children or adolescents can be treated with statins safely. The cholesterol management of these children should never be done without supervision, nor should their screening or treatment be postponed.

A large body of evidence suggests that a maternal elevated blood cholesterol level during pregnancy increases the risk of future coronary artery disease in offspring, even if the children become adults with normal blood cholesterol levels. One plausible explanation is that some oxidized LDL particles or their by-products trespass through the placenta and enter the fetal bloodstream where they may initiate the very early stages of the coronary quartet (Chapter 1). These oxidants may also change or damage the genetic makeup of the endothelial cells of the coronary artery, and reduce their resistance to injury during adult life. The obvious point here is that all pregnant women must have their blood cholesterol tested (as they do the blood sugar to rule out gestational diabetes). If the maternal blood cholesterol is abnormal, various measures listed in previous chapters (except for cholesterol-lowering drugs which are dangerous during pregnancy) should be considered to lower the mother's blood cholesterol as much as possible. Supplemental vitamin E is not only safe during pregnancy but also has the potential to reduce the risk of catastrophic cardiovascular events in the offspring of these affected mothers.

Older Persons and Cardiovascular Diseases

The world population is aging. Over a hundred years ago, only one out of six people lived to be seventy-five. Today, four out of six do. The average life span at that time was approximately fifty years. Today, it is about seventy-eight years for women and seventy-four years for men and is steadily rising. Indeed, we are moving towards a world where older people will soon outnumber children and adolescents.

In the United States, there are more than 50 million Americans sixty-five years of age or older. Table 67 below illustrates the aging of populations around the world, with 10 to 18 percent of the respective populations now over the age of sixty-five. Although aging is inevitable, age-associated diseases, disabilities, and premature death should not be. The role of science and medicine is to delay the aging process and prevent age-related disease. However, prevention of all age-related chronic disease must start twenty to forty years before the disease has set in. This simple fact escapes most people until they are stricken by an age-related disease. Predictably, age is seen as the culprit.

Table 67
World Populations Over 65 Years of Age

COUNTRY	TOTAL POPULATION (MILLIONS)	% >65
AUSTRALIA	18	12
CANADA	28	12
FRANCE	59	15
GERMANY	81	15
ISRAEL	5	10
ITALY	58	16
JAPAN	125	14
POLAND	39	11
RUSSIA	150	12
SPAIN	39	15
SWEDEN	9	18
UNITED KINGDOM	58	16
UNITED STATES	270	18

In the United States, a vast amount of our resources is spent for the care of age-associated chronic diseases. Yet very little is being done to prevent or preempt these mostly preventable diseases. Diet and exercise, diabetes and high blood pressure awareness, smoking cessation, seat belt and cholesterol-lowering campaigns, and breast cancer screenings are all primarily directed at young and middle-aged people. Yet all of these measures will benefit older persons at least as much, if not more.

Older women are even more affected by this negative "ageism." In the United States, a third of women past the age of sixty-five have overt, or undiagnosed, coronary artery disease. Cardiovascular diseases are the leading cause of death in women, resulting in over 500,000 deaths each year. There has been an unintentional gender bias on the part of health-care providers and women themselves, which has resulted in the pervasive under-treatment of cardiovascular diseases in women.

Like humans, all animals (including the higher primates) age and die. But unlike humans, animals rarely develop common diseases associated with aging such as cancers, cardiovascular diseases, and diabetes. In humans, the total death rate for cardiovascular diseases, chronic respiratory diseases, and cancers of the lung and digestive tract is over a thousand times greater in the elderly than in young people. This generational inequity need not be inevitable.

Age-associated diseases are not programmed into human genes to blossom at a later date. They are consequences of long-term exposure to a host of risk factors over a period of years. Although old age may be associated with chronic diseases, old age does not cause them. Positive and healthy aging is possible, but it requires active participation as well as an informed health care system, long before many of these cardiovascular, degenerative, or cancerous diseases have set in. It would be morally reprehensible to exclude screening for chronic diseases in older persons solely on the basis of their date of birth. The health, quality of life, and preferences of older persons should be the determining factors in deciding on safe, practical, and cost effective interventions to deal with health-related risk factors.

Older Persons and Cardiovascular Risk Factors

For older persons, the major risk factors for cardiovascular diseases are just as relevant as they are for young or middle-aged people. The individual impact of some of these risk factors, however, may be somewhat different. For example, systolic hypertension, sedentary lifestyle, smoking, elevated homocysteine level, chronic infection with c. pneumonia, low HDL cholesterol, and estrogen deficiency (in women) are more relevant in older persons than other risk factors. More importantly, as people live longer their longevity itself becomes a major determinant of cardiovascular or other acquired degenerative diseases.

Blood Cholesterol Levels in Older Persons

Over the past several years a large number of studies has greatly clarified the relevance of abnormal cholesterol values to cardiovascular diseases among older people. As people age beyond seventy, the blood levels of both LDL and HDL cholesterol tend to go down. Nevertheless, for older people acceptable cholesterol values are essentially the same as for their middle-aged counterparts (Table 3).

Several studies have shown that beyond the age of eighty, slightly elevated LDL cholesterol levels are, paradoxically, associated with less risk of overall deaths than are low LDL cholesterol levels. One reason for this "paradox" has to do with why LDL levels of older persons drop in the first place. Malnutrition due to chronic diseases, poor appetite, or depression will contribute to lower LDL levels. Understandably, older people not afflicted with concurrent diseases that could lower their blood cholesterol levels are healthier, and therefore tend to live longer. In this setting, a higher LDL cholesterol level is a surrogate for better health or, perhaps more accurately, less concurrent diseases. In a recent ten-year study of people over eighty-five (from the Netherlands), higher cholesterol levels were associated with longevity, primarily due to lower mortality from cancers and various infections.

Another reason why elevated LDL cholesterol levels in persons over eighty do not seem to increase the risk of cardiovascular events is that at this age most of the LDL particles are of the large variety which, unlike the small dense variety, are not so harmful. And, by this age, many older persons with high cholesterol levels would have already developed atherosclerosis if they were ever going to develop it. Among older people (over sixty-five), one out of three with elevated cholesterol has overt coronary artery disease. Thus, the older person with high LDL cholesterol and no apparent coronary artery disease may well belong to the other two out of three who are resistant to the negative impact of elevated cholesterol. In addition, as time goes by the independent effect of each risk factor is overshadowed by other age-associated risk factors. Thus, in advanced age the contribution of each risk factor tends to diminish or merge with other risk factors.

Unlike the oldest of the old, for people between the ages of sixty-five and eighty the impact of elevated blood cholesterol is still significant, but not as severe as for younger people. In a recent multicenter study enrolling cases from Massachusetts, Connecticut, and Iowa, four thousand men and women over sixty-five years of age were followed up for four years. After adjustments for other risk factors and markers of poor health and nutrition (such as blood albumin and iron levels), an elevated LDL cholesterol was associated with a 50 percent increase in the risk of death from coronary artery disease.

A recent five-year Scandinavian study of 4,444 men and women with coronary artery disease showed that the use of a cholesterol-lowering drug (Zocor, in this study) reduced major coronary events by about 34 percent. Importantly, the benefits were similar for individuals who were between sixty and seventy at the beginning of the study when compared with those who were younger. Similarly, in another five-year study, 1,283 men and women ages sixty-five to seventy-five who had mildly elevated blood cholesterol levels and a previous heart attack were treated with either a cholesterol-lowering drug (Pravachol) or a placebo. Among those who were given Pravachol, major coronary events were reduced by 32 percent. In this study, older women who were treated with the cholesterol-lowering drug benefited to a much greater extent than men.

Regrettably, in spite of these and other reports which clearly have shown the benefits of cholesterol-lowering in older persons, elevated blood cholesterol in this huge population is still undertreated and misunderstood. A recent study of five hundred men and women with coronary artery disease showed that among persons between the ages of sixty and eighty who had elevated blood cholesterol levels, only a dismal 7 percent used cholesterol-lowering drugs! In the Cardiovascular Health Study, investigators followed up 5,888 healthy men and women sixty-five and older for six years. Among persons with high blood-cholesterol levels who were eligible for cholesterol-lowering drugs after a period of diet therapy, only about 18 percent were ever started on these drugs; for the other eligible 82 percent, their physicians did not prescribe them. Why not?

In older people, the relation between coronary artery disease mortality and low levels of HDL cholesterol is even stronger than it is for elevated LDL cholesterol. At HDL levels between 35 and 49 mg/dl, the risk of coronary artery disease is increased by about 25 percent. But at HDL levels below 35 mg/dl, the risk of suffering a coronary event is more than 200 percent higher than it is at levels above 60 mg/dl. A low HDL cholesterol level is also a significant risk factor for stroke and atherosclerosis of the legs in older persons.

In a recent study, 220 men with an average age of sixty-four and a history of coronary artery disease, were examined by ultrasound to detect thickening of the wall of their carotid arteries (the arteries in the neck that carry blood to the brain). Although LDL cholesterol levels of these men were "desirable," their HDL cholesterol levels were low (an average of 32 mg/dl). In spite of their "desirable" LDL cholesterol levels, more than 80 percent had significant atherosclerosis of their carotid arteries, a precursor of stroke. Several other studies have also shown a significant association between both elevated LDL cholesterol or a low HDL cholesterol level and the risk of stroke.

Recent data have shown that noninvasive measurements of the thickness of the wall of the carotid arteries using ultrasound provide valuable information about the future risk of a cardiovascular event in older persons. In a multicenter study, 4,476 men and women sixty-five or older without previous cardiovascular diseases were followed up for an average of six years. Those with the highest thickness of their carotid arteries at entry into the study had a risk of heart attack or stroke that was more than three times greater than older persons with the lowest thickness. In other words, vascular wall thickness is indicative of a silent or hidden atherosclerotic process that involves many arteries and not just the carotids.

What You Should Do

You should have thorough, annual physical examinations to find out whether you have any evidence of atherosclerosis of the carotid or coronary arteries and poor circulation in the lower extremities, or high blood pressure. Necessary blood tests should include LDL cholesterol, HDL cholesterol, triglycerides, blood sugar, kidney and liver function tests, along with a blood count to make sure you are not anemic or do not have a high hematocrit. Since the presence of an underactive thyroid gland in the elderly is quite variable and may include elevated LDL cholesterol or low HDL cholesterol levels, you should also have a TSH test (the most accurate test to detect an underactive or overactive thyroid gland) every year.

As noted above, an ultrasound measurement of the thickness of the carotid artery wall should be obtained by an older person at least every two years. If you have developed thickened arterial walls, you will require a more aggressive treatment to reduce as many coronary risk factors as possible.

The treatment of abnormal cholesterol levels in the elderly cannot be done without regard to other medical problems. For example, an elevated blood cholesterol level in a person with dementia or multiple chronic medical problems may not need treatment, whereas in an otherwise healthy elderly person or one with coronary artery disease who is still functional and enjoys his or her life, it should be vigorously treated.

As with all other medical decisions, the management of cholesterol disorders in older persons must be individualized without regard to someone's birthdate. The treatments of cholesterol disorders in older persons are not appreciably different from those recommended for young or middle-aged persons. Rigid and impractical programs have even less relevance to older persons.

Although the late Arthur Fiedler's remark "He who rests, rots!" applies to older persons better than all other age groups, exercise regimens for older persons must begin with low-impact, low-intensity workouts and advance slowly over many weeks to months. In fact, if you do nothing else, exercising on a regular (hopefully daily) basis is the best thing you can do to reduce your risk of a disabling or fatal cardiovascular event by at least 50 percent. Recent data have shown that for this age group, mild to moderate weight training or resistance exercises not only increase strength by 25 to 100 percent, they also increase the bone density and lower the blood pressure and LDL cholesterol. Even one set of ten to fifteen repetitions of eight to ten different exercises several times a week may be adequate for older persons.

The adoption of a TRF diet with daily scores of about +30 provides older persons with varied choices and a dietary regimen that is suitable for almost any coexistent disease they might have. Almost all older persons should also take a low-dose aspirin (81 mg), vitamin E (400-800 IU), and folic acid (800 mcg or higher) on a daily basis. The use of cholesterol-altering or other cardio-protective drugs requires judicious and thoughtful consideration for each individual. In general, the approach to prevention or treatment of coronary risk factors of an older person should be the same as if they were in their fifties or sixties. In preventing coronary artery disease, we should learn to ignore birthdates.

(18) Premature Coronary Artery Disease in a Close Family Member

Among the twenty major risk factors for coronary artery disease listed in Chapter 1, at least half are fully or partially inherited disorders. Many of the nongenetic risk factors are also influenced by such factors as family environment, culture, lifestyle, and diet. Overall, nearly 80 percent of people with coronary artery disease have at least one inherited disorder that interacts with other nongenetic coronary risk factors. More than 50 percent of the relatives of coronary artery disease cases also have at least one genetic risk factor for the disease.

Some genetic disorders are easy to detect and understand, provided they are looked for. Examples are elevated LDL cholesterol and triglycerides, low levels of HDL cholesterol, diabetes, and hypertension. Others need further prodding such as elevated lipoprotein(a), homocysteine, fibrinogen, and the preponderance of small, dense LDL particles. But a vast number of genetic disorders involving various antioxidants, enzymes, and receptors are still only in the research stage.[27]

What You Should Do

No matter what kind of unfriendly genetic "baggage" you are saddled with (see Table 68), they are all at least partially modifiable. In other words, even though someone is genetically programmed—a high blood cholesterol or homocysteine level, for example—many ways exist to counteract these familial risk factors. A family history of premature coronary artery disease before the age of fifty-five in one or more first-degree relatives is a strong indicator of an inheritable, familial disorder which almost always can be identified with appropriate tests. If you have such a strong family history, even in the absence of other personal risk factors, you must be thoroughly evaluated. All coexistent risk factors, even the minor ones, should be looked for and addressed. Preemptive intervention must be started as early, and carried out as consistently, as possible.

In Part III, I have introduced a valid tool with which you can calculate your risk of a future heart attack. The goal is not to frighten you into submission, but to highlight your risks and encourage you to be more proactive with preemptive intervention. Because the impact of genetic factors is lifelong, short-term interventions provide very little or no protection. Lowering your homocysteine or blood cholesterol for two months, or treating hypertension and diabetes for six months, cannot be expected to offer lasting protection against coronary artery disease and its catastrophic complications. Once the familial predisposition to coronary artery disease has been established, intervention and treatment will always be long term.[28] In addition, if you have any genetic risk factors, all your siblings and children should be screened for similar coronary risk factors. Children can be screened beginning at the age of ten.

Table 68
Genetic Factors and Coronary Artery Disease
(Per 1 oz)

GENETIC DISORDERS	WHAT THEY CAUSE
LDL-RECEPTOR MUTATIONS	ELEVATED LDL CHOLESTEROL
LDL-RECEPTOR DEFICIENCY	ELEVATED LDL CHOLESTEROL
APOPROTEIN E4	ELEVATED LDL CHOLESTEROL
APOPROTEIN E2	LOW LEVELS OF LDL CHOLESTEROL
GENE FOR SMALL, DENSE LDL	SMALL, DENSE LDL PARTICLES
MUTATIONS IN APOPROTEIN A-1	LOW HDL CHOLESTEROL LEVEL
PARAOXONASE AA	EFFICIENT HDL CHOLESTEROL
PARAOXONASE BB	INEFFICIENT HDL CHOLESTEROL
MUTATIONS IN CHOLESTEROL-TRANSFER PROTEIN	ELEVATED LDL & VLDL CHOLESTEROL
MUTATIONS IN LIPOPROTEIN LIPASE	ELEVATED TRIGLYCERIDES
FAMILIAL GENE FOR LIPOPROTEIN(A)	ELEVATED LIPOPROTEIN(A)
MUTATIONS IN ENZYMES RESPONSIBLE FOR BREAKDOWN OF HOMOCYSTEINE	ELEVATED HOMOCYSTEINE LEVEL
FAMILIAL DIABETES	MATURITY-ONSET DIABETES
FAMILIAL HYPERTENSION (MULTIPLE GENES)	HIGH BLOOD PRESSURE
LOW BIRTH WEIGHT (MULTIPLE GENE MUTATIONS)	MULTIPLE CORONARY RISK FACTORS
VARIOUS KIDNEY-RELATED GENES	HYPERTENSION

(19) Personal History of Cardiovascular Disease

In people who have suffered heart attacks or have angina, the issue is no longer prevention of coronary artery disease. They already have it. Intervention for these people is entirely different, more urgent, and must be more aggressive in order to:

(1) stabilize their coronary plaques

(2) prevent a new coronary event

(3) slow down or stop further progression of their disease and involvement of other segments of the coronary artery

Regression or shrinking of coronary lesions is a desirable goal, but it takes time. Recent studies using ultra-fast CAT scans have shown that as the LDL cholesterol level is lowered to less than 100 mg/dl, the size of many coronary lesions decreases within one to two years. The reduction occurs almost exclusively by cutting down both the number of foam cells (the white blood cells stuffed with LDL cholesterol) and the amount of cholesterol they contain.

Of course, when regression occurs, it is not universal throughout the length of the coronary artery or other blood vessels. This is because plaques in different segments of an artery have different structures and vary in severity. Some lesions have developed severe scarring and are packed with immovable debris made of trapped cholesterol, white and red blood cells, fibrous tissue, smooth muscle cells, and a host of mineral deposits. This nearly ossified or bone-like structure of plaques also explains why chelation therapy is useless.

Other plaques may have less fibrous material, overgrown smooth muscle cells, or calcium deposits, but they may be more fatty and more inflamed. This combination makes the plaques quite unstable and vulnerable to rupture, setting the scene for a heart attack. Although these unstable plaques account for only about 20 percent of coronary lesions, they are responsible for 80 percent of all heart attacks. On angiograms—pictures obtained after injecting dye into a coronary artery through a catheter—these lesions may not be picked up, or may not be large enough to cause a substantial obstruction to coronary blood flow. Yet they are the true "fox in the chicken coop." This is one major reason why angioplasties of flow-obstructing lesions do not significantly reduce the risk of future heart attacks.

An established coronary artery disease is nearly always the end result of multiple coexisting coronary risk factors which have created havoc in the arterial wall for many years. As long as the process of the coronary quartet (Chapter 1) continues, so does the instability of plaques and the high probability of a new heart attack. In the Scandinavian study of 4,444 men with coronary artery disease and multiple risk factors, among those who were treated with a rigid low-fat, low-cholesterol diet, 28 percent suffered a heart attack during the five-year follow-up period. Treatment with cholesterol-lowering statins lowered the risk by a third (20 percent of treated individuals suffered a recurrent event compared to 28 percent of those not treated with cholesterol-lowering drugs). Among participants in two other studies of men and women with coronary artery disease, but with a relatively lower risk profile than the subjects in the Scandinavian study, recurrent events were considerably lower. These contrasting findings point out the primacy of reducing or eliminating as many risk factors as possible if the goal is to drastically reduce the chance of a future heart attack.

What You Should Do

People with preexisting coronary artery disease do not have the luxury to procrastinate or to manage their life-threatening disease in a piece-meal fashion. Whatever time they have should not be wasted on useless low-fat, low-cholesterol diets, half-measures, herbal supplements, or worse, doing nothing.

If you have already had a coronary event (angina, heart attack, angio-plasty, or bypass surgery), you should ask your doctor to check you for all twenty major and twenty minor coronary risk factors. Almost surely you need a variety of interventions to correct, or at least modify, your risk factors. A monothematic approach, such as cholesterol-lowering alone, is insufficient no matter how successful it may appear in the short term. These simplistic approaches are the reason why nearly one out of five with coronary artery disease treated solely with low fat, low-cholesterol diets and cholesterol-lowering drugs will still suffer a fatal or nonfatal heart attack within five years. What is heartbreaking is that most of these disabilities and deaths are completely preventable.

Sometimes when people find out that they have coronary artery disease in the course of routine examinations, stress tests, echocardiograms, thalium studies, heart scans, or angiograms, they proudly announce, "fortunately my heart problem was detected before I had a heart attack." Although these individuals have not suffered a heart attack, the goal must never be to wait until they have their first one. These people must be treated just as vigorously as if they had already suffered a heart attack. This is where prevention and preemption is paramount, because for many, the difference between primary intervention (in the case of those who have not yet had a heart attack) and secondary intervention (in the case of those who have suffered a previous heart attack) may be a matter of hours! That's why quibbling about primary versus secondary intervention is a frivolous and myopic argument among doctors and health care managers.

In the United States more than 60 percent of men and over 50 percent of women eventually die of cardiovascular diseases. The tragedy is that many of these—certainly the majority of the premature disabilities and deaths from cardiovascular disease—are preventable. But effective prevention requires early, all-inclusive, multifaceted, and continuous lifelong intervention. Shortcuts, undertreatment, or belated, half-hearted attempts at treating only one or two risk factors should no longer be accepted as adequate intervention.

At the dawn of the twenty-first century, we should not allow nearly one million Americans, many of them in the prime of life, to die each year, while countless others become disabled, from cardiovascular disease.

(20) A Typical Western Diet

What's wrong with a typical Western diet? It is true that no single meal, no matter how high its TRF Score, can cause irreparable harm to anyone's coronary artery. But the long-term consequence of frequent dietary intemperance is a significant increase in the risk of coronary artery disease, stroke, dementia, abdominal obesity, and diabetes, as well as breast, colon, and prostate cancers.

The problem with a Western diet is not just its overabundance of salt, saturated fat, and cholesterol. It is all of these plus vastly too many trans fatty acids, hydrogenated vegetable fats (margarines and shortenings), carbohydrates, and calories. This dietary imbalance is made even worse by inadequate intake of monounsaturated fat, omega-3 polyunsaturated fat (mainly seafood), antioxidants, and anti-carcinogens (mainly deeply colored fruits and vegetables).

And the typical Western diet is getting worse. In the past several years, for example, the number of steakhouses in the United States has mushroomed. Fifteen and twenty ounce T-bone or New York steaks are commonly featured in these restaurants, often accompanied by baked potatoes with butter and sour cream, large orders of french fries, or fried onion rings. By the time you have finished the desert, the total TRF score of your meal is well over +120. This equals the total scores of four days on a prudent diet.

Our increasing reliance on fast food makes the nutritional landscape even more dire. At Burger King, a double Whopper with cheese plus a king-size order of fries provides you with 97 grams of fat (38 grams of which are saturated), several grams of trans fatty acids, and 1,880 calories. Since the total daily intake of saturated fat should be less than 15 gm and the total of trans fatty acids less than one gm, this single meal packs the equivalent of two to three days worth of these undesirable fats. Burger King is certainly not the only culprit. Nearly all other fast food eateries, cafeterias (including those at schools and military bases), and restaurants are also guilty of similar nutritional assault and battery. Any other public health threat of similar magnitude would quickly be outlawed.

Obviously, all Western meals are not 20 ounce steaks or Double Whoppers. In fact, the main problem is not the red meat but the fat: primarily saturated fat, partially hydrogenated fat, and trans fat. Unfortunately, fatty meats, pizzas, deep-fried dishes, hot dogs, sausages, and greasy fast foods are staples of the American diet (and most Western diets). We further compound the problem by consuming snacks and desserts laden with hundreds of unneeded calories and plenty of trans fatty acids and saturated fats (such as chips, pastries, cakes, cookies, donuts, pies, and chocolate). This unbalanced dietary overload combined with the epidemic of sedentary lifestyle is not only coronary-unfriendly but carcinogenic as well. The dramatic rise in the number of Americans suffering from obesity and type 2 diabetes (Part II) is primarily a consequence of unhealthy diets and sedentary lifestyles which start during childhood or adolescence and continue into adult life.

What You Should Do

As noted in Part II, food is not the enemy, as long as you choose properly. Although a typical Western diet is not the sole cause of coronary artery disease, it paves the way for all the other risk factors and sabotages your effort to control them. Pills and supplements are not substitutes for good nutrition. The Twenty Risk Factor Diet provides you with a vast number of healthy choices that can serve as alternatives to standard Western fare.

Part III:
How to Estimate Your Own Risk of a Heart Attack

How to Estimate Your Own Risk of a Heart Attack

As noted in previous chapters, more than 50 percent of men and women in the United States die of cardiovascular diseases. Many of these deaths and cardiovascular disease-related disabilities occur in people who are in their forties or fifties. Although you can argue that "we all have to die of something," it is a defeatist and irrational argument. Why would anyone in his or her prime want to suffer a disabling or fatal heart attack?

Unlike strep throat, pneumonia, or appendicitis, which are almost always random events, people are not suddenly struck by heart attacks. A heart attack is the culmination of long-term exposure to multiple risk factors. Eliminate or greatly modify these risk factors, and you can prevent practically *every* heart attack.

Because coronary artery disease is multifaceted, the risk profile of an individual depends on the number and strength of each risk factor. Thus, to forecast someone's long-term probability or risk of heart attack accurately, most, or preferably all, of the risk factors should be considered.

Among the twenty major risk factors for coronary artery disease, ten can be determined on the first visit to a health care provider who is interested in the prevention and management of coronary artery disease. (Among the twenty minor risk factors, thirteen can be determined just as easily.) Age, gender, weight, abdominal obesity, smoking, dietary habits, level of physical activity, birth weight, family history of coronary artery disease, personal history of coronary artery disease, negative affect, and blood pressure are all readily determined. Six more major risk factors (blood levels of triglycerides, HDL cholesterol, LDL cholesterol, hematocrit levels, platelet count, and blood sugar) along with four minor risk factors (kidney and thyroid function, blood type, and a test for lupus) can all be determined with routine blood tests which are available everywhere. Thus, of the forty major and minor risk factors, only four major and three minor risk factors require additional testing. The remaining four major risk factors are: blood levels of lipoprotein(a), homocysteine, fibrinogen, and c. pneumoniae antibody along with C-reactive protein indicating a smoldering inflammatory or infectious process. All of these require special testing.

Tables 69 and 70 provide a comprehensive risk assessment tool that can be used at home or by health care providers to estimate accurately the ten-year probability of a coronary event for a person with a given set of risk factors. To improve the accuracy of risk estimates, data from numerous long-term studies of coronary risk factors have been pooled and incorporated into this model. Thus, the risk-estimate charts introduced here represent the most thorough and accurate tool that has *ever* been developed. Although the precision of risk estimates is improved by the inclusion of all major risk factors, enough flexibility is built into these estimates to allow an accurate assessment of the ten-year probability of a coronary event even if some are not included.

Ideally, the estimated ten-year risk of a coronary event for both men and women under sixty years of age should be close to zero. But since at least one-half of men between fifty and sixty (and one-third of women) have some degree of coronary artery disease, the average risk for the general population is much higher, ranging from 10 to 20 percent. When the ten-year risk of a coronary event is 20 percent or higher, vigorous intervention is essential. A doctor's assurance that "your risk is no higher than the average" is no longer acceptable, since this "average" risk reflects the failure to curb the epidemic of coronary artery disease. We must, and we can, do much better.

Even if you eliminate a few risk factors (such as smoking, abdominal obesity, sedentary lifestyle) and start a diet with TRF scores of under +30 per day, you can lower your risk of a coronary event by more than 80 percent. If you control other risk factors such as high cholesterol of homocysteine levels, you will be rewarded with even greater protection against coronary events or strokes. As an example, let us estimate the ten-year probability of a heart attack for Mr. Richard W, a fifty-year-old man (+6), nonsmoker (0), with abdominal obesity (+2) and sedentary lifestyle (+3), whose blood pressure and blood sugar are normal (0). His father and uncle had heart attacks in their midfifties (+5). His diet is essentially "meat and potatoes" (+3), and his recent blood tests showed LDL cholesterol of 151 (+3), HDL of 37 (+2), and normal triglycerides (0), with homocysteine level of 15 mmol/dl (+3), and a C-reactive protein level of 0.90 mg/dl (+3). His total score is +27. The accompanying graph shows that Mr. W's ten-year probability of having a heart attack is about 60 percent, an enormously high risk. Fortunately, most of his risk factors are modifiable and his risk can be dramatically reduced if he adheres to the group of interventions recommended to him. Do you know what your coronary risk factors are? Not knowing them will not make them go away. Every day you procrastinate, you fall farther and farther behind.

Table 69
Scores for Coronary Risk Factors

AGE	MALE	31-33	-1
		33-35	0
		36-38	+2
		39-40	+3
		40-45	+4
		46-50	+6
		51-55	+8
		56-65	+10
		>65	+12
	FEMALE	30-35	-5
		36-38	-2
		39-40	0
		40-45	+2
		46-50	+3
		51-55	+5
		56-65	+8
		>65	+10
SMOKING			+3
ABDOMINAL OBESITY			+2
EXERCISE LEVEL		SEDENTARY	+3
		LIGHT	-1
		MODERATE	-2
		HIGH	-3
DIABETES			+5
HYPERTENSION			+2
FAMILY HISTORY OF CAD (IN MEMBERS <55 YEARS OF AGE)			+5

Table 69 continued on next page

Table 69 continued

PERSONAL (PREVIOUS) HISTORY OF CAD			+10
DIET: DAILY TRF SCORES		>+40	3
		+30 to +40	1
		<+30	-3
		<+20	-5
REACTION PROTEIN		>0.40 MG/DL	+3
	LDL	100-130 MG/DL	+1
		131-160 MG/DL	+2
		>161 MG/DL	+3
		<30	+5
BLOOD LEVELS:	HDL	31-35	+3
		36-40	+2
		41-45	+1
		46-55	-1
		56-65	-3
		>65	-5
	TRIGLYCERIDES	<150	0
		150-200	+1
		>100	+3

Elevated blood fibrinogen, homocysteine, lipoprotein(a), and hematocrit >48%, each counts as +3.

Table 70
Comparison of Estimated 10-Year
Probability of a Future Heart Attack

Score		% Risk of Coronary Event
0		0
0-5		10
6-10		20
11-15		30
16-20		40
21-25		50
26-30		60
31-35		70
36-40		80
41-45		90
>46		100

Average 10-Year Risk* of a Coronary Event in General Population

AGE	MEN	WOMEN
30-35	3%	<1%
36-40	5%	1%
41-45	6%	2%
46-50	10%	5%
51-55	15%	10%
56-60	20%	15%
61-65	25%	20%
>65	35%	25%

* These unacceptably high risks reflect the presence of multiple coronary risk factors in general population.

Appendix A
Non-herbal Supplements and Cardiovascular Health

DHEA: Dihydro-Epi-Androsterone

DHEA is an androgenic (testosterone-like) hormone produced in the adrenal glands of both men and women. DHEA (and DHEAS, produced when a sulfate molecule is added to DHEA in the liver) has recently achieved stardom in the realm of supplement therapy. It is credited to do whatever the seller and the consumer want it to do. The long list includes: prevention of heart attacks, cancers, Alzheimer's disease, diabetes, aging, and osteoporosis; strengthening of the immune system; improving libido and curing sexual dysfunctions in both men and women; improving memory, relieving depression, burning off fat, and helping to build lean body mass and to improve athletic performance.

The wide-ranging "benefits" of DHEA are often the creation of advertisers, or the testimonials of well-paid celebrities. Very few rigorous scientific studies are available to support most of these claims. In fact, the Food and Drug Administration banned the sale of DHEA in 1985 based on false advertising claims. In 1994 the ban was lifted under the poorly conceived law that was heavily lobbied for by the supplement industry, the Dietary and Supplement Health and Education Act of 1994.

DHEA is present in the bloodstream principally in its sulfated version, DHEAS. Its concentration peaks at about age twenty and declines thereafter, so that by age sixty, its blood levels are about one-third what they were at age twenty. There are, of course, considerable variations; in some the decline is much less than in others.

Depression, cardiovascular diseases, diabetes, cancers, and many other acute and chronic diseases lower blood levels of DHEA and DHEAS. In other words, these various diseases are the cause and not the result of low blood concentrations of DHEA/DHEAS.

A troubling concern with supplemental DHEA is the possibility that at higher doses it may increase the risk of prostate cancer. Among people who take DHEA at doses of 25-50 mg daily, blood levels of a biologically active protein called "IGF-1" (insulin-like growth factor-1) rises by as much as 50 percent. A recent Harvard University study showed that men with high levels of IGF-1 had a more than 400 percent increase in their risk of developing prostate cancer. Even more alarming, in men over sixty years of age (those who are targeted most by advertisers and promoters of DHEA), the risk was 800 percent higher. Another concern is that heart rhythm irregularities can also occur in men and women who take DHEA. Thus, far from being cardio-protective, high doses of DHEA may actually be cardio-toxic.

DHEA at doses of 25-50 mg per day may have some minimal androgenic effects that might improve libido, fatigue, and perhaps memory during treatment. Since DHEA supplements will suppress the body's own production of these hormones, their use is quite inappropriate in persons from fifty to sixty years of age, quite irrational in those under the age of fifty, and even more so in those younger than forty. DHEA is an androgenic sex hormone, and if you have a family or personal history of breast, ovary, or prostate cancers, you should use the lowest doses (5-10 mg per day), if at all. Also, doses exceeding 25-50 mg per day may result in oily skin, acne, hair loss, irritability, fatigue, testicular atrophy, insulin resistance, hypertension, elevated LDL cholesterol and triglycerides, or lower HDL levels, hepatitis, and, if used by adolescents, short stature. It can also cause facial hair growth and male-pattern baldness in women. In athletes, bodybuilders, or overweight persons, contrary to misinformation, there is no evidence to suggest that DHEA, by itself and without vigorous exercises, has any impact on increasing lean body mass or "melting" body fat. The concern over DHEA's role in promoting coronary artery disease and the development of prostate cancer strongly argue against its use in doses exceeding 5-10 mg per day.

Certain DHEA products are promoted as "natural plant DHEA," with the misleading impression that because they are plant-source DHEA, they are better and safer. These products invariably use Mexican yam or wild yam which contains a compound that in the laboratory can be converted to DHEA. The problem is that such a chemical conversion does not occur in the body, making these so-called natural products totally useless. Beyond the narrow indications noted above, DHEA has no other significant virtue and may well be cardio-toxic and carcinogenic. Most certainly, DHEA is not the "fountain of youth."

Androstenedione

Androstenedione (often called "andro" and popularized by Mark McGwire, the "home run king") is very close to DHEA. Although a small portion of andro is converted to testosterone by the liver, a larger part is actually converted to the female hormones estradiol and estrone, which contribute to breast enlargement in men. Testosterone itself may help to strengthen muscles in athletes who exercise vigorously, but it does very little muscle building in a sedentary person. A recent study from Iowa State University showed that androstenedione, even in high doses (300 mg per day) did not strengthen muscles any more than a placebo, but reduced the HDL cholesterol level by 12 percent.

There is no doubt that long-term use of andro, by raising the LDL and lowering the HDL, will have a negative cardiovascular impact, especially among those with cholesterol disorders. A recent Australian study showed that exposure to androgenic hormones increases the adhesion of white blood cells (monocytes) to the endothelial lining of the arteries. As noted in Chapter 1, one of the prerequisites of coronary artery disease is the adhesion of monocytes to, and their subsequent trespassing through, the inner lining of the arterial wall, where they gobble up oxidized LDL and trigger coronary plaques.

Other adverse effects in men include acne, decreased production of natural testosterone by testicles and adrenal glands, infertility, testicular atrophy, enlarged breasts which may be irreversible, and the increased risk of prostate cancer. In women, it can cause a deeper voice which may be permanent, facial and body hair growth, which may also be irreversible, and acne, baldness, and coarsening of the skin, all of which may last for a long time even after the andro is stopped.

If you are an athlete, short-term use of small doses of andro may be harmless, and may help to strengthen the muscles when combined with bodybuilding exercises. However, in youngsters who have not completed their physical growth, andro may cause early termination of bone growth and result in short stature, testicular atrophy, acne, and many of the other undesirable side effects listed for DHEA. Overall, there is little justification or indication for using any amount of andro, especially for more than three to four months.

Andro is a drug far more potent than DHEA and has multiple side effects that should prohibit its sale as a nutritional supplement. The International Olympic Committee, the National Collegiate Athletics Association, the National Football League, and other athletic organizations should be given credit for banning the substance. Hopefully the baseball leagues will do likewise.

Appendix B
Estrogen Replacement Therapy and Cardiovascular Health

Over the past century, the average lifespan of women in the United States has increased by more than thirty years. This dramatic increase has not been the result of any notable genetic or physical changes in the human body: such changes require thousands of years. In fact, this impressive increase in longevity is the direct consequence of better medical care, management of infections, and public health advances, all of which are extraneous to genetics.

One consequence of longevity is longer exposure to a multitude of disease-producing or degenerative risk factors from which humans do not necessarily have an innate resistance. A passive attitude turns what should be a healthful aging process into an unhealthy cascade of age-associated diseases: from coronary artery disease and strokes, to degenerative bone and joint diseases, osteoporosis, cancers, and dementia.

Women have the good fortune to live longer than men by an average of five to ten years. But genetically, women are programmed to cease ovulating and producing estrogen from their ovaries by the time they are about forty-five years of age, while their male counterparts continue to have functioning testicles and producing testosterone and sperm into old age. Because most women now live thirty to forty years beyond their forced menopause, their programmed estrogen starvation seems to be a grand biological error.

Long-term estrogen-deprivation contributes to a large number of age-associated diseases and degenerative processes, including coronary artery disease, osteoporosis, macular degeneration of retina, depression, and dementia. Fortunately, Mother Nature's seeming blunder can be countered by estrogen-replacement therapy (or hormone replacement therapy, as it is often referred to).

It is now clear that coronary artery disease is gender blind. As seen in Table 71, cardiovascular diseases claim more lives among women than the next seven most common causes of death.

Table 71
Most Common Causes of Death
(Per Year)

MEN	#	WOMEN	#
CARDIOVASCULAR DISEASES	436,000	CARDIOVASCULAR DISEASES	505,000
CANCER	280,000	CANCERS (BREAST: 43,000)	250,000
ACCIDENTS	61,000	CHRONIC LUNG DISEASES	47,000
CHRONIC LUNG DISEASES	55,000	PNEUMONIA & INFLUENZA	45,000
SUICIDES & HOMICIDES	46,000	ACCIDENTS	31,000
PNEUMONIA & INFLUENZA	38,000	DIABETES	31,000
HIV INFECTION	32,000	KIDNEY DISEASE	21,000

The evidence favoring estrogen replacement therapy in women to lower the risk of coronary artery disease is now quite compelling:

In a recent multicenter study, 9,704 women who were sixty-five years of age or older were followed up for an average of six years. These women were from four separate communities: Portland, Oregon; Minneapolis, Minnesota; Baltimore, Maryland; and Pittsburgh, Pennsylvania. Overall, 1,258 women were taking estrogen replacement therapy, primarily to prevent or treat osteoporosis. During the six year follow-up period, cardiovascular deaths were 70 percent lower among current estrogen replacement therapy users when compared with those who had never used it. Death rates due to all cancers were also 40 percent lower as compared to those who didn't use estrogen. Beyond the age of seventy-five, the benefit of estrogen replacement therapy gradually fell, so that there was practically no net benefit for women over the age of eighty-five.

In the United States Nurses Health Study, 121,700 women between thirty and fifty-five years of age were followed up for eighteen years. Among them, there were 3,637 deaths during the course of the follow-up. Each woman who died was matched against ten who lived. Current estrogen users had a death rate 37 percent lower than nonusers. The greatest benefit was seen among women with one or more coronary risk factors; these had a 49 percent lower risk of dying from coronary artery disease. Estrogen replacement therapy benefits gradually decreased after ten years of continuous use, but women who used estrogen replacement therapy for more than ten years still had a 20 percent risk reduction. The lower mortality from coronary artery disease was, as expected, less apparent in women who had no coronary risk factors.

Breast Cancer and Estrogen Replacement Therapy

Although estrogen replacement therapy can reduce the risk of a heart attack among women who do not have advanced coronary artery disease, millions of women do not take it. The primary concern of almost all of them is the risk of breast cancer associated with long-term estrogen replacement therapy. Most people confuse the *incidence* (or the risk of developing) breast cancer with *mortality* (or death) from breast cancer. They are actually quite distinct.

The Impact of Hormone Replacement Therapy on Breast Cancer Incidence

In an analysis of fifty-one studies conducted in North America and Europe, nearly 54,000 women with breast cancer were compared with 108,400 women without breast cancer. The average incidence of breast cancer for women fifty and seventy years of age who did not take estrogen replacement therapy was 45 per 1,000 women. After five years of estrogen replacement therapy, only two additional cases of breast cancer per 1,000 women were seen, a 0.2 percent absolute increase. Among women who had used estrogen replacement therapy for ten to fifteen consecutive years, 6 to 12 additional cases per 1,000 developed breast cancer, a 0.6 to 1.2 percent increase. This massive study, along with other data collected from women who had used high-dose estrogen replacement therapy (high doses, the standard practice before the mid-1990s, are no longer used), show that there is a slight increase in the rate of breast cancer *incidence* among long-term users of high-dose estrogen replacement therapy. Even among these high-dose users, the absolute risk was extremely small: an increase of 0.2 percent after five years, and 0.6 percent after ten years. Moreover, a large majority of these women were taking a combination of estrogen and progesterone. Recent studies suggest that the combination is more likely to increase the risk of breast cancer than estrogens alone.

The Impact of Estrogen Replacement Therapy on Breast Cancer Mortality

Unlike its incidence, *mortality* from breast cancer declines as a percentage of overall deaths as women age. For example, out of one thousand women in their forties and fifties, about nine are likely to die of breast cancer and another nine from cardiovascular diseases. But in their sixties and seventies, eighteen will die of breast cancer compared with 105 from cardiovascular diseases.

In the United States each year, 500,000 women die of cardiovascular diseases and 65,000 from complications due to osteoporosis, as compared to 43,000 from breast cancer (see Table 71). Although the incidence of breast cancer among women has increased in the past twenty-five years (from 85 cases per 100,000 in 1975 to about 115 per 100,000 in 1999) mortality has continuously declined. Between 1990 and 1999, for example, breast cancer deaths in the United States and Great Britain decreased by 20 percent, mainly because of early detection and more effective treatment options. If we make the most conservative assumption that estrogen replacement therapy can reduce cardiovascular- and osteoporosis-related deaths by 20 percent (most studies suggest a more than 40 percent risk reduction), each year approximately 110,000 lives can be saved if women at risk for cardiovascular diseases take estrogen replacement therapy. On the other hand, if we make a gross overestimation that 2 percent of breast cancer deaths could be attributed to estrogen replacement therapy (by assuming that all post-menopausal women take it for more than ten years), 860 more lives would be lost from breast cancer. Saving 110,000 lives each year seems to argue in favor of estrogen replacement therapy. Of course, these numbers do not even include all the other benefits of estrogen replacement therapy as summarized in Table 72.

The other good news is that a number of studies have shown that breast cancers discovered in estrogen replacement therapy users are less advanced and associated with much *lower* mortality than breast cancers found among nonusers. For example, a recent study sponsored by the American Cancer Society showed *lower* mortality rates from breast cancer among estrogen replacement therapy users. These data were based on a nine-year follow-up of more than 422,000 post-menopausal women who were cancer-free when they began estrogen replacement therapy. Highlights of this study were:

The risk of breast cancer deaths decreased with younger age when estrogen replacement therapy was started. Women who started estrogen replacement therapy before the age of forty had a 34 percent *lower* risk of dying of breast cancer than women who had never used it. In women who were between forty and forty-nine years of age when they started estrogen replacement therapy, the risk was 16 percent *lower*, and among those over fifty, the risk was 11 percent *lower* than it was for those who never used estrogen replacement therapy.

Among women with a family history of breast cancer, estrogen replacement therapy users showed the same benefits that it showed in those without a family history of the disease.

The lower mortality from breast cancer among women on estrogen replacement therapy has a number of plausible explanations. Women who take estrogen replacement therapy seem to be more health-conscious, smoke less, exercise more regularly, and are less obese. They also see their physicians more frequently so that their breast lesions are detected earlier.

Does estrogen replacement therapy increase the risk of uterine cancer? Although estrogens without progesterone can increase the growth of uterine lining and theoretically can contribute to a few cancers, women with an intact uterus are practically never placed on estrogen alone. In fact, the incidence of uterine cancer in the United States has actually declined slightly since the 1970s, even though progressively larger numbers of women have taken estrogen replacement therapy during the same period.

Overall, uterine cancers account for only 2 percent of all cancer deaths in women (about 3 cases per 100,000 women); colon cancer deaths are six times more common. Estrogen replacement therapy can reduce colon cancer deaths among women dramatically while its role in contributing to uterine cancer is minimal.

Table 72
Potential Impact of Hormone Replacement Therapy

BENEFITS	**REDUCES:**
	LDL CHOLESTEROL BY >10%
	LIPOPROTEIN(A) BY >20%
	RISK OF CARDIOVASCULAR DISEASES BY 40-50%
	ALL-CAUSE DEATHS BY 40%
	OSTEOPOROSIS-RELATED DEATHS BY 50%
	RISK OF ALZHEIMER'S DISEASE BY 60%
	RISK OF CLINICAL DEPRESSION BY 30%
	RISK OF DEGENERATIVE OSTEOARTHRITIS, DIABETES, AND PREMATURE AGING
	SIGNS & SYMPTOMS OF MENOPAUSE
	COLO-RECTAL CANCER BY 35%
	DEATH RATE FROM BREAST CANCER BY 34% AMONG WOMEN <40 YEARS OF AGE, BY 16% IN THOSE 40-49 YEARS, AND BY 10% IN THOSE >50 YEARS OF AGE
POSSIBLE SIDE EFFECTS	**INCREASES:**
	HDL CHOLESTEROL BY 10%
	BONE MINERAL DENSITY BY >5%
	LIBIDO, VIGOR, AND SENSE OF WELL-BEING
	BREAST "CONGESTION" OR TENDERNESS (LESS WITH LOWER DOSES)
	RECURRENCE OF MONTHLY MENSTRUAL CYCLES (AVOIDABLE WITH CONTINUOUS ESTROGEN & PROGESTERONE THERAPY)
	POSSIBLE SIDE EFFECTS MAY INCREASE THE RISK OF BREAST CANCER AFTER 10 YEARS OF CONTINUOUS USE BY 0.6% (WITH HIGHER DOSES)
	MAY INCREASE THE RISK OF UTERINE CANCER SLIGHTLY (BUT NOT IN THOSE ON ESTROGEN & PROGESTERONE THERAPY)

Plant Estrogens (Phyto-estrogens) vs. Estrogens

Although about forty million American women are candidates for estrogen replacement therapy, only one-third take it. Misinformation and fear about possible side effects of estrogens have contributed to a new growth industry in plant estrogens.

Plant or phyto-estrogens are a group of naturally occurring chemical compounds in many edible plants, with chemical structures and biological actions similar to estrogen hormones. Recent data from experiments on primates (and a limited number of studies on humans) have suggested that plant estrogens may have some health-promoting benefits without significant adverse effects on the breast or uterus.

Among developed countries, Japanese women have the lowest rates of breast and uterine cancers. Recent studies have shown that Japanese women produce as much as eighty-five times more phyto-estrogens in their urine than white American women. This tremendous difference reflects the very high intake of phyto-estrogens (on average about 200 mg per day, mostly from soy products) of Japanese women, resulting in phyto-estrogen blood levels that are usually a few thousand times higher than their natural estrogens produced by ovaries. Although phyto-estrogens are given credit for the lower breast cancer rate among these women, Japanese women also have a number of other genetic and lifestyle factors that lower their risk of coronary artery disease and certain cancers.

Two recent studies from Singapore and Japan showed that high intake of soy foods (which contain isoflavones) reduces the risk of breast cancer among premenopausal women by 30 percent, but does not provide any protection in post-menopausal women. One plausible explanation is that soy's phyto-estrogens have an anti-estrogenic impact on breast tissue in women under fifty years of age. After menopause, when the ovaries stop producing estrogens, they begin to have an estrogen-like effect on breast tissue. Indeed, there is very little evidence that high soy intake decreases the risk of breast cancer in post-menopausal women, the group most likely to take these products as alternatives to estrogen replacement therapy. Also, there is no convincing evidence that soy's phyto-estrogens improve bone mineral density, preventing or correcting osteoporosis. Although the lower rate of hip fractures among Japanese women when compared with women in the United States is often cited as evidence that phyto-estrogens play a protective role, hip-bone density in Japanese women is actually the same or lower than it is in American women. In addition, Japanese women have a much higher rate of vertebral fracture than American women.

The evidence suggests that phyto-estrogens provide a slight to moderate decrease in the hot flashes associated with menopause without increasing the risk of breast or uterine cancer. There are no long-term data, however, that demonstrate the effectiveness and safety of Western-style soy products or over-the-counter phyto-estrogens at high doses, or whether they have significant cardio-protective, anti-carcinogenic, or anti-osteoporosis benefits (see Table 73).

Rich sources of phyto-estrogens include soy products, whole grains (such as wheat, rye, rice, and flaxseed), all legumes (such as chick peas, lentils, green peas, and beans), black cohosh, berries, and many other deep-colored fruits and vegetables. Even milk from free-range cows that graze on pastures overgrown with cloves contain high levels of phyto-estrogens. Although cattle and hogs fed soy meal products may contain a small amount of phyto-estrogens in their flesh, it is not significant. In fact, the vast majority of dairy products and meats sold in the United States contain almost no phyto-estrogens.

Products claiming to have high levels of phyto-estrogens derived from black cohosh or dong quai are sold for treatment of menopausal symptoms at exorbitant prices in many health food stores or through mail and internet retailers. A recent randomized double blind study of seventy-one post-menopausal women showed that after six months of daily treatment with 4.5 gm of dong quai, women had as much flushing, irritability, and heat intolerance as women who took the placebo. Supplements of black cohosh or dong quai may cost up to eighty dollars a month. As is true with all other herbs and nutritional supplements, there is no assurance that the ingredients listed on the bottle are indeed inside.

Phyto-estrogens are a collection of isoflavones, four of which are responsible for most of their estrogen-like effects. An individual food may contain one or two isoflavones while lacking the others. Concentration of phyto-estrogens may also vary widely even for the same products. For soybean, for example, these variations are due to differences in species, geographical areas they are grown in, extent and method of processing, and shelf life. Also, the composition of phyto-estrogens in various soy proteins available in the Far East is quite different from what is available in the United States and other Western countries. Many of the soy foods eaten in the Far East are highly fermented and may contain 50- to 100-fold greater concentrations of free "unconjugated" phyto-estrogens than their Western counterparts. These differences reduce the health impact of various soy products available outside the Far East. It is also quite possible that long-term exposure to free phyto-estrogens from an early age may have a totally different health impact than eating some Western-style soy products for six to twelve months as an adult. In fact, no short-term dietary intervention or supplement provides a long-term dividend. By providing a false sense of security, it may even be counterproductive.

How Do Phyto-estrogens Work?

Estrogens can enter only those cells in the body that contain estrogen-receptors on their cell surface. There are two types of human estrogen-receptors: alpha receptors (which are present primarily in the breast and reproductive system) and beta receptors (which are present mainly in the liver, bones, and blood vessels). Phyto-estrogens have very poor affinity for alpha receptors, and therefore cannot enter breast or uterus tissues to promote their growth or proliferation. Estrogen pills and patches, on the other hand, are nonselective, and will enter all tissues with either alpha or beta receptors (including bones, liver, breast, uterus, and coronary and cerebral arteries).

Phyto-estrogens also stimulate the liver to produce a protein that attaches to natural estrogens. Protein-bound estrogens do not have the same impact as free estrogens on breast or uterus tissue because they are no longer recognizable by estrogen-receptors, and therefore cannot enter these cells. By reducing the overall blood concentration of free estrogens, phyto-estrogens may decrease the impact of a person's own hormone on the breast and uterus. A recent study from the University of California, however, showed that women sixty-five or older with high blood levels of free estrogen had a 70 percent lower risk of cognitive decline when compared with those who have lower concentrations. This is an important drawback of phyto-estrogens, which lower the blood level of free estrogens.

Recent long-term studies have shown that low-dose estrogen replacement therapy (such as 0.3 mg of natural estrogens per day) has all of the benefits of larger doses (usually 1.25 to 2.5 mg per day) and fewer side effects, especially when used for fewer than seven consecutive years. Even at high doses, phyto-estrogens are unlikely to significantly reduce the risk of coronary artery disease, stroke, osteoporosis, or Alzheimer's disease, and can cause significant cognitive decline.

The available data suggest that concerns about the use of estrogen replacement therapy must be reconsidered. The aging population in

Table 73
Impact of Different Estrogenic Drugs

	IDEAL ESTROGEN	LOW-DOSE ERT*	HIGH-DOSE PHYTO-ESTROGENS	RALOXI-FENE
BONE DENSITY	+ + +	+ + +	+	+ +
LDL LEVEL	- - -	- - -	-	-
HDL LEVEL	+ + +	+ + +	?	?
LIPOPROTEIN(a) LEVEL	- - -	- - -	?	?
RISK OF CAD	- - -	- - -	-	?
DEPRESSION	- - -	- - -	?	?
RISK OF ALZHEIMER'S	- - -	- - -	?	?
MENOPAUSE SYMPTOMS	- - -	- - -	- -	+ +
UTERUS CANCER	- - -	+?**	-	- -
BREAST CANCER	- - -	+?***	- -	- - -
COLON CANCER	- - -	- - -	?	?
RISK OF BLOOD CLOTS	- - -	?	?	+ +

+ = Increase   - = Decrease   ? = Very little or no impact

* ERT = Estrogen Replacement Therapy
** Unopposed estrogen may increase the risk slightly, but estrogen plus progesterone will not.
*** Short-term (<10 years) : No increased risk. Long-term (>10 years): A small increase.

almost all developed and developing countries is increasing dramatically. Millions of women in the United States are expected to live well beyond their seventies. Low doses of estrogen replacement therapy provide a large variety of health benefits, including a lower risk of coronary events, osteoporosis, Alzheimer's disease, degenerative osteoarthritis, colon cancer, diabetes, depression, and the many adverse effects of estrogen deficiency.

The single most important rule with regard to estrogen replacement therapy is to use the *lowest* dose of estrogens whenever possible. Nearly all of the long-term studies of estrogen replacement therapy so far have used either high doses, sometimes combined with progesterone, and sometimes with a small amount of testosterone. As noted earlier, long-term progesterone therapy may increase the risk of breast cancer more than estrogens alone, especially when used for more than five years. One possible way of avoiding the potential side effects of combined estrogen-progesterone therapy is to use only small doses of progesterone at infrequent intervals (every four to six months, for example) to reduce the risk of uterine cancer without increasing the risk of breast cancer. Low-dose estrogen replacement therapy (such as 0.3 mg per day of Premarin or 5 mcg of ethinyl estradiol) provides all the benefits with minimal increased risk of major side effects, especially when used for less than seven years.

Although transdermal estrogen patches are effective in controlling estrogen deficiency symptoms and osteoporosis, their cardioprotection is considerably less than that of estrogen pills. This is because when you take an estrogen, it quickly travels to the liver where it helps to lower LDL and lipoprotein(a) while increasing HDL production. Oral estrogens also improve the function of endothelial cells and have a potent antioxidant role which contributes to their cardio-protective benefit. Estrogen patches release estrogen slowly into the blood stream and their concentration in the liver is too small to have significant cardiovascular benefits.

To obtain the recommended 70-80 mg of phyto-estrogens daily, you would have to eat a huge variety of soy products such as tofu, tempeh, soy flour, and soy meal. For most women in Western societies, this is not a practical, long-term option. The best-motivated women may find these products tasteless and boring, even after spending a good deal of time and effort preparing them with various spices to give them some flavor. At lower doses, phyto-estrogens are even less likely to have a significant beneficial impact on menopausal symptoms, vaginal dryness, skin aging, abdominal obesity, coronary artery disease, osteoporosis, and Alzheimer's disease, and may even contribute to cognitive decline.

For those who are still concerned about the possible side effects of estrogen replacement therapy, taking one or two tablets of phyto-estrogens (each containing 30-40 mg of the four major isoflavones), and folic acid (400-800 mcg), vitamin E (400 IU), and selenium (200 mcg), should lower the risk of breast cancer while allowing estrogen replacement therapy to provide its benefits.

An estrogen "substitute" such as raloxifene (Evista) is another option for the prevention of osteoporosis. Raloxifene actually decreases the risk of breast cancer by more than 90 percent. Its major drawback is that it increases some post-menopausal symptoms such as sweating and hot flashes. It also increases the risk of blood clot formation, but this may be effectively blocked by daily intake of vitamin E and a low dose of aspirin (81 mg per day), something that all post-menopausal women should do anyway. Although raloxifene lowers LDL cholesterol by a few percentage points, it has no HDL-raising benefit. Overall, low-dose estrogen replacement therapy provides twice the cardiovascular benefits of raloxifene.

As with any intervention, estrogen replacement therapy is not a prevent-all or cure-all drug. Some women on estrogen replacement therapy may still have a cardiovascular event, breast cancer, or osteoporosis. In fact, preliminary results of the recent Heart and Estrogen/Progesterone Replacement Study showed that in the first year, estrogen replacement therapy provided no protection against a recurrent coronary event. By the fourth and fifth year, however, women on estrogen replacement therapy had significantly lower rates of new coronary events. This is quite understandable, since the progression of the coronary quartet (see Chapter 1) cannot be stopped in a short time by estrogen replacement therapy alone. This takes us back to the vital importance of dealing with *all* coexisting coronary risk factors as early as possible to prevent coronary artery disease.

The decision concerning whether to use estrogen replacement therapy should never be based on scare tactics, misinformation, or misunderstanding of its risks and benefits. Why should we condemn millions of post-menopausal women, without breast cancer, to estrogen-starvation by withholding estrogen replacement therapy from them?

Two recent position papers by scientific panels in the United States and France have not objected to the use of estrogen replacement therapy even for women prone to breast cancer. Just as there continues to be a need for prudence in prescribing drugs for high blood pressure, diabetes, and other disorders, there is also a need for thoughtful and scientific consideration of estrogen replacement therapy for women who need it.

Since estrogens can cause some "congestion" and an increase in breast density, the older "one-view" mammograms are not very accurate. To avoid missing a lesion or overinterpreting the findings, two practical recommendations are timely:

Estrogen replacement therapy should be stopped for two to four weeks prior to a mammographic examination.

The attending physician ordering the test should request a two-view mammogram and inform the radiologist (who performs the test) about the individual's status as a current hormone user.

Table 74 below provides rational guidelines for health care providers and consumers when considering the use of estrogen replacement therapy versus alternatives such as estrogen-like compounds.

Table 74
Guideline for Choosing Hormone Replacement Therapy or Estrogen-like Compounds Like Raloxifene

RISK LEVEL			DRUG OF CHOICE	
OSTEOPOROSIS	CAD	BREAST CANCER	HRT	RALOXIFENE
LOW	LOW	LOW	+	
LOW	LOW	HIGH		+
LOW	HIGH	LOW	+	
LOW	HIGH	HIGH	+	+
HIGH	LOW	LOW	+	
HIGH	HIGH	HIGH		+
HIGH	LOW	LOW	+	
HIGH	HIGH	HIGH		+

High risk of osteoporosis = family history, low bone density, malnutrition, sedentary lifestyle, tall or slender women, history of long-term use of cortisone, and chronic kidney, liver, or digestive diseases and estrogen deficiency.

High risk of CAD (coronary artery disease) = coexistence of two or more major coronary risk factors (see Chapter 2).

High risk of breast cancer = personal or family history of breast or ovarian cancer in first degree relatives under the age of 55, obesity and sedentary lifestyle, excessive alcohol intake, i.e., three or more drinks per day, age at start of menstruation <12, age at first childbirth >30, two or more previous breast biopsies, age >50, and Ashkenazi (Jewish) ancestry.

Notes

Part 1: *Nutrition and Disease*

1. How do liver cells know when to increase or decrease the number of LDL-receptors? The most important signal for regulating the production of LDL-receptors is how much unattached or "free" cholesterol each liver cell has. When liver cells have an adequate amount of free cholesterol, they determine that they no longer need cholesterol and stop producing LDL-receptors. On the other hand, when the concentration of free cholesterol inside liver cells is low, they go into overdrive and make more LDL-receptors to bring in cholesterol from the blood circulation. The discovery of LDL-receptors and how they work to regulate blood cholesterol was so important in understanding the role of blood cholesterol in cardiovascular diseases that two American scientists, Drs. Joseph Goldstein and Michael Brown, were awarded the Nobel Prize for Physiology and Medicine in 1985 for their pioneering research in this area.

What is a free cholesterol? As soon as cholesterol is absorbed from the intestine, a single molecule of fatty acid may attach to it, a process called "esterification." Esterified cholesterol particles are no longer the "free" cholesterol the liver cells are interested in. Thus, the liver cells begin to look for cholesterol elsewhere and produce more LDL-receptors to bring in what they need. Dietary saturated fats (Chapter 2, "Saturated Fat") and trans fatty acids (Chapter 2, "Trans Fatty Acids") cannot attach to cholesterol particles. Consequently, plenty of free cholesterol reaches the liver cells, quenching their needs, so they stop producing LDL-receptors. As a result of this LDL-receptor deficiency, blood cholesterol goes up. Monounsaturated fats (Chapter 2, "Monounsaturated Fat") and polyunsaturated fats (Chapter 2, "Omega-6 Polyunsaturated Fat" and "Omega-3 Polyunsaturated Fat") readily attach to cholesterol particles, leaving very little free cholesterol to reach liver cells. Thus, liver cells produce more LDL-receptors to trap LDL cholesterol particles from the bloodstream, lowering the blood cholesterol.

The potential of monounsaturated fats to esterify cholesterol particles can be used effectively in dietary interventions. For example, omelettes prepared in olive or canola oil (Chapter 2, "Monounsaturated Fat") have very little potential to raise blood cholesterol levels. In contrast, omelettes prepared with butter or margarine (which may contain up to 30 percent saturated fat and as much as 20 to 30 percent trans fatty acids) may raise blood cholesterol level. Similarly, shellfish, such as clams, oysters, or shrimp, prepared in olive oil, do not have a significant impact on blood cholesterol levels.

2. How does saturated fat raise blood cholesterol levels? As noted in Chapter 2, "Should We Fear Dietary Cholesterol?" the presence of free cholesterol within the interior of liver cells dictates whether liver cells produce new LDL-receptors and how much. Since saturated fat cannot latch onto cholesterol particles, liver cells receive a good amount of free cholesterol and shut down their production of LDL-receptors. With fewer LDL-receptors around, LDL particles return to the bloodstream and raise the LDL level.

For several hours following a fatty meal containing butter, cheeses, creams, stick margarines, or shortening (all of which contain high concentrations of saturated fat or trans fatty acids) (Chapter 2, "Trans Fatty Acids"), blood levels of triglycerides may rise by more than 60 percent. This may interfere with the normal function of the arteries. Moreover, high triglyceride levels can also decrease the good HDL cholesterol level by more than 10 percent.

An often ignored but nasty habit of saturated fats is that they increase the tendency of blood platelets to clump together and adhere to the inner lining of the arteries, setting the stage for a heart attack or stroke. Thus, excessive amounts of saturated fat have four undesirable consequences: they (1) raise blood levels of the "bad" LDL cholesterol; (2) raise triglyceride levels; (3) lower the "good" HDL cholesterol; and (4) promote clot formation which may result in a sudden heart attack or stroke.

Is saturated fat always harmful? Not necessarily, for saturated fat plays an important role in maintaining the health and integrity of the vascular system and other organs, including the brain and the liver. This important virtue of saturated fat may be due to its resistance to oxidization, a property shared by monounsaturated fats but not polyunsaturates or trans fatty acids. Moreover, not all saturated fats are equally bad. Stearic acid, which accounts for nearly one-half of saturated fat in most lean meats, acts very much like monounsaturates and is not coronary-unfriendly. This helps explain why lean red meats do not raise blood cholesterol levels and are therefore included in the Twenty Risk Factors Diet.

Although consumers frequently assume that coronary-unfriendly saturated fat comes only from animal sources, a large proportion of dietary saturated fat is derived from plant sources. Coconut and palm kernel oils, for example, contain the highest concentrations of saturated fatty acids (92 percent and 82 percent, respectively), most of which are coronary-unfriendly.

Does saturated fat have any other benefits? Recent studies suggest that saturated fat may actually protect liver cells against damage caused by alcohol. Thus, it is possible that certain saturated fats can be used to treat acute alcohol-induced hepatitis in humans. This might also explain why alcohol taken with meals is less likely to cause liver damage. There are no adequate studies at this stage, however, to show whether the benefits of saturated fat seen in experiments with animals can be duplicated in humans.

Saturated fat also plays a major role in protecting the integrity of the brain's arteries. Recent studies have shown that low-saturated fat diets are associated with a 50 percent higher risk of stroke.

3. Monounsaturated fat lowers blood LDL cholesterol. This is because monounsaturated fatty acids readily attach to cholesterol particles, so that few free cholesterol particles reach the liver. As noted earlier, a low concentration of free cholesterol inside liver cells is a signal for these cells to produce more LDL-receptors. The result is a significant reduction in LDL cholesterol level (by about 10 percent). As seen in Figure 12, when dietary intake of monounsaturated fat increases, the activity and the number of LDL-receptors also rises. The response to saturated fats is the exact opposite.

Monounsaturated fat increases the good HDL cholesterol by about 5 to 10 percent.

Both monounsaturated fats and polyunsaturated fats are readily incorporated into LDL particles. The difference is that LDL particles enriched with mono-unsaturated fat are remarkably resistant to oxidization, which is an essential element in the initiation and progression of coronary artery disease. This often-ignored benefit of monounsaturated fat is the exact opposite of what polyunsaturated fats do. Even if monounsaturated fat does nothing else, reducing the oxidization of LDL cholesterol provides enormously important protection for the heart. This benefit is even more relevant to diabetics who have a greater tendency to oxidize the LDL.

Long-term use of monounsaturated fat can reduce the risk of a stroke by about 50 percent. The importance of dietary fat in prevention of a stroke was recently reported in a twenty-year follow-up study of 832 men from the Framingham Heart Study. These healthy individuals were between forty-five and sixty-five years of age at the beginning of the study. Contrary to prevailing views, higher dietary fat intake conferred a significant protection against stroke. The risk of a stroke by those with the highest total dietary fat, dietary monounsaturated fat, or even dietary saturated fats—but not polyunsaturates—was one-half to two-thirds lower than those who followed a very low-fat diet. A similar inverse relationship between dietary fat intake and the risk of stroke was recently reported among both Japanese living in Japan and Japanese living in Hawaii. The stroke prevention role of dietary fat is further supported by experiments in a certain strain of stroke-prone rats that develop fewer strokes when their food contains a high percentage of fat.

Why should a high-fat diet cause atherosclerosis in large arteries (such as the heart's coronary arteries and the carotid arteries in the neck that carry the blood to the brain) but protect smaller arteries of the brain? In humans, only 10 to 15 percent of all strokes are caused by large vessel disease (or clogging of carotid arteries). The rest (85 to 90 percent) are due to small vessel disease within and around the brain tissue. Numerous studies suggest that the brain's small arteries require sufficient amounts of fat to maintain their integrity and pliability so that they do not crack or rupture readily, especially during periods of emotional or physical stress.

Figure 12
The Impact of Dietary Fats on Activity of LDL Receptors*

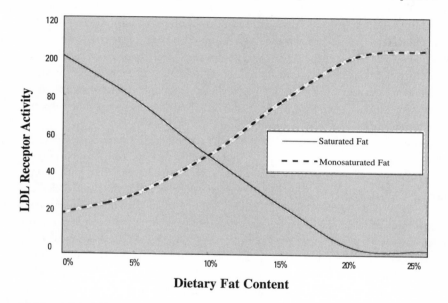

Dietary Fat Content

* As the activity (and number) of LDL receptors increases, more LDL particles are cleared out of the blood stream, resulting in lower blood cholesterol.

4. We see the term "polyunsaturated fat" on food labels almost on a daily basis. Although this will not be a lesson in biochemistry, it is helpful to know what these fats are, what they do, and what to make of all the propaganda surrounding vegetable oils, margarine, and shortenings.

The molecule of all fatty acids resembles a chain bracelet; the chain or rope of the bracelet is made up of carbon atoms lined side by side to which hydrogen atoms are attached like charms on a bracelet (Figures 13-A and 13-B). Fatty acids could have as few as three or as many as twenty-five carbons in their chains. Those with three to five carbons are called "short-chain"; those with six to eleven "medium"; those with twelve to twenty "long"; and those with over twenty carbons in their chain are referred to as "longer-chain" fatty acids.

One of the most important structural distinctions of fatty acids is whether both sides of their carbon atoms are fully occupied by hydrogen atoms. If they are fully occupied or "saturated," they are called saturated fatty acids. Otherwise, they would be "unsaturated." In the latter, carbon atoms have one less hydrogen atom dangling from them. This unsaturation forces the carbons missing a hydrogen atom to form a double bond (shown as =) with each other. The number of double bonds, and their positions along the chain of fatty acids, is enormously important and changes the entire character and function of fatty acids.

Figure 13-A
Various Types of Fatty Acids

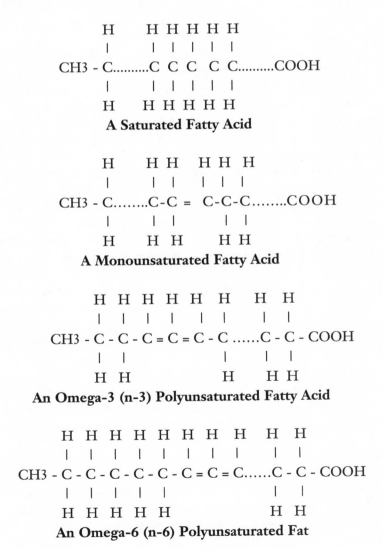

A Saturated Fatty Acid

A Monounsaturated Fatty Acid

An Omega-3 (n-3) Polyunsaturated Fatty Acid

An Omega-6 (n-6) Polyunsaturated Fat

When all the carbon molecules are fully occupied (they have *single bonds*, shown as -), the fatty acid is saturated.

When the carbon molecules are not fully occupied (they have *double bonds*, shown as =), the fatty acid is unsaturated.

If one carbon molecule is unsaturated, the fatty acid is *mono*unsaturated. If more carbon molecules are unsaturated, the fatty acid is *poly*unsaturated.

Oleic acid, the principal fatty acid of olive oil, canola oil, and hazelnut oil, has eighteen carbons in its chain with one double bond. Thus, oleic acid is called a monounsaturated fatty acid. Linoleic acid, the main fatty acid of many vegetable oils such as corn, safflower, sunflower, and soybean has two double bonds. Linoleic acid and all other fatty acids with two or more unsaturated carbons are called polyunsaturated fatty acids.

The reason that nearly all fat molecules are called fatty acids is because they are in reality very weak acidic compounds with a COOH at one end. But when they join together or to other compounds, they lose their acidic status.

What are omega-3 and omega-6 polyunsaturated fats? They are two distinctly different types of polyunsaturated fats with vastly different roles in human health. Structurally, if the first unsaturated double bond carbon, shown as =, is at the third carbon, counting from left to right, it is called an omega-3 polyunsaturated fat. When the first unsaturated carbon of a polyunsaturated fat is at carbon 6 of the chain, it is called an omega-6 polyunsaturated fat.

The cardio-protective fatty acids found in seafood are omega-3 polyunsaturated fatty acids with twenty or twenty-two carbons in their chains. These longer-chain polyunsaturated fatty acids are not present in any plant, and cannot be produced in the human body. For this reason, they are referred to as essential fatty acids, meaning that they must be supplied from outside sources. Linolenic acid is an 18-carbon omega-3 polyunsaturated fat which is present to varying degrees in certain seed oils such as flax seed, canola oil, soybean, and Persian walnuts. A small amount of this plant-source omega-3 (no more than 1 to 2 percent) may be elongated and converted into longer-chain fatty acids. In people who do not eat any seafood, this may be their only source of omega-3 polyunsaturated fat. Omega-6 polyunsaturated fats are plentiful and are present in all vegetable oils or fats, including margarine, shortenings, and cooking fats. The usual dietary intake of omega-3 polyunsaturated fat in the United States and many Western countries is about .5 to 2.5 grams per day, compared to twenty or more grams per day for omega-6 polyunsaturated fat.

5. The single most notable beneficial effect of vegetable oils or fats is that, as a replacement for dietary saturated fats, they can help lower blood cholesterol level by about 5 to 10 percent. This is because omega-6 polyunsaturated fatty acids can bind to cholesterol whereas saturated fatty acids cannot. As noted in Chapter 2, "Should We Fear Dietary Cholesterol?" when there is less free cholesterol within liver cells, more LDL-receptors are produced by these cells to enhance their ability to trap and remove LDL particles from the bloodstream, which lowers the LDL cholesterol level.

Aside from a small LDL-lowering effect, the case for increasing dietary omega-6 polyunsaturated fat is quite weak, and very difficult to justify. Unlike monounsaturates which have a three-thousand-year history of safety combined with proven cardio-protective benefits (Chapter 2, "Monounsaturated Fat"), omega-6 polyunsaturated fat has a short history with many unanswered questions.

Some of the main concerns about omega-6 polyunsaturated fat include:

Dietary omega-6 polyunsaturated fat will lower HDL cholesterol by approximately 5 to 10 percent. Lowering the HDL, especially in people who already have a low level, is a big step in the wrong direction.

Omega-6 polyunsaturated fat is more susceptible to oxidization than saturated fats or monounsaturates. Dietary fats, including polyunsaturated fat, are readily integrated into LDL cholesterol particles. Unfortunately, LDL particles enriched with omega-6 polyunsaturated fat are highly oxidizable. As noted in Chapter 1, it is the oxidized LDL that contributes to coronary artery disease, not the native or nonoxidized LDL. This concern over the increased potential for LDL oxidization is especially troublesome at higher levels of omega-6 polyunsaturated fat consumption. A recent study of 393 men with elevated blood cholesterol levels showed that dietary omega-6 polyunsaturated fat, without supplementation with antioxidants such as vitamin E, was the most important determinant of LDL susceptibility to oxidization. Clearly, in people with elevated LDL cholesterol levels, it makes no sense to put something in their diet, even if it is "all natural and cholesterol-free," that can increase oxidization of their cholesterol.

Increased oxidization of LDL cholesterol, and the resulting damage to various tissues (oxidative stress), is even more problematic in diabetics who already have a greater tendency for cardiovascular diseases. For this reason, diabetics should actually reduce dietary omega-6 polyunsaturated fat (all vegetable oils, margarine, and shortenings) in their diet as much as possible, and replace them with monounsaturates which stabilize their LDL particles and decrease oxidative stress.

Repeated heating of omega-6 polyunsaturated fat at high temperatures such as deep frying at home, or in fast food restaurants, causes degradation of these fats and produces a number of oxidized by-products. Recent studies have shown that consumption of foods containing these degradation products of previously heated omega-6 polyunsaturated fat makes the endothelium (inner lining) of the arteries dysfunctional, a precursor to coronary artery disease. Pretreatment of individuals consuming these products with antioxidant vitamins C and E blocks or decreases the endothelial dysfunction caused by repeatedly heated fats.

6. *"Designer" Margarines*

Recently several margarine manufacturers in the United States, following the lead of European countries, have marketed soft margarines with very little or no trans fatty acids. Some of these spreads (such as Benecol and Take Control) contain certain plant additives which can reduce the absorption of cholesterol from the intestine. Each serving of Benecol contains 1.5 gm of stanol (extracted from pine). Several studies have shown that stanol, 3 grams per day in divided doses and taken with food, can lower blood cholesterol by 5 to 10 percent. Other newer spreads contain different kinds of plant additives. For example, Take Control contains a plant sterol (chemically different from stanol) derived from soybean. It is less efficient in cholesterol-lowering than stanol. None of the plant additives has any impact on HDL cholesterol or triglyceride levels.

Most of the "designer" margarines have less total fat and calories (and more water) per serving than the conventional margarine spreads. They also have substantially less saturated fat and no trans fatty acids, making them a sensible substitute for other spreads, even though they are three to five times more expensive. Their main drawback is that they should be eaten three times a day with foods so that their additive can block or reduce the absorption of dietary cholesterol from the intestine. This is often impractical for most people, especially at breakfast and lunch and when they eat out.

7. The process of partial hydrogenation, however, is very imprecise. All fat molecules in the oil are not hydrogenated uniformly. In fact, only 30 to 50 percent of the fat molecules are hydrogenated, meaning they accept additional hydrogen atoms. Moreover, hydrogen atoms are added to fat molecules in a random fashion along the chain of fatty acids. The process is very much like adding one or more charm pieces, at random, to a large number of charm bracelets. When the job of adding new pieces is completed, not many bracelets would be alike. Similarly, during partial hydrogenation, at least twenty different new fatty acids (or "isomeres") of the original fat are produced. Each one of these new fat molecules may be different from the others depending on where and how many new hydrogen atoms have been added to the original fat molecule.

If the added hydrogen atoms are all on one side of the fatty acid chain, the new fat is called a "cis fatty acid." However, if the hydrogen atoms are distributed on both sides of the chain, the new fat is called a "trans fatty acid" (Figure 13-B below).

Figure 13-B
Other Fatty Acids

```
     H   H   H        H   H   H
     |   |   |        |   |   |
CH3 - C - C - C......C = C - C.......COOH
     |   |   |                |
     H   H   H                H
```
A Cis Fatty Acid

```
     H   H   H      H       H
     |   |   |      |       |
CH3 - C - C - C......C = C - C......COOH
     |   |   |          |   |
     H   H   H          H   H
```
A Trans Fatty Acid

The positions of the hydrogen atoms on the unsaturated carbons (double bonds) determine the cis or trans status. If the hydrogen atoms are on one side of the unsaturated carbon, it is a cis; if they are on both sides, it is a trans fatty acid.

Processing can also produce harmful saturated fats. For example, during hydrogenation of vegetable oils, small amounts of three long-chain saturated fatty acids (arachidic, behemic, and lignoceric) are produced which are coronary-unfriendly, even in small quantities.

What makes trans fatty acids distinctly different from cis fatty acids is that the cis varieties (such as fatty acids in natural vegetable oils) are "wiggly" and flexible at their double bonds, and therefore are liquid. On the other hand, the double bond in the molecule of a trans fatty acid is not wiggly and keeps the chain stiff, which contributes to keeping these fats solid at room temperature. These partially hydro-genated new fats now act a lot more like saturated fat than the polyunsaturated fat they used to be. In ruminating animals such as cows, sheep, goats, deer, and camels, a small amount of trans fat is produced by bacterial action in their rumen. Some of this trans fat will eventually appear in their flesh and milk (Table 8).

8. Recently, conjugated linoleic acid has gained a good deal of popularity as an over-the-counter supplement for preventing cancers, heart attacks, and obesity. Unfortunately, these claims are all extrapolated from studies on rodents and rabbits and may have no relevance to humans.

Atherosclerosis in hamsters and rabbits has been partially blocked by conjugated linoleic acid feeding. In some animal models, conjugated linoleic acid has also reduced total body fat and increased lean body mass. These experimental data have contributed to the recent popularity of conjugated linoleic acid among obese individuals. There is no valid study, however, to show that it has a weight-reducing effect in humans.

How and why conjugated linoleic acid accomplishes these beneficial effects is still unclear. Moreover, long-term safety of commercial conjugated linoleic acid in humans has yet to be established. These uncertainties argue against the use of supplemental conjugated linoleic acid, especially for "trimming the fat off" and "adding strong lean muscles."

9. There are two distinctly different types of omega-3 polyunsaturated fat: plant-derived, and the marine variety from fish, shellfish, and fish oil supplements.

Plant-derived Omega-3 Polyunsaturated Fat

The most abundant form of plant omega-3 polyunsaturated fat is alpha linolenic acid, which is present in high concentrations in flax seed oil (more than 50 percent), canola oil (10 percent), Persian or English walnuts (about 8 percent), soybean oil (about 7 percent), and to a much smaller degree in pistachios, filberts, almonds, and dark green leafy vegetables and herbs.

In a ten-year follow-up study of more than seventy-six thousand nurses, high intake of plant omega-3 polyunsaturated fat was associated with a 50 percent lower rate of fatal heart attacks, almost exclusively the result of reducing irregular heart rhythms.

In the landmark Lyon Diet Heart Study (from Lyon, France), more than six hundred individuals with a previous heart attack followed either a Mediterranean diet (with a high intake of monounsaturated fat and plant as well as seafood omega-3 polyunsaturated fat) or the American Heart Association (low-fat, low cholesterol) diet. After nearly five years, those who adhered to the new Mediterranean diet had a 70 percent lower risk of experiencing a new heart attack than those who were on the American Heart Association diet.

Seafood Omega-3 Polyunsaturated Fat

Seafood is a rich source of two omega-3 polyunsaturated fats: EPA, a twenty-carbon fatty acid, and DHA, which has twenty-two carbons. Both share the same healthful characteristics and both are almost always present together in all seafoods and shellfish. Although a small amount of the plant omega-3 polyunsaturated fat is converted to EPA in the human liver, only 1 to 2 percent of it can be converted to DHA.

Concentrations of omega-3 polyunsaturated fat vary in different seafoods (Tables 10 and 11). Even the same fish, such as salmon or tuna, may have higher or lower levels of omega-3 polyunsaturated fat depending on which season and where they were caught, their habitat, and their long-term food sources.

For example, a tuna caught off the Pacific Northwest of the United States may have three to five times more omega-3 polyunsaturated fat than a tuna caught off the coast of the Carolinas or Florida. For the same reason, farm-raised fish (such as rainbow trout and others) have substantially less omega-3 polyunsaturated fat than wild fish.

10. For a variety of reasons, some people do not eat enough seafood. For them, fish oil supplements are a reasonable alternative to seafood, especially if they have high triglyceride levels, or are at risk of arrhythmias.

Unfortunately, not all fish oils are pure and entirely safe. Many fish oil capsules contain a high concentration of trans fatty acids produced during processing. In addition, fish oil may undergo partial oxidization during storage and shelf life. At present, the weight of the evidence suggests that seafood EPA and DHA are the active agents in fish oil. Newer products containing a higher concentration of these two fatty acids without other impurities are on the horizon, which should make pure omega-3 polyunsaturated fat more readily available.

In diabetics, with or without cardiovascular diseases, the most promising dietary intervention is to increase their consumption of monounsaturated fat along with at least three or four seafood meals per week. As noted previously, the single most important aspect of preparing seafood is to make sure that, both at home and in restaurants, vegetable oils, margarine, shortening, mayonnaise, or cooking fats are not used. A can of tuna or a tuna fish sandwich once or twice a week for lunch (definitely without mayonnaise), plus one or two seafood dinners per week are practical dietary adjustments that can be associated with enormous benefits.

What About Mercury Exposure?

Mercury (Hg) is an elemental mineral present in the earth's crust, but certain industrial activities such as coal burning and trash incineration increase human exposure. Organisms in fresh or sea water convert mercury to methyl mercury which is then eaten by fish or shellfish and stored in their flesh. When these contaminated fish are eaten by other fish, they, in turn, pass on the contamination of the aquatic food chain.

There is no doubt that methyl mercury at high concentrations is toxic to human embryos. For adults, the World Health Organization has set a limit of 0.47 mcg/kg body weight per day of mercury over a lifetime as safe or nontoxic. However, the United States Environmental Protection Agency has set a limit that is 80 percent below the World Health Organization, or 0.1 mcg/kg of body weight per day.

During the third trimester of pregnancy, the human fetus needs plenty of omega-3 polyunsaturated fat in order for its brain cells to grow. Thus, for pregnant women, total avoidance of seafood for fear of mercury poisoning is counterproductive. Nearly all fish contain some mercury. But consumption of certain wild fish such as salmon, rainbow trout, snapper, and flounder once or twice per week during the third trimester is not only safe, it is essential to the development of the fetus's brain. A recent developmental study of children exposed to methyl mercury through maternal fish consumption, and an analysis of brain mercury concentrations in infants who died of unrelated causes in the same geographic area, found no nerve toxicity or excessive brain mercury levels. Even if some wild or farm-raised fish are contaminated with mercury, the amount of mercury per one or two servings of seafood per week almost always falls within the "safe" range. For nonpregnant adults eating two to three servings of seafood or shellfish, mercury contamination is essentially a nonissue.

However, since there are no adequate standards or Food and Drug Administration controls over the production and packaging of fish oils, their level of impurity or contamination with mercury is often unknown. For this reason, fish oil supplements should not be used by pregnant women unless the product is indeed free of mercury contamination.

Even with effective measures to reduce air and water pollution today, the concern over the contamination of seafood with mercury will not disappear in the near future because of the enduring nature of mercury in the seafood chain. We should remember, however, that more than 500,000 people die of heart attacks in the United States each year. Yet not a single person has died in the past two decades of mercury poisoning from eating seafood. Assuming that regular consumption of seafood can reduce the risk of cardiac death by about 30 percent, eating two or three seafood meals per week could have saved 3.4 million lives during the same twenty years.

Although mercury contamination is a source of concern for pregnant women, it does not follow that all people have an equal risk with low levels of exposure. We should all try to safeguard the purity and healthfulness of our foods, but we must not allow contentious and emotional outbursts by alarmists who see poison in every food to dissuade us from enjoying the vast health benefits associated with seafood.

What About Allergies to Seafood?

Approximately 1 to 2 percent of adults may have certain food allergies, primarily to peanuts, fish, pork, and strawberries. It is rare for anyone to be allergic to all items in a particular food group. For example, someone who is allergic to shrimp is unlikely to be allergic to all other shellfish or fish. Or if someone is allergic to tuna, there are a vast number of other fish to which he or she is not allergic.

A problem arises in restaurants when different fish are handled by the same person, the same cutting utensil or cutting surfaces, and often the same sautéing pan without proper or thorough washing each time. Cross-contamination by allergens from one seafood to another is common under these circumstances. All of these difficulties are certainly avoidable at home. When dining out you should always notify the server of specific food allergies—for example, shrimp or peanuts—then request that the cooking staff pay special attention to washing the cooking pans and cutting surfaces used. Since the heat of the grill will denature any residual allergens, the grill rack would not pose any problem. The important point is that food allergy is not an "all or nothing" proposition. Almost everyone who is allergic to one or two seafoods can tolerate the rest without any allergic reaction.

What About the Cholesterol Content of Seafoods?

As noted in Chapter 2, "Should We Fear Dietary Cholesterol?" dietary cholesterol is far less important in raising blood cholesterol than is saturated fat or trans fatty acids. Furthermore, the cholesterol content of fish is similar to, or even lower than, that of chicken or turkey. With the exception of squid, the remainder of shellfish do not necessarily have high concentrations of cholesterol (Tables 10 and 11). More importantly, because shellfish have an extremely low fat content (usually less than 2 percent) and since their level of saturated fat is almost negligible, their cholesterol content is essentially a nonissue. In fact, a recent study showed that although daily consumption of 10 ounces of shrimp for three weeks raised the LDL cholesterol by approximately 7 percent, it also increased the HDL by 12 percent. Thus, the net effect was a more favorable LDL/HDL ratio, and a more coronary-friendly cholesterol profile.

11. *Dietary Carbohydrates*

Simple carbohydrates are the three edible sugars: fructose, glucose, and galactose. In foods, sugars may be present individually, such as fructose in many fruits, or collectively, such as both glucose and fructose in honey. However, frequently, two sugar molecules join together to form a larger one. Examples include table sugar (dextrose), in which glucose and fructose are attached, or milk's sugar (lactose), in which glucose and galactose are attached.

Plants store glucose as a complex substance called "starch," but humans store glucose in the liver and muscles as glycogen. Glycogen molecules contain hundreds of glucose units attached to one another like branches of a tree. An average-sized person can store no more than one kilogram of carbohydrates in the form of glycogen at any given time. This amount of glycogen can last for two to three hours of intense physical activities, and somewhat longer during less strenuous exercises. As glycogen is broken down in the liver and muscles to release glucose, it is usually replenished within several hours with carbohydrate feeding. Unused carbohydrates are readily stored as fat and contribute to obesity.

The heart, brain, and muscles use glucose preferentially over protein and fats. For this reason, an adequate supply of carbohydrates, whether simple or complex, is essential for the health of these and other organs. Aside from providing adequate fuel for the function of various organs, dietary carbohydrates can reduce the need for dietary fat, especially saturated fat. One beneficial consequence of this exchange is a lower LDL cholesterol level (by about 5 to 10 percent). Unfortunately, this benefit is often negated by a similar percentage or even a larger reduction in HDL cholesterol. In other words, there is a limit to dietary carbohydrates: up to a point they are helpful; beyond that point they become counterproductive.

An analysis of twenty-five recent studies dealing with the impact of dietary fats and carbohydrates on coronary artery disease showed that replacing dietary saturated fat with carbohydrates consistently lowered the HDL cholesterol levels. In contrast, HDL levels were unchanged or actually increased when monounsaturates were substituted for saturated fat. In a recent British study of 1,420 adults, consumption of simple carbohydrates (or complex carbohydrates readily broken down into simple carbohydrates in the intestine) consistently lowered the HDL level. Even among children and adolescents, a high intake of dietary simple carbohydrates resulted in a significant lowering of HDL cholesterol.

The review of data from twenty studies (which included more than 95,000 nondiabetic individuals) showed that a fasting blood glucose level of 110 mg/dl increased the risk of cardiovascular events by 33 percent compared to those with a fasting blood glucose of 75 mg/dl. Since high carbohydrate intake (more than 50 to 55 percent of dietary energy intake) contributes to hyperglycemia (elevated blood glucose), it may indeed be counterproductive, and result in a significantly higher risk of heart attacks and strokes.

12. A good example of this disciplined approach is oxidization of the LDL cholesterol within the wall of the coronary artery. The first line of antioxidant defense is an internally produced antioxidant called "ubiquinol-10," followed by alpha-tocopherol (the most potent form of vitamin E), and, if needed, other antioxidants. Beta-carotene, a close member of the vitamin A family, is the last and the least potent defender.

13. *Vitamin E*
Vitamin E is the collective name for eight naturally occurring compounds: four are called tocopherol and the other four are tocotrienols. Synthetic vitamin E almost always is made up of alpha-tocopherol which is the most abundant and most potent form of vitamin E. Biological potencies of tocotrienols are much less than their tocopherol counterparts. In fact, there are no studies to show that these compounds have a significant health impact, and for this reason, they are often not included in various formulations of vitamin E.

14. *Vitamin C*

The two-way elimination pathway for vitamin C makes the use of mega doses (more than 1000 mg per day) unwise, wasteful, and associated with a number of side effects. In fact, excessive doses of vitamin C can increase urinary excretion of oxalate and uric acid, the principal components of most kidney stones. High doses of vitamin C may also contribute to digestive problems, including ulceration of the esophagus or stomach, and diarrhea or bloating. Vitamin C can also increase the absorption of iron from the intestine, in particular in persons with diseases related to too much iron in the blood, a condition referred to as "iron overload" or "hemochromatosis." Approximately one out of every four hundred Americans has this inherited disorder. The concern is that indiscriminate use of vitamin C in these individuals, especially when accompanied by multivitamin-mineral supplements containing iron, may result in accumulation of iron and severe injuries to several organs, including the liver, pancreas, heart, and brain. Moderate to high doses of vitamin C (more than 500 mg) can also interfere with the absorption of chromium, an important trace mineral (Chapter 2, "Supplemental Vitamins and Minerals").

Antioxidant potency of lycopene from tomato products is nine times, and that of alpha-tocopherol is eight times, greater than vitamin C in coping with a host of oxidants. On the other hand, since not all diseases are caused by the same group of oxidants, the availability of various antioxidants (including vitamin C) is essential for the health of many organs. For example, in some organs (such as the eyes, adrenal glands, and stomach), vitamin C has a prominent role, while in others its role is relatively small. This preferential action site explains why for those with high vitamin C intake (about 500 mg per day), the prevalence of cataracts is just one-fourth that in persons with a low intake (less than 125 mg per day).

15. The cardiovascular protection of the B family of vitamins is exclusively limited to B-3 (Niacin), B-6 (Pyridoxine), B-9 (folic acid), and B-12 (Cobalamin). Vitamin B-1 (thiamine) deficiency, a common finding among heavy drinkers, can cause a flabby heart muscle and heart failure, but it is not involved in the process of coronary artery disease or atherosclerosis of other arteries.

High doses of niacin (1500-3000 mg per day) can have a significant impact in reducing the risk of cardiovascular diseases. In fact, if it were not for its side effects, niacin would have been an ideal cholesterol-lowering drug, superior to all other modern (and far more expensive) drugs. At high doses, niacin lowers the LDL cholesterol and triglycerides by more than 30 percent, while it increases the cardio-protective HDL by the same percentage.

Even more importantly, niacin can significantly reduce the number of small, dense LDL particles and lower the risk of coronary artery disease. And niacin is the only drug (other than estrogens) currently available which can lower blood levels of lipoprotein(a) by 20 to 30 percent.

Niacin also decreases the risk of intra-arterial clot formation (thrombosis) and helps dissolve tiny clots that may form inside coronary arteries. Recent studies have shown that niacin expedites the repair of damaged lining of the arteries and restores its function. No other cholesterol-altering drug can do all this.

16. Vitamins B-6, folic acid (B-9), and vitamin B-12 taken together reduce the risk of cardiovascular events by helping to break down and lower blood levels of homocysteine, a blood protein that increases the risk of cardiovascular diseases several fold. The body breaks down homocysteine through two pathways: folic acid and vitamin B-12 work in tandem in one pathway, and vitamin B-6 works through another pathway.

17. For maximum effectiveness, folic acid and vitamin B-12 must always be used together. Folic acid plays an essential role in converting homocysteine into a harmless amino acid called methionine, and vitamin B-12 is a facilitator of this process. Even at very high doses, co-therapy with folic acid and vitamin B-12 is quite safe and devoid of any unpleasant side effects. About 10 to 20 percent of older persons may have various degrees of vitamin B-12 deficiency. Folic acid alone may improve the anemia that is often associated with vitamin B-12 deficiency. Unfortunately, unrecognized and untreated vitamin B-12 deficiency may result in irreversible neurological damage. This is another reason why folic acid, especially at high doses, should always be used with vitamin B-12 (in doses of 1 to 2 mg per day).

18. *Selenium*

Although selenium is a potent antioxidant there are very few scientific studies to show that it has a major impact on cardiovascular health. This paucity of information may be in part due to the fact that the role of antioxidants in cardiovascular health is judged primarily by whether they reduce oxidization of LDL cholesterol and improve endothelial function. Since selenium is not fat soluble, it is not readily transported into the wall of the arteries to prevent oxidization of LDL particles. In addition, there is no clinical study in which the impact of selenium on endothelial function has been explored.

A recent study focused on a potent antioxidant enzyme, glutathione, which is extremely dependent on selenium for its activity. Samples of atherosclerotic plaques from carotid arteries removed at surgery showed a more than 300 percent lower activity (and in some cases no activity at all) in glutathione enzymes when compared to normal arteries. It is not yet clear whether such a dramatic dysfunction of the selenium-dependent antioxidant enzyme is due to an overwhelming oxidant load, or occurs after the plaques are already formed. Either way, this antioxidant deprivation adds to the burden of the plaque. At present, a reasonable case can be made for using supplemental selenium to restore or increase the activity of glutathione enzymes in coronary or other vascular plaques and thus slow down the progress of coronary artery disease.

19. *Chromium*

Chromium helps insulin work more efficiently to control the blood sugar. Insulin must enter the cells through special receptors on the cell surface to help them break down carbohydrates. Recent studies have shown that chromium can double the number of insulin receptors in muscles and liver cells and improve insulin's effectiveness. Conversely, chromium deficiency reduces the number of insulin receptors, making insulin less effective. Insulin resistance raises the blood sugar and lowers the high blood HDL cholesterol level. For this reason, a large number of individuals with impaired sugar metabolism, including sedentary people, obese people, and diabetics, may benefit from chromium supplementation. Since impaired sugar metabolism and diabetes constitute a major risk factor for all cardiovascular diseases, including heart attacks, strokes, and peripheral vascular disease, the importance of adequate chromium intake becomes even more compelling.

20. As the process of coronary artery plaque formation develops, minerals present in blood (such as calcium, magnesium, iron, and copper) can become trapped within the plaque. These mineral deposits become part of the hardened structure of the arterial wall, and may further expand the inflammatory process that is at the core of atherosclerosis.

Calcification is an almost universal feature of advanced atherosclerosis. Coronary plaques with their ongoing inflammatory process create the right environment for the depositing of calcium or other minerals present in blood circulation. But there is no relationship between dietary calcium intake, the level of blood calcium, cholesterol levels, and calcification within the wall of coronary arteries.

Because vitamin D is fat soluble, supplemental vitamin D, either added to milk, cereals, or in multivitamin pills, is carried by lipoproteins and may accumulate within the arterial wall along with cholesterol. The concern is whether this excess vitamin D in people who have other coronary risk factors could be counterproductive, especially in post-menopausal women. It is quite plausible that the accumulated vitamin D can contribute to calcium deposits in the arterial wall. Unlike the vitamin D present in various foods and supplements, the vitamin D that is produced in the skin through sun exposure is carried by proteins (rather than fat) throughout the body, and therefore has very little or no risk of accumulating in the arterial wall and contributing to arterial calcification.

21. Of course the body does not absorb all flavonoids in foods efficiently. For example, quercetin in onions is in the form of quercetin glucoside, which the body absorbs at a rate of about 50 percent. On the other hand, quercetin in tea is in the form of quercetin rutinoside which is absorbed at a rate of about 17 percent. The higher concentration of quercetin in a cup of brewed, dark tea compensates for its slower absorption rate.

Part II: *The Twenty Risk Factors: One by One*
22. C. pneumoniae lives and replicates within the lungs' alveolar cells, and white blood cells carry them into the arterial wall. Among other things, these germs provoke the endothelial cells of the arteries into producing and releasing a compound called "tissue factor." Tissue factor is one of the most potent clotting agents, and, by promoting aggregation (clumping) of platelets, it may initiate tiny blood clots inside the arteries and contribute to the turmoil in the wall of coronary, carotid, or cerebral arteries that leads to strokes and heart attacks.

23. HDL "Milano"
Scientists have discovered a special HDL cholesterol called "Milano" (named after the city where it was first diagnosed) that is associated with longevity and freedom from coronary artery or other vascular diseases. Paradoxically, people with HDL Milano have a low level of HDL, usually in the range of 20-25 mg/dl.

When researchers gave HDL Milano to mice with experimentally induced atherosclerosis, they saw a dramatic decrease in, and even reversal of, the rodents' arterial disease. (Whether a similar result will be seen in humans given synthetic HDL Milano awaits further study.) In effect, HDL Milano particles are extremely efficient in removing cholesterol from the vessel wall, unloading it in the liver, and returning for more. HDL Milano also has a potent antioxidant effect, so that it almost completely blocks oxidization of LDL cholesterol in the arterial wall. Unfortunately, this type of HDL is quite uncommon; so far it has been seen only among some Mediterraneans and Japanese. Thus, for all practical purposes, a low HDL level almost always has an unfavorable cardiovascular impact.

HDL's antioxidant effect is due to an enzyme it carries called "paraoxonase." Nearly everyone has some paraoxonase; this enzyme can detoxify the poison gas sarin and dioxin if humans are exposed to them. In a recent study, investigators removed the gene responsible for producing the paraoxonase enzyme from a certain strain of mice. When they then tested the HDL cholesterol of these rodents, it failed to act like a normal HDL; instead of preventing oxidization of LDL cholesterol, it actually increased it.

The ability of the HDL cholesterol of different people to protect LDL cholesterol against oxidization varies greatly. This is because there are three different paraoxonase enzymes: AA, AB, and BB, each different in only a single amino acid in its chemical structure. The AA type enzyme provides a potent protection against LDL oxidization for several hours. In contrast, the BB variety is very weak and loses whatever potency it has within a few hours. The AB type is somewhere in between AA and BB. This genetic difference in HDL's paraoxonase also explains why some people with normal or even low HDL levels are protected against coronary artery disease, while others with normal or even relatively high levels of HDL are not.

Testing for HDL's paraoxonase is not widely available. However, in the near future it should be quite enlightening to learn about the paraoxonase type (AA, BB, or AB) of people with low HDL cholesterol, especially if they have multiple risk factors for coronary artery disease.

Are High HDL Cholesterol Levels Always Cardio-protective?

High HDL cholesterol provides substantial protection against coronary artery disease whether the LDL cholesterol is elevated or not. But this protection is at best about 50 percent. Since there are twenty major risk factors for coronary artery disease, we cannot expect one single protective measure to deal effectively with so many countermeasures. This fundamental reality of coronary artery disease once again emphasizes why prevention and treatment of coronary artery disease always require a variety of interventions, not just one or two.

Another problem with placing inordinate importance on a high HDL level is the existence of five subclasses, of which only HDL2 and HDL3 are cardio-protective. Also, in several disorders, HDL particles, even when there are plenty of them around, cannot function properly. To unload cholesterol in the liver, the HDL requires an unloading specialist called "cholesterol transfer protein." Several mutations (alterations in the amino acid sequence) of cholesterol transfer protein have been discovered that make this enzyme dysfunctional. As a result, HDL particles become like pick-up trucks loaded with debris (cholesterol), but are essentially useless because they cannot dump their load.

24. Why do some people have small LDL particles? There are several plausible explanations:

As blood triglyceride levels rise, the proportion of small, dense LDL particles increases progressively. When triglyceride levels exceed 300 mg/dl, a disproportionate number of LDL particles (more than 50 percent) are the small type B. Conversely, when triglycerides are under 100 mg/dl, most of the LDL particles are large or type A. When triglycerides are between these two levels, it is no longer so clear-cut. Since a large percentage of people have triglyceride levels that hover in the range of about 100-300 mg/dl, it is not possible to put these people accurately into one category or the other without the actual measurement of their LDL particle size.

People with diabetes or insulin resistance (the latter associated with abdominal obesity and sedentary lifestyle, with or without low HDL levels) also tend to have a high number of small, dense LDL particles. In a recent Canadian report (the Quebec Cardiovascular Study), investigators showed that the combination of raised LDL cholesterol level with a predominance of small, dense LDL particles, and an elevated fasting blood sugar level, was associated with a twentyfold increased risk of coronary artery disease in men. Of particular interest was the finding that adjustments for levels of other blood lipids (VLDL, HDL, or triglycerides) did not alter the results significantly.

People with a family history of premature coronary artery disease (before the age of fifty-five) whose LDL level is "normal" may have inherited the trait that produces more small LDL particles (type B). These individuals may or may not have elevated triglycerides, but often they have low HDL levels. In spite of their "normal" LDL level, their risk of experiencing a cardiovascular event is still three to five times greater than that of people with type A LDL. Several recent studies have confirmed that type B LDL exerts a powerful influence on the progression of coronary artery disease.

Individuals with coronary artery disease whose LDL pattern can be improved (from B to A), show far less progression, and may show regression, of their coronary artery disease than those whose pattern B remains unchanged.

As shown in Figure 14 below, when dietary fat provides 30 percent of energy intake, approximately 40 percent of LDL particles are of the small, dense (type B) variety. However, when total dietary fat is reduced to about 10 percent, nearly two-thirds of the LDL particles are type B. The transformation of large (type A) LDL particles to small (type B) particles which are highly atherogenic, provides another powerful argument against very low-fat, high-carbohydrate diets.

Figure 14
The Relation of Dietary Fat Intake to LDL Particle Size

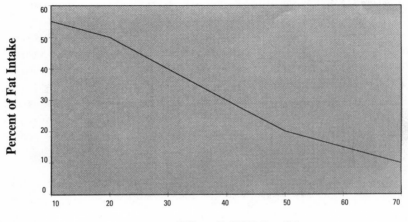

Percent of Type B LDL Particles

As the total dietary fat intake is *decreased*, a substantially higher percentage of LDL particles become smaller and denser (type B). Thus, very low-fat (and high-carbohydrate) diets often convert a type A (predominantly large LDL particles) to the more atherogenic type B (predominantly small, dense LDL particles).

25. *Safety and Side Effects of Statins*

In the past ten years, millions of people throughout the world have been treated with various statins with a high level of safety. Indeed, when used judiciously, all statins are quite safe. On rare occasions, someone who takes statins might develop minor "abnormalities" in his or her liver-function tests. Most often, this is not due to any damage to the liver, but is the result of a slight increase in the liver cells' permeability, allowing some liver-made compounds to leak into the bloodstream and be picked up by blood tests. This is a harmless effect, and gradually goes away as use of the statin is continued. The distinction between a harmless short-term biological event and a true toxic effect is important, because many people are unduly frightened by the possibility of liver damage with the use of any drug. Each year, nearly half a million people in the United States die of coronary artery disease, but very few have ever had a serious or fatal side effect from these drugs. Overall, fewer than one out of five hundred people who take statins at average doses show any minor abnormalities in liver function tests. Extremely rare cases of acute or chronic hepatitis have been reported in some users, but the risk is miniscule. For this reason, frequent monitoring of liver tests is unnecessary.

Occasionally, people who take statins may experience muscle pain, especially when statins have been used at high doses. Muscle pain occurs in approximately one out of five hundred cases with average doses of statins. There is no evidence to suggest that any one statin is more likely to cause muscle pain than others. In these situations, stopping the drug for one to two weeks is all that is required. You can almost always resume the same statin (or a different statin) at a slightly reduced dose within two weeks. To avoid recurrence of muscle pain, it is advisable to have a two-day "drug holiday" (for example, no statin on weekends), or even use it every other day for two to three months before the daily dose is resumed.

Although the manufacturers of statins recommend a blood test called "creatine kinase" to detect muscle injury in those who experience pain, this test is rarely useful. To register on the CK test as abnormal, the measurement would have to exceed ten times the normal level. More than 95 percent of the people who experience muscle pain while on statins do not have any change in their CK levels, or their levels are far less than ten times the norm.

Except for Pravachol, statins can react with a number of drugs taken concurrently, which can significantly increase the risk of muscle pain. Some of these include anti-fungal drugs, calcium channel blockers (taken by many patients with cardiovascular disease), and certain antibiotics such as erythromycin or Biaxin. For these individuals, Pravachol is clearly preferable to other statins. The alternative is to stop the statin during treatment with the above drugs, something that is neither practical nor desirable.

Recent long-term data from four large studies, which included more than ten thousand individuals who were treated with statins for over five years, have shown no evidence that statins cause cancers, psychiatric disorders, or any other chronic side effects. Approximately 1 percent of those who take statins may develop an allergic reaction to them. However, an allergic reaction to one drug does not mean a similar reaction to other statins.

Several recent studies have shown that statins not only lower LDL cholesterol and triglycerides, but are extremely effective in preventing or treating osteoporosis. This is an immensely important new finding since a large number of people who take these drugs are over the age of fifty, when osteoporosis usually starts. New studies have also shown that statins may have an important role in preventing certain cancers such as colon, breast, or prostate.

26. Lipoprotein(a) is present only in monkeys, apes, humans, and (for some inexplicable reason) hedgehogs. Blood levels of lipoprotein(a) are, to a great extent, genetically determined. Normal values should be under 30 mg/dl. People in the Far East (especially Japanese) and African Americans tend to have much higher blood levels. Recent studies have shown that there are over thirty-five different types (or isoforms) of lipoprotein(a), among which only isoforms with low molecular weight have atherogenic potential. Many African Americans with elevated lipoprotein(a), even in excess of 100 mg/dl, have very low levels of the low molecular weight isoforms, and therefore are not at a particularly higher risk of developing coronary artery disease. Because of its various isoforms and their biologically diverse functions, interpretation of lipoprotein(a) levels is not straightforward. Still, in those at high risk of coronary artery disease, lipoprotein(a) levels should be obtained. In the future, testing for lipoprotein(a) isoforms may prove more helpful than testing for total lipoprotein(a) level.

27. Although, for the sake of convenience and simplification, HDL cholesterol is often presented as a single entity, there are actually at least five different types of HDL, of which HDL-2 accounts for most of the cardio-protective function. It has long been known that one of the major functions of HDL cholesterol is to prevent oxidization of LDL particles. But this protective role may vary from person to person, even with the same blood level of HDL cholesterol. Recent studies have shown that HDL particles contain a potent antioxidant enzyme called paraoxonase. There are two different types of paraoxonases: A and B. People who are genetically programmed to have type AA (one gene from each parent) can protect LDL against oxidization for many hours. In contrast, the antioxidant potency of type BB HDL cholesterol is very weak. Approximately one-third of the population has type AA paraoxonase while another one-third has type BB. The remainder are AB types with intermediate antioxidant potentials. This, and other genetic differences between HDL particles, partially explains why some people with "normal" HDL levels may still develop coronary artery disease and heart attack, while others with relatively low HDL levels are protected.

Although people are often quick to blame diet for their elevated LDL cholesterol, the majority have an inherited disorder in which their liver cells are unable to produce enough healthy LDL-receptors. Admittedly, your diet and lifestyle can increase or decrease the number of LDL-receptors you have, but the basic problem is still a genetic defect inherited from parents or grandparents. So far, over 350 different mutations in the structure of LDL-receptors have been identified, each affecting the work of these receptors differently.

There is a constant exchange of cholesterol for triglycerides, and a give-and-take between HDL cholesterol, LDL cholesterol, and VLDL cholesterol in the bloodstream. This bartering is regulated by an enzyme called "cholesterol transfer protein." When cholesterol transfer protein is genetically defective, this bartering cannot take place efficiently, so the LDL and VLDL cholesterol and triglyceride levels go up. Another important enzyme called "lipoprotein lipase" is responsible for breaking down triglycerides so that they can enter the liver cells for disposal. Genetic mutations of this enzyme are often the main reason for a familial disorder in which blood triglyceride levels are very high.

The protein part of lipoproteins is called "apoprotein." HDL's important protein is apoprotein A-1, and LDL's is apoprotein B-100. Aside from apoprotein A and B, there are a number of other apoproteins (from C to H) that have various roles in cardiovascular health. Apoprotein E and its subgroups (apo E2, E3, and E4; apo E1 is extremely rare) have a significant role in a person's response to dietary fat and cholesterol.

Depending on which genetic form of apo E a person receives from each parent, there could be six variants or "isoforms" of apo E: E2-2, E2-3, E2-4, E3-3, E3-4, E4-4. People who have apo E4-4 are cholesterol and saturated fat responders: after a fatty meal, their blood cholesterol levels go up nearly three times as much as those who have the apo E2-2. People who have apo E4-4 also show a more dramatic fall in their blood cholesterol level in response to cholesterol lowering measures. On the other hand, those with apo E3-2 or E2-2 have much lower blood cholesterol levels, and do not show a significant response to dietary fat or cholesterol. Thus, the apo E status of an individual goes a long way toward explaining why some people with "terrible" eating habits do not have raised blood cholesterol levels or develop coronary artery disease.

Although carriers of a single genetic risk factor may not have a high risk for developing coronary artery disease, people who inherit several coronary risk factors have a much greater risk. Some examples of more ominous combinations of risk factors include: elevated homocysteine with hypertension and high LDL cholesterol; or elevated cholesterol with low HDL, diabetes, and sedentary lifestyle.

Of course, not all the genetic information we receive from our parents is harmful. For example, if we are lucky enough to receive the genes for a decent HDL level, apo E2-2, or large LDL particles, we are protected to a much greater extent against coronary artery disease. One of the clotting factors in our blood circulation is factor 7 (there are twelve clotting factors). People with mutations in their factor 7 which make it dysfunctional have a 50 percent lower risk of a heart attack because they are far less likely to develop blood clots in their coronary artery, even if they have coronary artery disease.

28. Gene Therapy

Because of the great influence of genetic factors on coronary artery disease, gene therapy may provide some of the most promising approaches to prevention and treatment. Although genetic manipulations are at various stages of research, many are currently being conducted in clinical settings among people suffering from coronary artery disease.

For example, the gene for the LDL-receptor has been identified and transferred to humans with severe LDL-receptor deficiency who have very high blood LDL cholesterol and severe coronary artery disease. Unfortunately, the technique is not yet sufficiently refined, and the genes do not survive for more than several weeks. More recently, independent groups of researchers have developed novel methods to inject genetic material into the heart muscle in order to promote the production of a protein called "vascular-endothelial growth factor." This protein stimulates the growth of new blood vessels for oxygen-starved portions of the heart muscle in people who have suffered previous heart attacks and have not responded to bypass surgery. Preliminary data suggest that a large number of these individuals respond, with the result of at least several months of relief from their angina.

In the future it may be quite possible to implant genetic materials prophylactically into the liver of people with low HDL, high LDL, or high triglycerides, long before they have suffered the devastating consequences of coronary artery disease. Other genetic manipulations might help repair endothelial damage, correct diabetes, or homocysteine disorder. Until then, we have to do what we can to counteract Mother Nature's misdeeds. The Twenty Risk Factors provides a wealth of information to keep your heart healthy until these technological advances have been refined and made practical.

Glossary

Angiography—Injecting a dye into an artery and taking X-ray pictures to check for narrowing or clogging of the arteries.

Angioplasty—Removing debris from the clogging and plaques in the arterial wall to open or at least widen the lumen of an artery. This is usually done through special catheters inserted into the arteries. At times, tiny balloons are passed through these catheters and placed within the narrow segments of the vessels. By gently dilating the balloons repeatedly, some narrow segments can be dilated to allow an adequate blood flow. This is called "balloon angioplasty."

Apoproteins—Also called apolipoproteins (or apo). These important proteins are the "managers" or the "drivers" of lipoprotein-cholesterol molecules. They direct where the good or bad cholesterol particles go, and what they do. The important apoproteins are: apo A-1, which is carried by HDL cholesterol and is cardio-protective, and apo B-100, which is carried by LDL cholesterol and is damaging to the inner wall of the arteries.

Arteriosclerosis—Hardening (= sclerosis), thickening, and loss of elasticity of the arteries, due to degenerative changes.

Atherogenic—Having the potential to cause atheroma formation (see atheroma).

Atheroma—An area of the arterial wall that is bulging with a collection or deposits of various substances. Atheroma is commonly made up of blood platelets, white blood cells that have gobbled up and are engorged with oxidized-cholesterol (foam cells), dysfunctional smooth muscle cells, and deposits of collagen fibers and various minerals, such as iron, calcium, copper, etc. Rupture of an atheroma is the principal cause of heart attack.

Atherosclerosis—When there are numerous atheromas along the arterial tree, especially in coronary arteries or brain arteries, the condition is referred to as atherosclerosis.

Cis and trans fatty acids—The molecules of fatty acids are arranged like bracelets or chains made up of carbon atoms. Hydrogen atoms dangle from these carbon atoms like charms on a bracelet. When hydrogen atoms are on one side (up or down) of unsaturated carbons in a polyunsaturated fat, it is called a cis form. Cis fatty acids are usually liquid at room temperature. When the hydrogen atoms are on both sides (up and down) of the chain, it is called a trans fatty acid (Figure 13-B). Trans fatty acids are produced during the hydrogenation process of vegetable oils, and are usually solid or semisolid at room temperature.

Cholesterol—One of many fatty substances in blood and tissues of all animals. No plant contains cholesterol.

Cholesterol look-alikes—These are plant versions of cholesterol that are called phytosterols (phyto=plant). Phytosterols are usually not absorbed by the human intestine. They also reduce or block the absorption of dietary cholesterol.

Coronary Artery Disease (CAD)—When any segment or branch of the heart's artery (= coronary artery) is distorted or clogged (either partially or more extensively), the condition is referred to as coronary artery disease or atherosclerosis of the coronary artery.

Coronary Heart Disease (CHD) (or ischemic heart disease)—When CAD has progressed and caused certain coronary events such as angina (chest pain), heart failure, or heart attack, it is called CHD. Since in CHD the damage to heart muscle is the result of poor circulation (ischemia), Europeans often refer to it as "ischemic heart disease."

Down-regulating—Slowing down, suppressing, inhibiting.

Endogenous—Produced within the human body.

Endothelium—The thin inner lining of arteries made up of a single layer of cells. Injury to, or dysfunction of, the endothelium is the first and the most important step in the development of coronary artery disease.

Enzyme—Important substance within the human body that facilitates a variety of functions, without which the body cannot function.

Essential—When used in the context of the human body, it implies that it must be provided through dietary intake, since the body cannot produce it. Some amino acids and fatty acids are "essential" for the body's function, but carbohydrates or most fats are not.

Exogenous—Provided from outside the body, such as through diet or in the form of medications or supplements (the opposite of endogenous).

Fatty Acids—These are the smaller by-products of the breakdown or digestion of various fats. There are several kinds of fatty acids. When one molecule of fatty acids is joined to one molecule of glycerol, it is called "monoglyceride." When two or three fatty acids are attached to one molecule of glycerol, they form "diglycerides" and "triglycerides." If the carbon molecules in fatty acids are fully occupied with hydrogen atoms, they are called saturated, otherwise they are unsaturated (Figure 13-A).

Foam cells—These white blood cells, called "monocytes," reside inside the wall of the arteries and gobble up large amounts of LDL cholesterol. When viewed under a microscope, the cholesterol-laden monocytes look foamy or bubbly, hence the name.

Free Radicals, also Oxygen Free Radicals, Superoxides, and Hydroxyl Radicals—Each living cell, especially in humans and higher animals, is a nonstop microscopic factory where hundreds of biochemical reactions are constantly taking place. During these activities, certain unstable and toxic by-products are produced which are referred to as "free radicals." Some free radicals have very unstable oxygen atoms, hence oxygen free radicals. Normally, almost all of these unstable by-products are immediately neutralized within the cells by other chemicals, enzymes, and reactions. Excessive production or inadequate neutralization of these free radicals may have important roles in certain cancers, damage to the heart muscle, liver, lungs, and many other organs (see Oxidize).

Hydrogenation—A processing technique in which hydrogen atoms are added to unsaturated fatty acids. This is done to convert a liquid fat (oil) into a solid fat which improves its stability and shelf life. During partial hydrogenation of natural oils, a number of trans fatty acids are produced which are actually harmful. Recent advances in food technology have enabled margarine manufactures to produce some spreads with very little or no trans fatty acids (see Cis and trans fatty acids).

Lipids—Various fatty substances, including those in blood circulation, such as cholesterol, lipoproteins, etc.

Lipoproteins—These are tiny pellets that contain various fats (lipids) and proteins (hence, lipo-proteins). Lipoproteins are nature's "limousines" for cholesterol to ride on and be transported throughout the body. The more protein they have the denser they are. Conversely, higher concentrations of various fats make them less dense, very much like lean versus fatty meats. Based on their density, they are classified as very low density lipoproteins (VLDL) with the highest fat, to intermediate density lipoproteins (IDL), low density lipoproteins (LDL), and high density lipoproteins (HDL) with the lowest amount of fat and highest concentration of protein (Figure 1).

Macrophages—see Monocytes.

Monocytes—These are specialized human white blood cells which often play the role of scavengers in various tissues. Larger monocytes are called macrophages and act like a biological "pac-man," clearing debris, oxidized cholesterol, etc. from various sites in the human body.

Morbidity—Complications and disabilities of a disease.

Mortality—Death rate from a given disease. Mortality can be expressed per 100, 1,000, or 10,000 cases depending on how common the death rate is for a given disease.

N-3 and N-6 polyunsaturated fatty acids (PUFA)—also called omega-3 and omega-6 PUFA (Figure 13). If the first double bond (unsaturated carbon) of a PUFA is three carbons away from the left end of the chain, it is called an n-3, or omega-3 PUFA. If the first double bond is six carbons away, it forms an n-6 PUFA. The position of this first double bond confers profoundly different biological functions to PUFA (Chapter 2, "Omega-6 Polyunsaturated Fat" through "Omega-3 Polyunsaturated Fat").

Omega-3 and Omega-6 polyunsaturates—see above.

Oxidants (or Oxidizing Agents)—Any compound that gives up oxygen, or attracts hydrogen or electrons from another compound. Antioxidants inhibit or reduce these reactions.

Oxidize—To combine with oxygen, or to give up hydrogen or electrons. A compound is oxidized when it is combined with oxygen, or coerced to give up hydrogen or electrons. Oxidization should not be confused with oxygenation. The browning of an apple after a bite or rusting of a nail are examples of oxidization.

Oxygenation—The process of delivering oxygen to various tissues. Since oxygen is carried by red blood cells, uninterrupted blood circulation is essential for tissue oxygenation.

Polymerization—Most fats, especially polyunsaturated fatty acids, form larger molecules or polymers when exposed to relatively high temperatures. Polymerization reduces the bio-availability of polyunsaturated fatty acids, making them less absorbable.

Psyllium (pronounced silly-om)—A water soluble fiber from the husk of a plant. Psyllium is used as a supplement (or is in some cereals) to provide additional fiber to the diet.

Receptor Activity and Receptor Sites—To work properly in the human body, many chemical and biochemical substances must enter various cells through specific receiving docks or entrances. These entrances are called "receptors" or "receptor sites." If an adequate number of receptors are not available, or have already been occupied ("competitively") by other substances, then the receptor activity is low. For example, a low receptor activity for LDL cholesterol will prevent LDL particles from entering the liver and other tissues for disposal. Under these circumstances, LDL cholesterol particles have no place to "dock," so they return to blood circulation and raise the blood cholesterol level. In some cases, there are plenty of LDL-receptors, but because they are defective, or "mutants," they cannot allow LDL particles to enter liver cells. So far, over 350 mutant or abnormal types of LDL-receptors have been identified.

Responder and Nonresponder—In medicine, these terms are used to identify individuals who will or will not respond to a particular form of treatment or intervention. For example, many people are salt nonresponders, meaning that no matter how much salt they eat, it will not affect their blood pressure. Similarly, about 70 percent of the population are cholesterol nonresponders whose blood cholesterol levels will not rise appreciably with cholesterol feeding.

Sterols—The basic skeleton of certain chemicals made in animal or plant tissues. Cholesterol is a sterol that is produced in animal tissues only. The plant version of sterol or its cholesterol look-alike is called phytosterol (phyto = plant).

Superoxides—Potent oxidants that are generated within human tissues, usually under metabolic stress (see Oxidants).

T-lymphocytes or T-cells—Special white blood cells which are enormously important in defending against various bacterial and viral infections. When the number of T-cells is abnormally low, immune defenses are broken down, making an individual very susceptible to infections and certain cancers.

Thrombogenic—Having the potential to cause a thrombosis, or clotting of the blood inside the arteries or veins.

Thrombosis—Clotting of blood inside an artery or a vein. Thrombosis of a coronary artery chokes off the circulation, causing a heart attack. The same process in a cerebral artery results in a stroke, whereas a thrombosis in a vein results in phlebitis.

TPA Tissue Plasminogen Activator—One of the most potent clot-busting anti-coagulants. TPA is the drug used in emergency departments as soon as someone with a heart attack (or coronary thrombosis) arrives. The goal is to dissolve the clot and open up the artery's lumen before severe, irreversible damage to the heart muscle occurs.

Trans fatty acids—see Cis and trans fatty acids.

Selected References

PART I

Chapter 1

Verschuren Wm, Jacobs Dr, Boemberg BPM, et al. Serum total cholesterol and long-term coronary heart disease mortality in different cultures. Twenty-five-year follow-up of Seven Countries Study. JAMA 1995; 274: 131-36.

Kwiterovich PO. The anti-atherogenic role of high density lipoprotein cholesterol. Amer J Cardiol 1998; 82: 13Q-21Q.

Miller M, Seidler A, Moalemi A, Pearson TA. Normal triglyceride levels and coronary artery disease events: The Baltimore Coronary Observational Long-Term Study. J Amer Coll Cardiol 1998; 31: 1252-57.

Gaziano JM, Henneken CH, O'Donnell EJ, et al. Fasting triglycerides, high density lipoprotein and risk of myocardial infarction. Circulation 1997; 96: 2520-25.

Selwyn AP, Kinlay S, Creager M, et al. Endothelial cell dysfunction in atherosclerosis and ischemic manifestations of coronary artery disease. Amer J Cardiol 1997; 79 (5A): 17-23.

Kullo IJ, Edwards WD, Schwartz RS. Vulnerable plaque: pathobiology and clinical implications. Ann Intern Med 1998; 129: 1050-60.

Ross R. Atherosclerosis—An inflammatory disease. N Eng J Med 1999; 340: 115-26.

For "The Twenty Major Risk Factors," see references for Part II.

Chapter 2: "Should We Fear Dietary Cholesterol?" and "Saturated Fat"

West of Scotland Coronary Prevention Study Group. Influence of pravastatin and plasma lipids on clinical events in the West of Scotland Coronary Prevention Study. Circulation 1998; 97: 1440-45.

Sacks FM, Moye LA, Davis BR, et al. Relationship between plasma LDL cholesterol concentrations during treatment with pravastatin and recurrent coronary events. Circulation 1998; 97: 1446-52.

MacMahon S, Sharpe N, Gamble G, et al. Effects of lowering average or below-average cholesterol levels on progression of carotid atherosclerosis. Circulation 1998; 97: 1784-90.

Stein EA, Illingsworth DR, Kwiterovich PO, et al. Efficacy and safety of lovastatin in adolescent males with heterozygous familial hypercholesterolemia. A randomized controlled study. JAMA 1999; 281: 137-144.

Hu FB, Stampfer MJ, Manson JE. Dietary fat intake and the risk of coronary heart disease in women. N Eng J Med 1997; 337: 1491-99.

Dupuis J, Tardif JC, Cernacek P, et al. Cholesterol reduction rapidly improves endothelial function after acute coronary syndromes. Circulation 1999; 99: 3227-33.

Chapter 2: "Monounsaturated Fat" through "Omega-3 Polyunsaturated Fat"

DeCaterina R, Liao JK, Libby P. Fatty acid modulation of endothelial activation. Am J Clin Nut, 2000; 71: 213-223s.

Lichtenstein AH, Ausman LE, Jalbert SM, Schafer EJ. Effects of different forms of dietary hydrogenated fats on serum lipoprotein cholesterol levels. N Eng J Med 1999; 340: 1933-40.

Williams MJA, Sutherland WHF, McCormick MP, et al. Impaired endothelial function following a meal rich in used cooking fat. J Amer Coll Cardiol 1999; 33: 1050-55.

Willet WC. Specific fatty acids and risks of breast and prostate cancer: Dietary intake. Am J Clin Nutri 1997; 66: 15575-635.

Wolk A, Bergstrom R, Hunter D, et al. A prospective study of association of monounsaturated fat and other types of fat with risk of breast cancer. Arch Intern Med 1998; 158: 41-45.

Ascherio A, Katan MB, Stampfer MJ, Willett WC. Trans fatty acids and coronary heart disease. N Eng J Med 1999; 340: 1994-98.

Eritsland J. Safety considerations of polyunsaturated fatty acids. Am J Clin Nutr 2000; 71 (Suppl): 197-201s.

Hunter DJ, Spiegleman D, Adami HO, et al. Cohort studies of fat intake and the risk of breast cancer. A pooled analysis. N Eng J Med 1996; 334: 354-61.

Gillman MW, Cupples A, Millen BE, et al. Inverse association of dietary fat with development of ischemic stroke in men. JAMA 1997; 218: 2145-50.

GISSI—Prevenzione investigators. Dietary supplementation with n-3 polyunsaturated fatty acids and vitamin E after myocardial infarction: results of the GISSI-Prevenzione Trial. Lancet 1999; 354: 447-55.

Hu FB, Stampfer MJ, Manson JE, et al. Dietary intake of alpha-linolenic acid and risk of fatal ischemic heart disease among women. Am J Clin Nutr 1999; 69: 890-97.

Siscovick DS, Raghunathan TE, King I, et al. Dietary intake and cell membrane levels of long-chain N-3 polyunsaturated fatty acids and the risk of primary cardiac arrest. Am J Clin Nutr 2000; 71 (Suppl): 208-212s.

Daviglus ML, Stamler J, Orencia AJ, et al. Fish consumption and the 30-year risk of fatal myocardial infarction. N Eng J Med 1997; 336: 1046-53.

Goodfellow J, Bellamy MF, Ramsey MW, et al. Dietary supplementation with marine omega-3 fatty acids improve systemic large artery endothelial function in subjects with hypercholesterolemia. J Am Coll Cardiol 2000; 35: 265-70.

Egeland GM, Middaugh JP. Balancing fish consumption benefits with mercury exposure. Science 1997; 278: 1904-05.

Davidson PW, Myers GJ, Cox C, et al. Effects of prenatal and post-natal methylmercury exposure from fish consumption on neurodevelopment. JAMA 1998; 280: 701-07.

Albert CM, Hennekens CH, O'Donnell CJ, et al. Fish consumption and risk of sudden cardiac death. JAMA 1998; 279: 23-28.

Stoll AL, Severus E, Freeman MP, et al. Omega-3 fatty acids in bipolar disorder. A preliminary double blind, placebo-controlled trial. Arch G Psychiatry 1999; 56: 407-12.

de Lorgeril M, Salen P, Martin JL. Mediterranean diet, traditional risk factors, and the rate of cardiovascular complications after myocardial infarction. Final report of the Lyon Diet Heart Study. Circulation 1999; 99: 779-85.

Chapter 2: "Carbohydrates and Proteins"

Starc TJ, Shea S, Cohn LC, et al. Greater dietary intake of simple carbohydrates is associated with lower concentrations of high density lipoprotein cholesterol in hypercholesterolemic children. Am J Clin Nutr 1998; 67: 1147-54.

Stefanick ML, Mackey S, Sheehan M, et al. Effects of diet and exercise in men and post-menopausal women with low levels of HDL cholesterol and high levels of LDL cholesterol. N Eng. J Med 1998; 339: 12-20.

Hu FB, Stampfer MJ, Manson JE, et al. Dietary protein and risk of ischemic heart disease in women. Am J Clin Nutr 1999; 70: 221-27.

Chapter 2: "Supplemental Vitamins and Minerals"

Kushi LH, Folson AR, Prineas RJ, et al. Dietary antioxidant vitamins and death from coronary heart disease in post-menopausal women. N Eng J Med 1996; 334: 1156-62.

Stephens NG, Parsons A, Schofield PM., et al. Randomized controlled trial of vitamin E in patients with coronary disease: Cambridge Heart Antioxidant Study. Lancet 1996; 347: 781-86.

Keli So, Hertog MGL, Feskins EJM, Kromhout D. Dietary flavonoids, antioxidant vitamins and incidence of stroke. The Zutphen Study. Arch Intern Med 1996; 154: 637-42.

Motoyama T, Kawano H, Kugiyama K, et al. Vitamin E administration improves impairment of endothelium-dependent vasodilation in patients with coronary spastic angina. J Am Coll Cardiol 1998; 32: 1672-79.

Heinonen OP, Albanes D, Virtamo J, et al. Prostate cancer and supplementation with alpha tocopherol and beta carotene: incidence and mortality in a controlled trial. J Nat'l Cancer Institute 1998; 90: 440-46.

Miller ER, Appel LJ, Risby JH. Effect of dietary pattern on measures of lipid peroxidation. Results from a randomized clinical trial. Circulation 1998; 98: 2390-95.

Lionis C, Faresjo A, Skoula M, et al. Antioxidant effects of herbs in Crete. Lancet 1998; 352: 1987-88.

Paetau I, Khachik F, Brown ED, et al. Chronic ingestion of lycopene-rich tomato juice or lycopene supplements significantly increases plasma concentrations of lycopene and related tomato carotenoids in humans. Am J Clin Nutr 1998; 68: 1187-95.

Day AP, Kemp HJ, Bolton C, et al. Effect of concentrated red grape juice consumption on serum antioxidant capacity and low density lipoprotein oxidization. Ann Nutr Metab 1997; 41: 353-57.

Philipp CS, Cisar LA, Saidi P, Kostis JB. Effect of niacin supplementation on fibrinogen levels in patients with peripheral vascular disease. Am J Cardiol 1998; 82: 897-99.

Riggs KM, Spiro A, Tucker K, Rush D. Relations of vitamin B-12, vitamin B-6, folate, and homocysteine to cognitive function in the Normative Aging Study. Am J Clin Nutr 1996; 63: 306-14.

Giovannucci E, Stampfer MJ, Colditz GA. Multivitamin use, folate, and colon cancer in women in the Nurses' Health Study. Am Intern Med 1998; 29: 517-24.

Zhang S, Hunter DJ, Hankinson SE, et al. A prospective study of folate intake and the risk of breast cancer. JAMA 1999; 281: 1632-37.

Curhan GC, Willet WC, Speezer, et al. Comparison of dietary calcium with supplemental calcium and other nutrients as factors affecting the risk for kidney stones in women. Ann Intern Med 1997; 126: 497-504.

Ernest E. Chelation therapy for peripheral arterial occlusive disease. A systematic review. Circulation 1997; 96: 1031-33.

Dawson-Hughes B, Harris SS, Krall EA, Dallal GE. Effect of calcium and vitamin D supplementation on bone density in men and women 65 years of age or older. N Eng J Med 1997; 337: 670-76.

Baron JA, Beach M, Mandel JS, et al. Calcium supplements for the prevention of colorectal adenomas. N Eng J Med 1999; 340: 101-07.

Weinberg MH. The salt-blood pressure connection: data and implications. Contem Intern Med 1997; 9: 7-11.

Egan BM, Stepniakowski KT. Adverse effects of short-term very-low salt diets in subjects with risk factor clustering. Am J Clin Nutr 1997; 65: 671s-77s.

Clark LC, Dalkin B, Krongrad A, et al. Decreased incidence of prostate cancer with selenium supplementation: Results of a double blind cancer prevention trial. Br J Urol 1998; 81: 730-34.

Yoshizawa K, Willet WC, Morris SJ, et al. Study of prediagnostic selenium level in toenails and the risk of advanced prostate cancer. J Nat'l Cancer Inst 1998; 90: 1219-24.

Carti MC, Guralnik JM, Salive ME, et al. Serum iron level, coronary artery disease, and all-cause mortality in older men and women. Am J Cardiol 1997; 79: 120-27.

Sullivan JL. Iron and the genetics of cardiovascular disease. Circulation 1999; 100: 1260-63.

Liao F, Folsom AR, Brancati FL. Is low magnesium concentration a risk factor for coronary heart disease? The Atherosclerosis Risk in Communities Study. Am Heart J 1998; 136: 480-90.

Chapter 2: "Fruits, Vegetables, Herbs, and Nuts"

Cao G, Booth SL, Sandowski JA, Prior RL. Increases in human plasma antioxidant capacity after consumption of controlled diets high in fruits and vegetables. Am J Clin Nutr 1998; 68: 1081-87.

Miller ER, Appel LJ, Risby TH. Effect of dietary pattern on measures of lipid peroxidation. Results from a randomized clinical trial. Circulation 1998; 98: 2390-95.

Jacobs DR, Meyer KA, Kushi LH, Folsom AR. Whole grain intake may reduce the risk of ischemic heart disease death in post-menopausal women: The Iowa Women's Health Study. Am J Nutr 1998; 68: 248-57.

Joshipura KJ, Ascherio A, Manson JE, et al. Fruit and vegetable intake in relation to risk of ischemic stroke among men and women. JAMA 1999; 282: 1233-39.

Rimm EB, Ascherio A, Givannucci E, et al. Vegetables, fruit, and cereal fiber intake and risk of coronary heart disease among men. JAMA 1996; 275: 447-51.

Chapter 2: "Herbal Supplements"

Sheikh WM, Philen RM, Love LA. Chaparral-associated hepatotoxicity. Arch Intern Med 1997; 157: 913-19.

Larrey D. Hepatotoxicity of herbal remedies. J hepatol 1997; 26s: 47-51.

Mashour NH, Lin GI, Frishman WF. Herbal medicine for the treatment of cardiovascular disease. Arch Intern Med 1998; 158: 2225-34.

Chan JM, Stampfer MJ, Giovannucci, et al. Plasma insulin-like growth factor and prostate cancer risk. Science 1998; 279: 563-66.

Goldberg M. Dehydroepiandrosterone, insulin-like growth factor and prostate cancer. Ann Intern Med 1998; 129: 587-88.

Leder BZ, Longcope C, Ahrens B, et al. Oral androstenedione administration and serum testosterone and estrogen concentrations in young men. JAMA 2000; 283: 779-82.

Khatta M, Alexander BS, Kritchten CM, et al. The effect of coenzyme Q10 in patients with congestive heart failure. Ann Intern Med 2000; 132: 636-40.

Isaacsohn JL, Moser M, Stein E, et al. Garlic powder and plasma lipids and lipoproteins. Arch Intern Med 1998; 158: 1189-94.

Berthold HK, Sudhp T, Von Bergmann K. Effect of a garlic oil preparation on serum lipoproteins and cholesterol metabolism: A randomized, controlled trial. JAMA 1998; 279: 1900-02.

Superko HR, Krauss RM. Garlic powder (has no) effect on plasma lipids, post-prandial lipemia, low-density lipoprotein particle size, high-density lipoprotein, subclass distribution, and lipoprotein(a). J Am Coll Cardiol 2000; 35: 321-26.

Fugh-Berman A. Herb-drug interactions. Lancet 2000; 355:134-38.

Chapter 2: "Dietary Fiber"

Rimm EB, Ascherio A, Giovannucci, et al. Vegetable, fruit, and cereal intake and risk of coronary heart disease among men. JAMA 1996; 275: 447-51.

Jacobs DR, Meyer KA, Kushi LH, Folsom AR. Whole grain intake may reduce the risk of ischemic heart disease deaths in post-menopausal women: The Iowa Women's Health Study. Am J Clin Nutr 1998; 68: 248-57.

Wolk A, Manson JE, Stampfer MJ, et al. Long-term intake of dietary fiber and decreased risk of coronary heart disease among women. JAMA 1999; 281: 1998-2004.

Brown L, Rosner B, Willet WW, Sacks FM. Cholesterol-lowering effects of dietary fiber: a meta-analysis. Am J Clin Nutr 1999; 69: 30-42.

Fuchs CS, Giovannucci EL, Colditz GA, et al. Dietary fiber and the risk of colo-rectal cancer and adenoma in women. N Eng J Med 1999; 340: 169-76.

Schatzkin A, Lanza E, Corle D, et al. Lack of effect of a low-fat, high-fiber diet on the recurrence of colorectal adenomas. N Eng J Med 2000; 342: 1149-55.

Chapter 2: "Beverages"

Klatsky A, Armstrong MA, Friedman GD. Red wine, white wine, liquor, beer, and risk for coronary artery disease hospitalization. Am J Cardiol 1997; 80: 416-20.

Kiechl S, Willett J, Rungger G, et al. Alcohol consumption and atherosclerosis: What is the relation? Prospective results from the Bruneck Study. Stroke 1998; 29: 900-07.

Camargo CA, Hennekens CH, Gaziano M, et al. Prospective study of moderate alcohol consumption and mortality in U.S. Male Physicians. Arch Intern Med 1997; 157: 74-85.

Nigdikar S, Williams NR, Griffin BA, Howard AN. Consumption of red wine polyphenols reduces the susceptibility of low-density lipoprotein to oxidization in vivo. Am J Clin Nutr 1998; 68: 258-65.

Valmadrid CT, Klein R, Moss SE. Alcohol intake and the risk of coronary artery disease mortality in persons with older-onset diabetes. JAMA 1999; 282: 239-46.

Teyssen S, Lenzing T, Gonzalez-Calero G, et al. Alcoholic beverages produced by fermentation but not by distillation are powerful stimulants of gastric secretion in humans. Gut 1997; 40: 49-56.

Gaziano SM, Hennekens CH, Godfried SL, et al. Type of alcoholic beverage and risk of myocardial infarction. Am J Cardiol 1998; 83: 52-57.

Sacco RL, Elkind M, Boden-Albala B, et al. The protective effect of moderate alcohol consumption on ischemic stroke. JAMA 1999; 281: 53-60.

Tjonneland A, Gronbaek M, Stripp C, Overvad IC. Wine intake and diet in a random sample of 48,763 Danish men and women. Am J Clin Nutr 1999; 69: 49-54.

Curhan GC, Willett WC, Speizer FE, Stampfer MJ. Beverage use and risk of kidney stones in women. Ann Intern Med 1998; 128: 534-40.

Michaud DS, Spiegelman D, Clinton SK, et al. Fluid intake and risk of bladder cancer in men. N Eng J Med 1999; 340: 1390-97.

Day AP, Kemp HJ, Bolton C, et al. Effect of concentrated red grape juice consumption on serum antioxidant capacity and low-density lipoprotein oxidization. Ann Nutr Metab 1997; 41: 353-57.

Garzon P, Eisenberg MJ. Variation in the mineral content of commercially available bottled waters: implications for health and disease. Am J Med 1998; 105: 125-30.

Rubenowitz E, Axelsson G, Rylander R. Magnessium and calcium in drinking water and death from acute myocardial infarction in women. Epidemiology 1999; 10: 31-36.

Willett WC, Stampfer MJ, Mason JE, et al. Coffee consumption and coronary heart disease in women. A ten-year follow-up. JAMA 1996; 275: 458-62.

Leitmann MF, Willett WC, Rimm EB, et al. A prospective study of coffee consumption and the risk of symptomatic gallstone disease in men. JAMA 1999; 281: 2106-12.

Sesso HD, Gaziano JM, Buring JE, Hennekens CH. Coffee and tea intake and the risk of myocardial infarction. Am J Epidemiology 1999; 149: 162-67.

Chapter 3

Selwyn AP, Kinlay S, Creager M, et al. Endothelial cell dysfunction in atherosclerosis and ischemic manifestations of coronary artery disease. Amer J Cardiol 1997; 79 (5A): 17-23.

Kullo IJ, Edwards WD, Schwartz RS. Vulnerable plaque: pathobiology and clinical implications. Ann Intern Med 1998; 129: 1050-60.

Ross R. Atherosclerosis—An inflammatory disease. N Eng J Med 1999; 340: 115-26.

PART II

(2)

Calle EA, Thun MJ, Petrelli JM, et al. Body mass index and mortality in a prospective cohort of U.S. adults. N Eng J Med 1999; 341: 1097-105.

Davidson MH, Hauptman J, Foreyt JP, et al. Weight control and risk factor reduction in obese subjects treated for 2 years with Orlistat. A randomized controlled trial. JAMA 1999; 281: 235-42.

Daniels SR, Morrison JA, Sprecher DL, et al. Association of body fat distribution and cardiovascular risk factors in children and adolescents. Circulation 1999; 99: 544-45.

Frankel S, Elwood P, Sweetnam P, et al. Birthweight, body mass index in middle age, and incident coronary heart disease. Lancet 1996; 348: 1478-80.

Martyn CN, Gale CR, Jespersen S, and Sherriff SB. Impaired fetal growth and atherosclerosis of carotid and peripheral arteries. Lancet 1998; 352: 173-78.

Forsen T, Ericksson JG, Tuomilehto J, et al. Mother's weight in pregnancy and coronary heart disease in a cohort of Finnish men: follow-up study. Brit Med J 1997; 315: 837-40.

Neugebauer R, Hoek HW, Susser E. Prenatal exposure to wartime famine and development of anti-social personality disorder in early adulthood. JAMA 1999; 282: 455-62

Rich-Edwards JW, Colditz GA, Stampfer MJ, et al. Birthweight and the risk for type 2 diabetes mellitus in adult women. Ann Intern Med 1999; 130: 278-84.

Irving RJ, Belton NR, Elton RA, Walker BR. Adult cardiovascular risk factors in premature babies. Lancet 2000; 355: 2135-36.

(3)

Gueyffier F, Boutitie F, Boissel JP, et al. Effect of anti-hypertensive drug treatment on cardiovascular outcomes in women and men. A meta-analysis of individual patient data from randomized, controlled trials. Ann Intern Med 1997; 126: 761-67.

Berenson GS, Srinivason SR, Bao W, et al. Association between multiple cardiovascular risk factors and atherosclerosis in children and young adults. N Eng J Med 1998; 338: 1650-56.

Berlowitz DR, Ash AS, Hickey EC, et al. Inadequate management of blood pressure in a hypertensive population. N Eng J Med 1998; 339: 1957-63.

Forette F, Seux ML, Staessen JA, et al. Prevention of dementia in randomized double-blind placebo-controlled systolic hypertension in Europe. Lancet 1998; 352: 1347-51.

Van Den Hoogen PCW, Feskens EJM, Nagelkerke NJD. The relation between blood pressure and mortality due to coronary heart disease in different parts of the world. N Eng J Med 2000; 341: 1-8.

(4)

Gurfinkel E, Bosovich G, Daroca A, et al. Randomized trial of roxithromycin in non-Q wave coronary syndroms. Lancet 1997; 350: 404-07.

Mehta JL, Saldeen TGP, Rand K. Interactive role of infection, inflammation, and traditional risk factors in atherosclerosis and coronary artery disease. J Am Coll Cardiol 1998; 31: 1217-25.

Meier CR, Derby LE, Jick SS, et al. Antibiotics and risk of subsequent first-time acute myocardial infarction. JAMA 1999; 281: 427-31.

Bartels E, Maass M, Bein G, et al. Detection of chlamydia pneumoniae but not cytomegalovirus in occluded saphenous vein coronary artery bypass grafts. Circulation 1999; 99: 879-82.

Ridker PM, Hennekens CH, Buring JE, Rifai N. C-reactive protein and other markers of inflammation in the prediction of cardiovascular disease in women. N Eng J Med 2000; 342: 836-43.

(5) through (7)

Tunstall-Pedoe H, Woodward M, Tasendale R, et al. Comparision of the prediction by 27 different factors of coronary heart disease and death in men and women of the Scottish Heart Health Study. Brit Med J 1997; 315: 722-29.

Danesh J, Collins R, Appleby P, Peto R. Association of fibrinogen, c-reactive protein, albumin, or leukocyte count with coronary artery disease. JAMA 1998; 279; 1477-82.

Siegrist J, Peter R, Cremer P, Seidel D. Chronic work stress is associated with atherogenic lipids and elevated fibrinogen in middle-aged men. J Intern Med 1997; 242: 149-56.

Phillipp CS, Cisar LA, Saidi P, Kostis JB. Effect of niacin supplementation of fibrinogen levels in patients with peripheral vascular disease. Am J Cardiol 1998; 82: 697-99.

Weiss EJ, Bray PF, Tayback M, et al. A polymorphism of a platelet glycoprotein receptor as an inherited risk factor for coronary thrombosis. N Eng J Med 1996; 334: 1090-94.

Erikssen G, Thaulous E, Stormorken H, Erikssen J. Hematocrit: A predictor of cardiovascular mortality? J Intern Med 1993; 234: 447-51.

Verheught FWAS. Aspirin, the poor man's statin? Lancet 1998; 351: 227-28.

Husain S, Andrews NP, Mulchy D, et al. Aspirin improves endothelial dysfunction in atherosclerosis. Circulation 1998; 97: 716-20.

(8)

Graham IM, Daly LE, Refsum HH, et al. Plasma homocysteine as a risk factor for vascular disease. JAMA 1997; 277: 1775-81.

Stubbs PJ, Al-Obaidi MK, Conroy RM, et al. Effect of plasma homocysteine concentration on early and late events in patients with acute coronary syndromes. Circulation 2000; 102: 605-10.

Nygard O, Nordiehang JE, Refsum H, et al. Plasma homocysteine levels and mortality in patients with coronary artery disease. N Eng J Med 1997; 337: 230-36.

Ridker PM, Manson JE, Buring JE, et al. Homocysteine and risk of cardiovascular disease among post-menopausal women. JAMA 1999; 281: 1817-21.

Van Beynum IM, Seitink JAM, den Heijer M, et al. Hyperhomocysteinemia: A risk factor for ischemic stroke in children. Circulation 1999; 99: 2070-72.

Jacques P, Resenberg IH, Rogers G, et al. Serum total homocysteine concentrations in adolescent and adult Americans: results from the Third National Health and Nutrition Examination Survey. Am J Clin Nutr 1999; 69: 482-9.

(9)

Denollet J, Sys SU, Stroubant N, et al. Personality as independent predictor of long-term mortality in patients with coronary artery disease. Lancet 1996; 347; 417-21.

Siegrist J, Peter R, Cremer P, Seidel D. Chronic work stress is associated with athergenic lipids and elevated fibrinogen in middle-aged men. J Intern Med 1997; 242: 49-56.

Gullette EC, Blumenthal JA, Babyak M, et al. Effects of mental stress on myocardial ischemia during daily life. JAMA 1997; 277: 1521-26.

Blumenthal JA, Jiang W, Babyak M, et al. Stress management and exercise training in cardiac patients with myocardial ischemia. Arch Intern. Med 1997; 157: 2219-23.

Everson SA, Roberts RE, Goldberg DE, Kaplan GA. Depressive symptoms and increased risk of stroke mortality over a 29-year period. Arch Inter Med 1998; 158: 1133-38.

Ford DE, Mead LA, Change PP, et al. Depression is a risk factor for coronary artery disease in men. Arch Intern Med 1998; 158: 1422-26.

(10)

Celermajes DS, Adams MR, Clarkson P, et al. Passive smoking and impaired endothelium-dependent arterial dilatation in healthy young adults. N Eng J Med 1996; 334: 150-54.

Law MR, Hakksaw AK. A meta-analysis of cigarette smoking, bone mineral density, and risk of hip fracture: Recognition of a major effect. Brit Med J 1997; 315: 841-46.

Tribarren C, Tekawa IS, Sidney S, Friedman GD. Effect of cigar smoking on the risk of cardiovascular disease, chronic obstructive pulmonary disease, and cancer in men. N Eng J Med 1999; 340: 1773-80.

Hughes JR, Goldstein MG, Hurt RD, Shiffman S. Recent advances in the pharmacotherapy of smoking. JAMA 1999; 281: 72-76.

Jorneby DE, Leischow SJ, Nides MA, et al. A controlled trial of sustained-release bupropion, a nicotine patch, or both for smoking cessation. N Eng J Med 1999; 340: 685-91.

(11)

Lemaitre RN, Siscovick DS, Raghunathan TE, et al. Leisure time physical activity and the risk of primary cardiac arrest. Arch Intern Med 1999; 159: 686-90.

Bijnen FC, Caspersen CJ, Feskens EJM, et al. Physical activity and 10-year mortality from cardiovascular diseases and all causes. The Zutphen Elderly Study. Arch Intern Med 1998; 158: 1499-1505.

Kujala UM, Kaprio J, Sarna S, Koskenvuo M. Relationship of leisure-time physical activity and mortality. The Finnish Twin Cohort. JAMA 1998; 279: 440-44.

Lee CD, Blair SN, Jackson AS. Cardiovascular fitness, body composition, and all-cause and cardiovascular disease mortality in men. Am J Clin Nutr 1999; 69: 373-80.

Manson JE, Hu FB, Rich-Edwards JW, et al. A prospective study of walking as compared with vigorous exercise in the prevention of coronary heart disease in women. N Eng J Med 1999; 341: 650-58.

Wei M, Gibbons LW, Mitchell TL, et al. The association between cardiorespiratory fitness and impaired fasting glucose and type 2 diabetes mellitus in men. Ann Intern Med 1999; 130; 89-96.

Hambrecht R, Wolf A, Gielen S, et al. Effect of exercise on coronary endothelial function in patients with coronary artery disease. N Eng J Med 2000; 345: 454-60.

Zeni AI, Hoffman MD, Clifford PJ. Energy expenditure with indoor exercise machines. JAMA 1996; 275: 1424-27.

Thompson PD. Cardiovascular complications of vigorous physical activity. Arch Intern Med 1996; 156: 2297-02.

Samaras K, Kelly PJ, Chiaro MN, et al. Genetic and environmental influences on total body and central abdominal fat: the effect of physical activity in female twins. Ann Intern Med 1999; 130: 873-82.

(12)

Harris MI, Flegal KM, Cowie CC, et al. Prevalence of diabetes, impaired fasting glucose, and impaired glucose tolerance in U.S. adults. Diabetes Care 1998; 21: 518-24.

Rich-Edwards JW, Colditz GA, Stampfer MJ, et al. Birth weight and the risk for type 2 diabetes mellitus in adult women. Ann Intern Med 1999; 130: 278-84.

Wei M, Gibbons LW, Mitchell TL, et al. The association between cardiorespiratory fitness and impaired fasting glucose and type 2 diabetes mellitus in men. Ann Intern Med. 1999; 130: 89-96.

Starc TJ, Shea S, Cohn LC, et al. Greater dietary intake of simple carbohydrates is associated with lower concentrations of high-density lipoprotein cholesterol in hypercholesterolemic children. Am J Clin Nutr 1998; 67: 1147-54.

Solomon CG, Hu FB, Stampfer MJ, et al. Moderate alcohol consumption and risk of coronary heart disease among women with type 2 diabetes. Circulation 2000; 102: 500-05.

Ajani UA, Gaziano JM, Lotufo PA, et al. Alcohol consumption and risk of coronary heart disease by diabetes status. Circulation 2000; 102: 500-05.

(13) through (16)

LaRosa JC. Triglycerides and coronary risk in women and the elderly. Arch Intern Med 1997; 157: 461-68.

Gaziano JM, Hennekens CH, O'Donnell EJ, et al. Fasting triglycerides, high-density lipoprotein, and risk of myocardial infarction. Circulation 1997; 96: 2520-25.

Miller M, Seidler A, Moalemi A, Pearson TA. Normal triglyceride levels and coronary artery disease events: The Baltimore Coronary Observational Long-Term Study. J Am Coll Cardiol 1998; 31: 1252-57.

Stampfer MJ, Krauss RM, Jing M, et al. A prospective study of triglyceride level, low density lipoprotein particle diameter, and risk of myocardial infarction. JAMA 1997; 157: 961-68.

Kwiterovich PO. The anti-atherogenic role of high-density lipoprotein cholesterol. Am J Cardiol 1998; 82: 13Q-21Q.

Dwyer T, Iwane H, Dean K, et al. Differences in HDL cholesterol concentration in Japanese, American, and Australian children. Circulation 1997; 96: 2830-36.

Stefanick ML, Mackey S, Sheehan M, et al. Effects of diet and exercise in men and post-menopausal women with low levels of HDL cholesterol and high levels of LDL cholesterol. N Eng J Med 1998; 339: 12-20.

Starc TJ, Shea S, Cohn LC, et al. Greater dietary intake of simple carbohydrates is associated with lower concentrations of high-density lipoprotein cholesterol in hypercholesterolemic children. Am J Clin Nutr 1998; 67: 1147-54.

Mackness MI, Arrol S, Mackness B, Durrington PN. Alloenzymes of paraoxonase and effectiveness of high-density lipoproteins in protecting low-density lipoprotein against lipid peroxidization. Lancet 1997; 349: 851-52.

Scandinavian Simvastatin Survival Study (4s) Group. Randomized trial of cholesterol lowering in 4,444 patients with coronary heart disease. Lancet 1994; 344: 1383-89.

Shephard J, Cobbe SM, Ford I, et al. Prevention of coronary heart disease with pravastatin in men with hypercholesterolemia. N Eng J Med 1995; 333: 1305-12.

Sacks FM, Moye LA, Davis BR, et al. Relationship between plasma LDL concentrations during treatment with pravastatin, and recurrent coronary events in the cholesterol and Recurrent Events Trial. Circulation 1998; 97: 1446-52.

West of Scotland Coronary Prevention Study Group. Influence of pravastatin and plasma lipids in clinical events in the West of Scotland Coronary Prevention Study. Circulation 1998; 97: 1440-45.

Downs JR, Clearfield M, Weis S, et al. Primary prevention of acute coronary events with lovastatin in men and women with average cholesterol levels: results of AFCAPS/TEX CAPS. JAMA 1998; 279: 1615-22.

Long-term Intervention with Pravastatin in Ischemic Disease (Lipid Study Group). Prevention of cardiovascular events and death with pravastatin in patients with coronary heart disease and a broad range of initial cholesterol levels. N Eng J Med 1998; 339: 1349-57.

Rosenson RS, Tangny CC. Anti-athero-thrombotic properties of statins: implications for cardiovascular event reduction. JAMA 1998; 279: 1643-50.

Gardner CD, Formann SP, Krauss RM. Association of small low-density lipoprotein particles with the incidence of coronary artery disease in men and women. JAMA 1996; 276: 875-81.

Strong JP, Malcom GT, McMahan CA. Prevalence and extent of atherosclerosis in adolescents and young adults. JAMA 1999; 281: 727-35.

Stein EA, Illingworth DR, Kwiterovich PO, et al. Efficacy and safety of lovastatin in adolescent males with heterozygous familial hypercholesterolemia. JAMA 1999; 281: 137-44.

Furberg CD. Natural statins and stroke risk. Circulation 1999; 99: 185-88.

Brown L, Rosner B, Willett WC, Sacks FM. Cholesterol-lowering effects of dietary fiber: a meta-analysis. Am J Clin Nutr 1999; 69: 30-42.

Nilausen K, Meinertz H. Lipoprotein(a) and dietary proteins: Casein lowers lipoprotein(a) concentrations as compared to soy proteins. Am J Clin Nutr 1999; 69: 419-25.

de Lorgeril M, Salen P, Martin JL, et al. Mediterranean diet, traditional risk factors, and the rate of cardiovascular complications after myocardial infarction. Final report of the Lyon Diet Heart Study. Circulation 1999; 99: 779-85.

Dreon DM, Fernstrom HA, Williams PT, Krauss RM. A very-low fat diet is not associated with improved lipoprotein profiles in men with a predominance of large, low-density lipoproteins. Am J Clin Nutr 1999; 69: 411-18.

Davidson MH, Hunninghake D, Maki KC, et al. Comparison of the effects of lean red meat vs. lean white meat on serum lipid levels among free-living persons with hypercholesterolemia. A long-term randomized clinical trial. Arch Intern Med 1999; 159: 1331-38.

Doherty TM, Wong ND, Shavelle RM, et al. Coronary heart disease deaths and infarctions in people with little or no coronary calcium. Lancet 1999; 353: 41-42.

Bostom AG, Cuppler LA, Jenner JL, et al. Elevated plasma lipoprotein(a) and coronary heart disease in men aged 55 and younger. A prospective study. JAMA 1996; 276: 544-48.

Dangas G, Mehran R, Harpel P, et al. Lipoprotein(a) and inflammation in human coronary atheroma: association with the severity of clinical presentation. J Am Coll Cardiol 1998; 32: 2035-42.

(17)

Strong JP, Malcolm GT, McMahon CA, et al. Prevalence and extent of atherosclerosis in adolescents and young adults. JAMA 1999; 281: 727-35.

Kwiterovich PO, Barton BA, McMahon RP. Effects of diet and sexual maturation on low density lipoprotein during puberty: the dietary intervention study in children. Circulation 1997; 96: 2526-33.

Napoli C, Glass CK, Witztum JL, et al. Influence of maternal hypercholesterolemia during pregnancy on progression of early atherosclerotic lesions in childhood. Lancet 1999; 354: 1234-41.

Sinakiko AR, Donahue RP, Jacobs DR, Prineas RJ. Relation of weight and rate of increase in weight during childhood and adolescence to body size, blood pressure, fasting insulin, and lipids in young adults. The Minneapolis Children's Blood Pressure Study. Circulation 1999; 99: 1471-76.

Stein EA, Illingworth DR, Kwiterovich PO, et al. Efficacy and safety of lovastatin in adolescent males with heterozygous familial hypercholesterolemia. A randomized controlled study. JAMA 1999; 281: 137-44.

Starc TJ, Shea S, Cohn LC, et al. Greater dietary intake of simple carbohydrates is associated with lower concentrations of high-density lipoprotein cholesterol in hypercholesterolemic children. Am J Clin Nutr 1998; 67: 1147-54.

Wenger NK. Coronary heart disease: an older women's major health risk. Brit Med J 1997; 315: 1085-90.

Weverling-Rljnsburger AW, Blauw GJ, Lagaay AM, et al. Total cholesterol and risk of mortality in the oldest old. Lancet 1997; 350: 1119-23.

Coti MC, Guralnik JM, Salive ME, et al. Clarifying the direct relation between total cholesterol levels and death from coronary heart disease in older persons. Ann Intern Med 1997; 126: 753-60.

Miller M, Byington R, Hunninghake D, et al. Sex bias and underutilization of lipid-lowering therapy in patients with coronary artery disease in the United States & Canada. Arch Intern Med 2000; 160: 343-47.

Lewis SJ, Moye LA, Sacks FM, et al. Effect of pravastatin on cardiovascular events in older patients with myocardial infarction and cholesterol levels in the average range. Ann Intern Med 1998; 129: 681-89.

O'Leary DH, Polak JF, Kronmal RA, et al. Carotid artery intima and media thickness as a risk factor for myocardial infarction and stroke in older adults. N Eng J Med 1999; 340: 14-22.

Lloyd-Jones DM, Larson MG, Beiser A, Levy D. Lifetime risk of developing coronary heart disease. Lancet 1999; 353: 89-92.

(18) through (20) and PART III

Prospective Studies Collaboration. Cholesterol, diastolic blood pressure, and stroke: 13,000 strokes in 450,000 people in 45 prospective cohorts. Lancet 1995; 346: 1647-53.

Burk AP, Farh A, Malcom GT, et al. Coronary risk factors and plaque morphology in men with coronary disease who died suddenly. N Eng J Med 1997; 336: 1276-82.

Gillum RF, Mussolino ME, Madans JH. Coronary heart disease incidence and survival in African American women and men: The NHANES 1 Epidemiologic Follow-up Study. Ann Intern Med 1997; 127: 111-18.

Durington PN, Prais H, Bhatnagar D, et al. Indications for cholesterol-lowering medication: Comparison of risk assessment methods. Lancet 1999; 353: 278-81.

Tunstall-Pedoe H, Woodward M, Tasendale R, et al. Comparison of the prediction by 27 different factors of coronary heart disease and death in men and women of the Scottish Heart Health Study. Brit Med J 1997; 315: 722-29.

Lowe LP, Greenland P, Ruth KJ, et al. Impact of major cardiovascular disease risk factors, particularly in combination on 22 year mortality in women and men. Arch Intern. Med 1998; 158: 2007-14.

Wilson PWF, D'Agostino RB, Levy D, et al. Prediction of coronary heart disease using risk factor categories. Circulation 1999; 97: 1837-47.

Lloyd-Jones DM, Larson MG, Beiser A, Levy D. Lifetime risk of developing coronary heart disease. Lancet 1999; 353: 89-92.

Pahor M, Elam MB, Garrison RJ, et al. Emerging noninvasive biochemical measures to predict cardiovascular risk. Arch Inter Med 1999; 159: 237-45.

Stamler J, Stamler R, Neaton JD, et al. Low risk-factor profile and long-term cardiovascular and noncardiovascular mortality and life expectancy. Findings from 5 large cohorts of young adult and middle-aged men and women. JAMA 1999; 282: 2012-18.

Nabel EG. Coronary heart disease in women—An ounce of prevention. New Eng J Med 2000; 343: 572-74.

Appendix B

Grodstein F, Stampfer MJ, Colditz GA, et al. Post-menopausal hormone therapy and mortality. N Eng J Med 1997; 336: 1769-75.

Mendelsohn ME, Karas RH. The protective effects of estrogen on the cardiovascular system. N Eng J Med 1999; 340: 1801-11.

Recker RR, Davies M, Dowd RM, Heaney RP. The effect of low-dose continuous estrogen and progesterone therapy with calcium and vitamin D on bone in elderly women. A randomized controlled trial. Ann Intern Med 1999; 130: 897-04.

Collaborative Group on Hormonal Factors in Breast Cancer: Breast cancer and hormone-replacement therapy: Collaborative reanalysis of data from 51 epidemiological studies of 52,705 women with breast cancer and 108,411 without breast cancer. Lancet 1997; 350: 1047-59.

Sellers TA, Mink PJ, Cerhan JR, et al. The role of hormone replacement therapy in the risk of breast cancer and total mortality in women with a family history of breast cancer. Ann Intern Med. 1997; 127: 973-80.

Phillips KA, Glendon G, Knight JA. Putting the risk of breast cancer in perspective. N Eng J Med 1999; 340: 141-44.

Grodstein F, Martinez C, Platz EA, et al. Post-menopausal hormone use and risk of colorectal cancer and adenoma. Ann Intern Med 1998; 128: 705-12.

Messina MJ. Legumes and soybeans: Overview of their nutritional profile and health effects. Am J Clin Nutr 1999; S70: S439-S50.

Ingram D, Sanders K, Kolybab M, Lopez D. Case-control study of phytoestrogens and breast cancer. Lancet 1999; 350: 990-94.

Burke W, Daly M, Garber J, et al. Recommendations for follow-up care of individuals with an inherited predisposition to cancer. BRAC1 and BRAC2: Cancer Genetics Studies Consortium. JAMA 1997; 277: 997-1003.

Eisinger F, Alby N, Bremond A, et al. Recommendations for medical management of hereditary breast and ovarian cancer: The French National Ad HOC Committee. Ann Oncol 1998; 9: 939-50.

Kavanagh AM, Mitchell H, Giles GG. Hormone replacement therapy and accuracy of mammographic screening. Lancet 2000; 355: 270-74.

Setchell KDR. Phytoestrogens: the biochemistry, physiology, and implications for human health of soy isoflavones. Am J Clin Nutr 1998; 68: 1333s-46s.

Potter SM, Baum JA, Teng H, et al. Soy protein and isoflavones: their effects on blood lipids and bone density in post-menopausal women. Am J Clin Nutr 1998; 68: 1375s-79s.

Willett WC, Colditz G, Stampfer M. Post-menopausal estrogens—opposed, unopposed or none of the above. JAMA 2000; 283: 534-35.

Yaffe K, Lui LY, Grady D, et al. Cognitive decline in women in relation to non-protein-bound estradiol concentrations. Lancet 2000; 356: 708-12.

Acknowledgments

I owe a great debt of gratitude to Miss Hillary Trowell for her reassuring patience while preparing countless revisions of this book.

Many thanks to Ms. Elizabeth Frost-Knappman of New England Publishing Associates for her thoughtful guidance in nurturing the manuscript to its publication.

And my thanks also to Mr. Brian Robertson at Lifeline/Regnery Publishing for editing and rearranging the manuscript, and (almost) convincing me that he was right.

Index